MOVING WITH THE I

MOVING WITH THE MOON

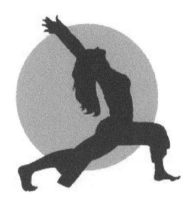

Nurturing Yoga, Movement and Meditation for
Every Phase of your Menstrual Cycle and Beyond

ANA DAVIS

Illustrated by Sophie Duncan

1st Edition 2018, paperback.
ISBN: 978-1-925764-49-9
EPUB: 978-1-925764-50-5
MOBI: 978-1-925764-51-2
Publishing services by: PublishMyBook.Online

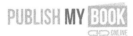

Cover image by Kellie Knight
Fluid Retention poem reproduced with the kind permission of the poet.
A catalogue record for this book is available from the National Library of
Australia.

DEDICATION

I dedicate this book to my yoga students and teacher trainees. To the new wave of women who seek natural, empowered ways to connect with their bodies, and their unique feminine psyches; who seek to step out of the masculine paradigm and establish new ways to practise yoga and to live their lives creatively, joyfully, and most importantly, authentically.

May we all grow wiser, calmer and more grounded in our femininity within this crazy world, in order to better support ourselves and those around us.

And in special memory of my paternal grandmother, Toni Davis, who was a force of nature. A remarkable woman inspiring in her abundant creativity, dynamism, and unflagging love, who shepherded me so delightfully through my first-bleed.

Praise for *Moving with the Moon*

'This book is a return to the feminine in yoga practice. A reminder that we are swayed by the tides and need to love and nurture ourselves. Thoroughly approachable and geared to the novice and experienced practitioner alike, *Moving with the Moon* is a call to reclaim your wellbeing. Ana writes with passion and clarity while bringing through quotes, stories and wisdom from many inspired female writers and cultural traditions. A treasure trove of practices and advice with a reminder that being a woman carries different shades of being and that tuning into yourself is to tune to your womb. As you explore the practices and suggestions throughout, you'll feel Ana's expert and sensitive guidance and come away with tools for any age or stage of life. *Moving with the Moon* is a gem for women!'

—RACHEL ZINMAN
Author of *Yoga for Diabetes, How to Manage your Health with Yoga and Ayurveda*,
and Global Yoga Teacher,
www.yogafordiabetesblog.com

'One of the most important and groundbreaking books of the 21st century for women. This is essentially a revolutionary bible for women's care of the womb. Ana Davis offers a powerful new voice and perspective in support of the rise of the Sacred Feminine without burnout. If you don't wish to suffer from the push that can so often come with being an ambassador for service to others as a yoga teacher, practitioner, coach or healer, or a woman on purpose, then this is the book for you. Being gentle with our-selves, being able to live more fully in our bodies and becoming a positive role model for slow, sustainable and longevity-enhancing yoga practices which are a mirror for how we 'do' life. These are all things that will change the world for the better. This book has it all and more and I can't recommend it more highly.'

—LISA FITZPATRICK
Author of *Healing the Heart of Your Business: Sustainable Success for Heart-Centred Women*,
and founder of Sacred Women's Business Coaching,
www.lisafitzpatrick.com.au

'In my 15 years of practice and 7 years of being completely immersed in the yoga industry through my work, I have never come across such a comprehensive yet gentle exploration of the issues female practitioners face in their asana practice and beyond. *Moving with the Moon* invites us to understand ourselves more intimately and modify our practices accordingly while at the same time celebrating our divine femininity. So accustomed to pushing ourselves to practise in a traditional, masculine style, the yoga world, consisting mostly of women these days, has been calling out for a book like this. A blessing to women in the growing yoga community, this book will evolve your practice and views about what it means to be a true yogini.'

—JESSICA HUMPHRIES
Editor *Australian Yoga Journal,*
www.jesshumphries.com

'*Moving with the Moon* is a comprehensive resource for understanding our menstrual cycle. Ana has reframed what women need from yoga and offers a thorough and very helpful guide for the necessary and different needs we have around our cycle within our yoga practice. She presents a feminine yoga practice for life, through each and every cycle, and beyond, past menopause. Ana's suggestions will help women become more in tune with their bodies, a very necessary and important thing. This feminine approach to yoga holds much medicine for us all.'

—JANE HARDWICKE COLLINGS
Midwife and Women's Mysteries teacher,
www.janehardwickecollings.com

'Here Ana Davis gives detailed and thoughtful instructions for yoga practices for each part of the menstrual cycle, and locates them in a holistic context of wise self-care, richly drawn from Western and Eastern traditions. In my own experience, establishing a simple yoga routine designed around changing needs throughout the cycle is a key to better menstrual health and wellbeing, and to developing access to a stable sense of embodied inner serenity. Restorative yoga practices alone can be a revelation for busy women, especially as we get older. This clearly written book makes it possible to develop such a practice in the comfort of your own home.'

—LARA OWEN
Author of *Her Blood Is Gold: Awakening to the Wisdom of Menstruation,*
www.laraowen.com

CONTENTS

Fluid Retention

Who is this
naked woman
striding in cyclically
to straddle me in my
own mirror? Is she
ignorant of nubile
fashion? She
is so
ludicrously
voluptuous and fecund,
she is so pendulous and undulating,
that I am ashamed to look at her. What is
she insinuating with her lascivious curves
piled so high that her flesh rolls?
Belly full, thighs
bulging,
hips protruding,
threatening to drown me in
their tidal swell. It's as if she is defining a
woman's space as huge and mountainous. A giant
jutting promontory…. Can we take up this much room?
Shouldn't we be starving ourselves into a tiny skeletal corner?
Suck in our breath, bite our tongues, strap up our breasts,
hide our blood, conceal the meaty clots. Cloak
ripening fruits in displays of charity. How

dare 'She' blithely   stride, blatantly
fertile, into   my mirror,
with her   mounds
of jelly   flesh
wobb-   ling,
as she reach-   ches for
my scraw-   ny hand.

—Shana Michele Matheson

FOREWORD

It's been a man's world, the yoga world, right back to yoga's beginnings. Centuries ago, classic yoga was a male-only practice. Today, we still employ a masculine approach to how we do yoga practices, even though the majority of practitioners are women. Styles such as 'Hot Yoga' and 'Power Yoga' don't allow for the changing cyclic needs of menstruating women or the transitions of antenatal and menopausal women. And most yoga teachers don't have the depth of experience to address these needs. They are unable to offer yoga sequences appropriate to a woman's cycle or stage of life.

When I first learned yoga in 1971, I took a male approach to doing yoga. That was the culture of the times. The man who taught me to teach yoga was as tough as they come. The atmosphere in which I learned to teach was ruled by the maxim, 'no gain without pain'. Those were the days of women's liberation and the sexual revolution. Women were clamouring for equality. In yoga classes, there was no real distinction between the practices performed by men or women. Women's yoga was unheard of.

The first time I participated in classes at the Ramamani Iyengar Memorial Yoga Institute in Pune in 1984, I was shocked. Some of the classes were men-only and women-only. To my Western mind, it seemed like such a backward notion. Yet I found I enjoyed the feminine atmosphere and pace of the 'ladies' classes'.

Taught by Geeta Iyengar, I saw there was a different way, a more organic way, a woman's way to do yoga. Geeta recognised the importance of women doing yoga appropriate to their biological cycles and stages. For the first time, I learned to modify my yoga practice to suit my menstrual cycle. For the first time, my periods became regular.

There is still a tremendous need for women to learn to adapt yoga practices to their cyclic needs. For this reason, I celebrate and recommend this new and, in many ways, revolutionary book, *Moving with the Moon*. What Ana Davis's book outlines is 'moving with your womb: a feminine approach to yoga'.

Why is the book revolutionary? Because we—men and women alike in modern society—are conditioned to believe that menstruation is at best a nuisance and at worst a curse. Instead of viewing the whole of a woman's cycle as the crucible of her fertility and potency, it is seen as something to be ignored, disdained or overcome. In *Moving with the Moon*, we are presented with the opportunity to reframe the negative paradigm and make a woman's bleeding time cause for healing and celebration.

As director of the Sydney Yoga Centre, I met Ana in 1996 when I became her teacher and mentor for teacher training. I felt fortunate when Ana joined our team of teachers at my second school, Simply Yoga. Ana was developing her own teaching style and was highly regarded by her students. Less than ten years after completing her yoga teacher training, Ana was directing her own school and developing the prototype of Bliss Baby trainings.

Ana has taken every opportunity to learn about and evolve her passion for working with women through yoga and meditation. Her own pregnancy led her to found Bliss Baby Yoga which specialises in Prenatal and Postnatal, Fertility Yoga, Women's Yoga, and Restorative Yoga.

This book, this 'baby' that has gestated through all the learning and teaching Ana has done, is needed and wanted by women of all ages.

For the most part, and I would include my younger self in this group, we women override our cycles to carry on with our family and work responsibilities. This is often to the detriment of our health. We have adopted the dominant cultural view that we are capable and should push ourselves to accomplish as much as possible. We are not only out of touch with the rhythms of our cycles and seasons, we are also unacquainted with them.

This disconnectedness leads to health problems on all levels: mental, emotional, physical and spiritual. Problems with menstruation, for instance, apart from pain or discomfort, can create difficulties with fertility and later in life with menopause.

Moving with the Moon is a tutorial on what it means to be a woman—in relation to nature, to our biology, to the planet. It's a book that encourages women to come home to themselves, to listen to the drum and thrum of their own biorhythms. Ana has given us a richly resourced book from which we learn to integrate many modalities and practices: Ayurveda, mudras, asana, pranayama, relaxation, visualisation, Yoga Nidra, restorative yoga. Through following the detailed holistic programs in the book, we can cultivate more awareness, sensitivity and freedom on the mat, and off the mat. This is the aim of yoga.

More than anything, the message of *Moving with the Moon* is one of empowerment. It comes from Ana's own experience of coming home to her own feminine being. The book is a beautiful roadmap on how we women can all live a life in tune with our natural rhythms, one that leads to fulfilment, creativity and a life of ease.

Eve Grzybowski

author of *Teach Yourself Yoga* and *The Art of Adjustment,*
and Yoga Teacher, www.eveyoga.com

April, 2018

PREFACE

Disconnection to the true feminine manifests with tightness at the heart-womb, blocking the giving and receiving of love. Living life in an emotional state, repressing, fearing true feeling, makes us ignorant of life's larger cycles. The fear of working with the essential wisdom of polarities and the disavowment of the dark or shadow aspects leads to disempowerment. Power is found in the darkness once you are brave enough to consistently venture into it and reclaim your power. In this wisdom you acquire the willpower to transform and empower self.

—PADMA AND ANAIYA AON PRAKASHA[1]

THE WOUND IN THE WOMB

In our fast-paced lives many people override the needs of their bodies. We are preoccupied with our computers and smartphones; we feel compelled to fulfil numerous stressful and conflicting demands. We are apt to submit ourselves to punishing exercise regimes, or no exercise at all; and indulge in unhealthy diets and abuse drugs; all of which can divorce us from a loving connection with our bodies.

In my twenty-plus years as a yoga teacher I have regularly witnessed this phenomenon of 'living in our heads'. Many yoga students seem to lack awareness of where their bodies are in space—something technically known as 'proprioception'. It can also be recognised in those students who insensitively try to push their bodies to obey their wills.

It follows that many women can go through their entire lives disassociated from the feminine core of their bodies—their wombs. For some women, if an awareness of their womb occurs at all, it's in a negative way, acknowledged only through the pain and discomfort of menstrual

---

1   Padma and Anaiya Aon Prakasha, *Womb Wisdom: Awakening the Creative and Forgotten Powers of the Feminine,* location 893 (Kindle version)

cramping or during childbirth. Of course there is the joy that a pregnant woman experiences when nurturing a new life in her womb, which is the first—and perhaps only—positive connection to the uterus she may ever enjoy, as she instinctively rubs her swelling belly.

A woman may mask her feminine cycles and any potential positive connection with the ebb and flow of her womb by popping contraceptive pills for years on end. Or she invades her womb with an IUD and stuffs her vagina with dioxin-bleached tampons. As an older woman traverses the rite of passage into menopause she will often quell the symptoms with HRT (Hormone Replacement Therapy). Additionally, many women bear the womb-scars of abortion, miscarriage, and even hysterectomy.

Why can't women enjoy a more sustained connection with the very centre of their feminine being? Like the tree roots I've just had removed from under the paving in my courtyard, the answer is deep, complex and interconnected.

Our contemporary culture has disconnected from the feminine, and by association, from a cyclical way of living that is the very definition of what it means to be a woman. Most women labour under a patriarchal hangover that denies and represses the messiness, juiciness, pure irrationality and unpredictability that characterises the feminine. Also, in the social change precipitated by feminism modern women have lost some of their essential femininity in their drive to be considered equal to their male counterparts.

In my work training yoga teachers, I often meet women who are at a crossroads in their lives. They are taking time out of their city-based daily grind to practise yoga intensively. Perhaps for the first time in their lives they are questioning who they are. They reflect on where they have come from, and where they are now headed. These women come up to me after my sessions and ask me 'why'?

Why have they not had their period for such a long time? Why do they suffer so much when they bleed? Why can't they get pregnant? The answer is often quite obvious to me. The women that stand before me are usually overly masculinised—their bodies are wiry and muscly, their faces chiselled, their eyes hard and sad. They speak quickly and furtively to me about their 'problem'. They obviously carry a deep wound in their womb.

'Honey,' I think to myself, 'you need to juice-up!' Many of these women need to round out their edges and reclaim their femininity. You can't get pregnant when your body and mind are like a man's. From a purely scientific point of view, a woman's monthly cycle depends on a certain level of oestrogen, and oestrogen needs fat cells in which it can flourish.[2]

The first thing I suggest to these women is to stop practising yoga like a man. I encourage them to listen more sensitively to the changing needs of their bodies and their emotions as they cycle through the fluctuations of their menstrual month. These women need to make space for a regular, nurturing, nourishing practice, rather than the strong, 'yang' practice that they may have been attached to. They will need to shift their intention so that no longer are they striving to be something, whether that something is for themselves or for others. Instead of trying to be something, embody the art of *being gentle with yourself*—I urge.

Moving with the Moon is my gift to women who have lost their way. My dearest wish is that if you are like these women and you have lost your connection to your deep, female woman-centre, the information in this book will help you. If you have lost your way in a man's world, and there is a niggling feeling that something is just not 'right', play with the ideas, practices and sequences in this book. It is my hope that you will make them your own, and in so doing, break new ground for yourself and ultimately find your way home to your womb and your deepest health and fulfilment as a woman.

---

2   'Fat cells (also) actually produce oestrogen. Therefore, the more fat cells present in the body, the more oestrogen is produced.' So writes Gabriella Rosa, researcher and natural fertility specialist in an online article: https://naturalfertilitybreakthrough.com/womens-health-female-fertility/ is-oestrogen-making-you-fat-and-impacting-fertility/

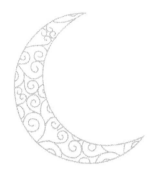

Part One

Context

INTRODUCTION
STRESSING THE FEMININE

*When the feminine returns to the female body, the
masculine is naturally inspired to reinvent the outer
structures (roles, relations, work, home) in a more
sustainable and life-giving manner. Natural systems are
self-regulating once the core balance is restored*

—TAMI LYNN KENT[3]

Are you tired too much of the time? Do you feel depleted and emotionally
overwhelmed? Do you feel ill-equipped to manage the stresses in your life?
Do you dread getting your period? Is your menstrual cycle something you
know little about or something you'd much rather ignore? Are you finding
the transition into menopause bewildering, frustrating and perhaps even
debilitating? If you answered yes to any, or all of these questions, you're not
alone, and it is likely stress has something, if not everything, to do with how
you're feeling.

The negative effects of stress are reaching epidemic proportions in our
modern lives and women are falling like flies—our bodies and souls are suffering. Even though it's across the board, burnout or 'adrenal fatigue' is more
common in women[4] and Chronic Fatigue Syndrome affects women at four
times the rate of men.[5] Co-founder and editor-in-chief of the Huffington

---

3   Tami Lynn Kent, *Wild Feminine: Finding Power, Spirit and Joy in the Female Body*,
    p. xxiv

4   'In fact, it is more common in women. This is due mainly to social—lifestyle changes.
    Many women now work outside the home and raise the children as well. Many
    are in single parent homes or both parents work just to pay the taxes. Women have
    more sluggish oxidation rates to begin with, so burnout may be less apparent in
    women, but it is just as common or more so than in men.'
    See: http://www.womenlivingnaturally.com/articlepage.php?id=6

5   Reference:
    http://www.medicinenet.com/script/main/art.asp?articlekey=149436&page=3

Post, Arianna Huffington, writes, 'women in highly stressed jobs have a nearly 40% increased risk of heart disease and heart attacks and a 60% greater risk for type 2 diabetes.' She goes on to say that women are also twice as likely to die of a heart attack in high-stress jobs and are also more vulnerable to alcoholism and eating disorders when stressed.[6] Also related to women's high stress levels is the rise in infertility[7] and menstrual disorders,[8] which points to the fact that the female hormonal system is like the canary in the mineshaft, signaling something is very wrong.

It's therefore evident that reducing stress is the first thing to be done to heal women's bodies. At the very least women need to learn how to become more 'stress resilient'. I remind my students it may not always be possible to eliminate many stressors from our lives, but the key lies in how we *respond* rather than *react* to so many of life's inevitable triggers.

It's little wonder that in the USA and Australia, 72–85% of yoga practitioners are women,[9] who flock to yoga for its feel-good, stress-

---

6   Arianna Huffington, *Thrive*, p.24. Huffington draws these statistics together from a number of disparate research studies that were conducted in developed countries that included the USA and Britain. See her notes section for the specific studies cited— pp. 285 and 288

7   '…in 2007 there were 56,817 ART treatment cycles (including fresh and thawed cycles) in Australasia, 92 per cent from Australia and eight per cent from New Zealand. This reflects an increase of approximately 40,000 cycles per year since 1991.' This is according to Dr Philip McChesney in PDF Doc, 'Demographics of Infertility', by MRANZCOG CREI Trainee, Spring, 2010

8   According to Marcelle Pick OB/GYN NP, in an online article, a common menstrual disorder, endometriosis is on the rise: https://www.womentowomen.com/sex-fertility/endometriosis-start-with-a-natural-approach/ Ayurvedic doctor Dr. Robert E. Svoboda writes: 'The modern woman, (however), goes through menarche earlier (thanks to better nutrition and artificial light) and commonly delivers only one or two children, whom she is usually able to nurse for a few months at best. She therefore has many more menstrual cycles, during which wide hormone swings dramatically affect the tissues of her ovaries, uterus, and breasts. Each of the swings, acts as an opportunity for an imbalance to occur, or for an imbalance that already exists to be exacerbated.'—Svoboda, *Ayurveda for Women*, pp. 70-71

9   According to a 2016 'Yoga in America' research survey conducted by *The Yoga Journal* and Yoga Alliance, 72% of practitioners in America are women: http://media.yogajournal.com/wp-content/uploads/2016_YIAS_American-Public_FactSheet.pdf. And, a national 'Yoga in Australia' survey conducted in 2012, found that women represented as many as 85% of the total yoga practitioner population— https://www.ncbi.nlm.nih.gov/pmc/articles/PMC3410203/

relieving benefits. However, the irony is that for many women, their yoga practice may be adding to their problems!

While it is definitely true that yoga can help women manage their stress levels, it may also add to them when practised in a way that doesn't support their feminine natures. I suggest that at the heart of women's health issues is an imbalance in the essential masculine/feminine duality. This imbalance is then perpetuated when women step on their yoga mat.

Many women live their lives from an overly masculinised perspective in which they drive themselves to exhaustion. As career women, co-parents, single parents, and general high achievers, women are suffering from relentless self and societal expectation to be constantly 'switched on', productive, outcome focused, to 'do', and to 'go, go, go!'. It all stems from the very context of modern society that values the masculine qualities over the softer, feminine ones. Author and Spiritual Business Coach Lisa Fitzpatrick explains this well:

> The world has reached a time where feminine wisdom is so needed to rebalance and address the dysfunctional bias towards patriarchal ways of being. Notice how the patriarchal structures of finance, politics, law and commerce are in trouble right now. Mother earth is groaning and suffering under the weight of a dominant paradigm which honours logic and denies intuition. The body's innate wisdom has been rejected in favour of a linear viewpoint which is dissociated and dissected from the whole story. The competitive, scientifically proven, masculine mainstream approach to life has also rejected the value of spontaneous, creative, sensual, playful and collaborative feminine ways of being which has cost the human race dearly. Both men and women are suffering from an epidemic of stress, overwhelm, depression, anxiety and autoimmune diseases as the vitality and life force of the feminine has been suppressed.[10]

HEALING THE WOUNDS: A FEMININE APPROACH TO YOGA

Reflecting this overemphasis on the masculine, many female yoga teachers and students are practising an inappropriate 'yang' style of yoga that is not serving their unique needs as women and can actually increase the stress placed upon their bodies.

---

10   Lisa Fitzpatrick—http://lisafitzpatrick.com.au

This is not surprising given the ancient tradition of yoga—as it is known today—was created by men for men. Even the term 'hatha' (as in 'Hatha Yoga', the branch of yoga concerned with the physical postures) can be translated as 'force', which represents a stronger, more masculine approach.

A more cohesive interpretation of Hatha Yoga is a *union of opposites*—'ha' means the sun, representing the more heating 'masculine' qualities, 'tha' means the moon, representing the cooling 'feminine' qualities. In fact, the word 'yoga' means 'yoking' or 'union', which encapsulates a more balanced and therefore more feminine approach to yoga. This more authentic interpretation incorporates both the masculine and feminine energies to create an organic interchange between the dark and light—the *yin* and *yang*— that naturally occurs in nature and in human monthly, seasonal and life cycles.

A more feminine, and therefore more balanced approach to yoga, negates an unhealthy focus on ego based pushing and striving within the posture practice which can perhaps be doubly destructive for women practitioners—as yoga teacher and author Nischala Joy Devi suggests:

> On an emotional level, a woman's sensitivity often shifts to more of a masculine 'ha' if she continually takes on challenges and engages in competition. Instead of experiencing feelings of compassion when confronted with a situation, we may first exhibit anger. Because of the emphasis placed on our more masculine side, our feminine qualities are depleted instead of enhanced. Both aspects need to be honoured.[11]

As female yoga practitioners it is important to remember that we are inherently cyclical. A woman's hormones are perpetually in flux throughout the monthly cycle as well as throughout her life cycle—from menarche (when she first menstruates) right through to menopause, and this has an undeniable impact both physically and emotionally. Yoga can support women more effectively if it fluidly reflects these changes.

Riding the 'third wave' of feminism, women now seek new ways to be, as women. In keeping with our inherently collaborative and consultative natures, we need to (re)learn to have *power with* rather than striving to have *power over*. If women can find a way to practise yoga that goes *with* rather than *against* their natural ebb and flow of energy, they can then carry this heightened awareness into all areas of their life—into their work, parenting, and all their relationships.

---

11 Nischala Joy Devi, *The Secret Power of Yoga*, p.228

MOVING WITH THE MOON: WHAT IS IT?

A woman can expect to menstruate up to 500 times during her fertile life. Month after month, for around 40 years—unless she is pregnant or breastfeeding—her energy levels, emotions and her physical sensations fluctuate, sometimes wildly.

Learning to 'move with the moon' involves using a Feminine Yoga practice to support and mirror the waxing and waning of the uterus as its lining builds and then sheds in an endless cycle. This process can help you fall in love with your cycle rather than resenting its irrevocable rhythms.

Considering we are essentially cyclical, why should we carry out our lives in a linear way like that of our male counterparts? Why should we keep doing the same thing all month long even when our bodies and emotions feel so completely different?

A Moving with the Moon approach to yoga offers tools to respond sensitively to the four energetic phases of a woman's monthly cycle, which I describe in detail in chapter two. This book will explore how you can move and flow with your monthly moon cycle. It's a creative and empowering process of adapting, changing, and crafting a yoga practice from day to day. Just as the moon waxes and wanes, so too does the energy of your body-mind. This book will unfurl and deepen your connection to this subtle internal rhythm as you learn to reflect this in a fresh approach to your yoga practice as a cycling woman.

A Moving with the Moon approach recognises the point in your cycle when you bleed—your Dark Moon phase—is a time of natural low ebb in your energy, so we support this with gentle Restorative Yoga. Post-menstruation and leading up to ovulation—during your Waxing Moon phase—you tend to feel stronger and have more energy, so your yoga practice becomes more dynamic. When you are ovulating—the Full Moon phase—your energy is outward and people focused, which suits a heart-opening yoga practice. Finally, leading up to your period—your Waning Moon phase—your energy begins to decline and moodiness sets in—the dreaded PMS phase—requiring a nourishing, grounding, and balancing yoga practice.

This philosophy of a feminine, cyclical approach to yoga is the Tao in action—an interplay between light and dark, *yin* and *yang*, masculine and feminine. Where there is movement there also needs to be its opposite—stillness. The Moving with the Moon approach detailed in this book explores the dance between activity and inactivity throughout women's monthly and life cycles, with an emphasis on honouring the beauty of stillness just as much as action. As Ayurvedic women's health expert Mother Maya (Maya Tiwari) says, there is great courage in 'taking pause'.[12]

MOVING WITH YOUR *WOMB*: A FEMININE YOGA PRACTICE FOR LIFE

A feminine approach to our yoga practice supports us as women not just throughout our monthly cycles, but also throughout the various unique transitions of our feminine lives.

Working with the key Feminine Yoga principles (discussed in chapter three) that underpin a cyclical, Moving with the Moon practice will help a woman become more in tune with her body and what it needs to get pregnant—the pre-conception phase.

If she becomes pregnant, this gentle, sensitive, *feminine* approach to yoga can accompany her as she moves into the prenatal phase, helping her adapt to doing 'yoga for two' throughout the three trimesters. Likewise, the tools of softening into self-awareness will also offer her an adapted, postnatal practice to support her into motherhood. Of course, while the general Feminine Yoga principles are transferable, prenatal, post-natal, and fertility yoga comprise a canon of specific, beneficial (and safe) postures and practices, which are the subject of a whole other book.

Finally, the same Moving with the Moon approach that can be practised during a woman's fertile years will provide a template for living that she can carry into menopause and beyond! I delve into yoga for menopause in detail in chapter nine.

A Moving with the Moon approach offers an evolving, juicy practice to support women throughout the 'womb-phases' of their uniquely feminine lives. It gifts you with an understanding that every time you step onto your yoga mat your practice may be different, and it's this understanding that will ultimately enhance your health, wellbeing and connection with your body and the cycles of nature.

---

12   From a talk, 'Living Ahimsa' given by Mother Maya (Maya Tiwari) February, 2012, Mullumbimby, Australia

WHAT DOES FEMININE YOGA LOOK AND FEEL LIKE?

*When we're in our flow, all we have to do is
walk across a room to be mesmerising.
We feel confident in ourselves because we're connected to the
earth and in harmony with her rhythms, cycles, and moods.*

—GABRIELLE ROTH[13]

Much of the yoga practised these days is angular, directional, and linear, reflecting the masculine principle. Women naturally love to move their bodies in fluid, sensuous ways, reflecting their physical curves and their cyclical nature. This means that a Feminine Yoga practice may look, and most definitely will *feel*, different from the traditional masculine approach.

I like to incorporate a lot of spinal rolls, hip circles (what I call 'Womb Circles'—see Figure 187, p.230), swaying, and flowing. These movements are all accompanied with sighing, releasing, and sometimes sounded, exhalations. The feel and intention is softness, surrender, conscious, luscious, and joyous savouring of the physical sensations of moving and releasing my body, of totally inhabiting the feminine body.

The spirit of a feminine practice is one of play and spontaneity. I like my body to guide me. *Where am I feeling tight and restricted? Where can I let go and soften more? When do I need to rest sweetly and nourish my nervous system?* Balancing this are questions like: *When do I feel like moving and flowing in a dynamic, stimulating way? Where do I crave more internal stability and support? Where do I want to feel strong and powerful?* Physical strength that I cultivate in my practice also comes from a deep place of internal listening. I never want to impose upon my body, or my psyche, a structure or challenge from the outside. Everything is from the *inside out.*

To create this juicy and potent mix, this work is inspired by many traditions and approaches that include Restorative Yoga, Viniyoga, Vinyasa Flow Yoga, Iyengar Yoga, Classical Yoga (Satyananda), somatic body work, Pilates, dance, Chi Kung and mindfulness meditation.

The Moving with the Moon practices that are detailed in this book were ultimately born of my own play and experimentation. I encourage you to go through the same creative process, with these practices serving just as a starting point for your own intuitively, evolving journey.

---

13   Gabrielle Roth, *Sweat Your Prayers*, p.51

WHO IS THIS BOOK FOR?

This book is for you if you already practise yoga but are feeling disenchant-ed with its effects and benefits—your yoga practice is not giving you the joy and vibrancy you crave. Equally, this book is for you if you're new to yoga and would like to give it a go, but you're intimidated by the idea of joining a local yoga class because there's some part of you that knows you need something more personal and supportive.

In a nutshell, this book is for you if you'd like to learn natural ways, through yoga, meditation, mindfulness, and movement, to boost your health and wellbeing as a woman. It doesn't matter what age you are; you will gain valuable tips and inspiration on therapeutic practices to give you more energy and vitality—whether you are a younger woman or are blossoming into menopause, the 'second spring' of your life.

If you are of menstruating age you will receive insights into employing the Moving with the Moon template (described in detail for each of the four phases of your menstrual cycle—in chapters four to seven); a template that works in synergy with your unique monthly cycle.

If you are menopausal and no longer menstruating, or if you are currently undergoing the rocky transition to menopause (perimenopause), you can work with the same Moving with the Moon practices, but rather than matching them to each phase of your menstrual cycle you can literally align with the cycles of the moon. You can also integrate the recommended practices in chapter nine into your life to support you in your 'wise woman' phase.

This book is appropriate for any level of yoga experience. That's the beauty of a feminine approach to yoga—it will meet you wherever you are! The practices are clearly illustrated and explained throughout the book as well as in the informative appendices.

However, if you are brand new to yoga, I advise that, alongside the prac-tices detailed in this book, you seek out some tuition with a well-qualified yoga teacher.[14] This will support you with your alignment awareness, so you don't fall into any 'bad habits' that could be counter-productive.

Once you have a foundational understanding of safe alignment, it's important to cultivate a regular home practice; this is the keystone to

---

14   Try a teacher from the Bliss Baby Yoga Directory of qualified yoga teachers (https://www.blissbabyyoga.com/directory/), or you can book a personalised (online) yoga session with myself or one of our Bliss Baby Yoga Feminine Yoga Facilitators (https://www.blissbabyyoga.com/one-on-one-sessions/)

the Moving with the Moon approach to yoga. For tips on setting up and staying motivated for a home practice see chapter three. You may also want to take advantage of the audio meditations and online video classes that accompany this book to support you in your Feminine Yoga home practice.[15]

In addition to providing home practice support and inspiration, this book is designed as a resource for both female and male yoga teachers and complementary health practitioners who would like to offer the Moving with the Moon, Feminine Yoga approach to their students or clients. Teachers will find a wealth of theoretical and practical information to support their students or clients with yoga throughout their menstrual cycle and into menopause.

If you're a younger yoga teacher or health practitioner, the information I share around menopause (see chapter nine) will be particularly useful, so you can meet your older female clients or students where they are— something that would otherwise be difficult if you yourself have not yet had the experience of perimenopause and menopause.

HOW TO USE THIS BOOK

Moving with the Moon is intended to offer a practical step-by-step guide for developing your own Feminine Yoga practice as well as a theoretical background to understanding the underlying motivations and principles of this unique approach to yoga, and in fact, for living as a woman.

In this book I share the scripts for a number of my favourite feminine meditation, relaxation and Pranayama (breath-work) practices. If you would like additional support in implementing these special practices, you may like to download the accompanying audio tracks that are available on my website.[16] In particular, for the Yoga Nidra (deep, guided relaxations) practices, I recommend either availing yourself of my recordings or making your own recordings of the scripts to play to yourself when you are doing them as part of your Feminine Yoga Practice.

In the spirit of the Moving with the Moon philosophy that honours a recognition of our *individual* needs, here are a few different suggestions for navigating your way around this book.

---

15   For more information on Moving with the Moon audio-visual materials, see: https://www.blissbabyyoga.com/online-yoga-classes/

16   See: https://www.blissbabyyoga.com/courses/moving-with-the-moon-audio/

If you're a menstruating woman and keen to dive into the Moving with the Moon practices and taste them first-hand, you could start by reading chapters two and three. This will give you an understanding of your cycle and the important principles for practice. You can then go straight to the relevant chapter of where you are in your cycle at that time (choosing from chapters four to seven). Read the background information on that particular phase or simply jump straight into practising the relevant sequences for that phase.

If you prefer to slowly digest the ideas and gain the broader picture of the Moving with the Moon approach—deeply exploring its history and context—you may want to read this book in its entirety before trying the practices.

If you have been suffering a particular menstrual imbalance, whether it be menstrual cramps, PMS (premenstrual syndrome), endometriosis, absent periods, polycystic ovary syndrome (PCOS) or fibroids, you may want to go straight to the information and tips for your relevant condition—all detailed in chapter eight. This will steer you towards a course of action in using yoga (and other practices) to support your return to health and balance.

If you're a perimenopausal or menopausal woman, you may want to go straight to chapter nine, which will then refer you back to other relevant sections of the book to support you during this often challenging feminine life-stage.

Above all, I urge you to follow your intuition—a recommendation that I have also tried to weave throughout this book. It is only when you connect with your intuition, as both the starting and finishing point for your self-development work through yoga, that you can hope to reconnect with your essential femininity and reclaim your wholeness as a woman.

CHAPTER ONE
HONOURING YOUR CYCLE

The Period is perhaps the most important rite and moment
in ALL of our Lives. Consider what it represents. It is a
time for CELEBRATION of the Life Force that is moving
through a Woman. When this is embraced, the dreaded
'PMS' becomes a cause for celebration, and those heavier
energies become the invitation to surrender to the FLOW.
Man and Woman together. It is miraculous and the cause
for Life. Men are largely responsible for this attitude
because of Fear, but it is not from men alone. It is from
a culture of shaming. This is denying Nature and childish.
Men, embrace this part of your Woman's life and you will
find your inner woman smile and greet you. PERIOD.

—MARK REILLY, YOGA TEACHER[17]

A BRIEF HISTORY OF MENSTRUATION

To begin let's delve into the 'her-story' of cultural attitudes towards menstruation to gain an understanding of the present situation.

Throughout human history menstruation has either been feared or revered, sometimes both at the same time! Many cultures have maintained taboos around menstruation. The word 'taboo' is Polynesian in origin and contains a dual meaning[18]—it means a particular practice, person, place,

---

17 Mark Reilly is a yoga teacher based in Tokyo, Japan. You can connect with him on Facebook here: https://www.facebook.com/mark.reilly.5817?ref=br_rs

18 According to Elissa Stein and Susan Kim in *Flow: The Cultural History of Menstruation* (p.38), the word 'taboo' comes from the Polynesian word 'tapua' and means 'sacred'.

or thing that is forbidden, yet, it also means something which is very sacred.[19]

The frightening power of a bleeding woman

Repressive views towards a woman's menstrual period have threaded through numerous cultures and religions over the centuries. An example can be found in these words from the Old Testament book of Leviticus:

> And if a woman have an issue, and her issue in her flesh be blood, she shall be put apart seven days: and whosoever toucheth her shall be unclean until the even.
>
> And every thing that she lieth upon in her separation shall be unclean: every thing also that that she sitteth upon shall be unclean.
>
> And whosoever toucheth her bed shall wash his clothes, and bathe himself in water, and be unclean until the even.[20]

Many religions have considered menstruating women as 'impure', 'dirty', and even 'dangerous'. Even today in some religions menstruating women are not permitted entry into temples and mosques; men are not allowed to sleep with their menstruating wives, and these 'cursed' women must not cook for others for fear of 'tainting' the food.[21]

Around A.D. 77, Roman philosopher Pliny the Elder propagated a number of absurdly negative and fearful theories around menstruation. He claimed a menstruating woman could sour wine, kill insects and flowers, cause fruit to drop from the trees, blunt knives, discolour mirrors, and make dogs rabid![22]

---

19 Thomas Buckley and Alma Gottlieb in *Blood Magic: The Anthropology of Menstruation* write: 'This etymology shows a lack of unilateral stress on either negative or positive dimensions, and Steiner accordingly suggested that concepts of 'holy' and 'forbidden' are inseparable in the many Polynesian languages,' p.7.

20 Leviticus 15:19–33. I found this quote from Leviticus in *The Curse: A Cultural History of Menstruation* by Janice Delaney, Mary Jane Lupton and Emily Toth, p.37

21 From an article entitled, 'Menstrual Taboos among Major Religions'. See: http://ispub.com/IJWH/5/2/8213

22 I first came across references to Pliny's attitudes towards menstruation in Ruth Trickey's, *Women, Hormones and the Menstrual Cycle: Herbal and Medical solutions from adolescence to menopause*, p.33; the full quotation from Pliny appears in *The Curse: A Cultural History of Menstruation* (Delaney, Lupton and Toth), p.9

Pliny was following on from Democritus, an ancient Greek Philosopher who in the Fourth Century B.C. wrote, 'a girl in her first menstruation should be led three times around the garden beds so that caterpillars there would instantly fall and die.'[23]

In nineteenth-century Saigon, women were not employed in the opium industry because it was believed that the proximity of a menstruating woman would ruin the opium, rendering it bitter![24]

These are just a few examples of the numerous strange and disturbing superstitions that have surrounded menstruation across the world's cultures.

The troublesome wandering uterus

Negative views of a woman's natural, bodily function carried through to a pathological fear of the female body in general which was exhibited in the long-standing belief that a woman's uterus was the source of all her problems.

The ancient Greek philosopher Plato wrote:

> The animal within them (the so-called womb or matrix) is desirous of procreating children, and when remaining unfruitful long beyond its proper time, gets discontented and angry, and wandering in every direction through the body, closes up the passages of the breath, and, by obstructing respiration, drives them to extremity, causing all varieties of diseases.[25]

This bizarre notion led to the invention of the so-called female disease, 'hysteria', which was attributed to this 'wandering uterus', purportedly causing all manner of health troubles. The faux-diagnosis of hysteria was perpetuated for centuries, reaching epic proportions during the Victorian era. Diagnosis of hysteria derived from an exhaustive list of physical and emotional symptoms, such as anxiety, sleeplessness, irritability,

---

23   Cited by Ruth Trickey in *Women, Hormones and the Menstrual Cycle: Herbal and Medical solutions from adolescence to menopause*, p.33

24   Found in an online article—http://facts.randomhistory.com/random-facts-about-menstruation.html—and also quoted in *The Curse* (Delaney, Lupton and Toth), p.9

25   This quote found in: Stein and Kim, *Flow: The Cultural History of Menstruation*, p.37

heaviness in the abdomen, and inexplicable emotional behaviour—to name just a few![26]

The creation of hysteria ultimately represented a twisted manifestation of the suppression of female sexuality that had continued for centuries. One method for relieving this 'disease' involved manual stimulation of the clitoris to stimulate what were called 'hysterical paroxysms',[27] now known as orgasms! Considering that women were not supposed to masturbate or enjoy sex with their husbands it's not surprising that this release of tension and therefore alleviation of the so-called 'hysteria' was considered necessary.

A more extreme treatment for hysteria was the removal of the reproductive organs—the ovaries and uterus. Elissa Stein and Susan Kim, authors of *Flow: The Cultural Story of Menstruation* write, 'patients were usually brought in by their husbands, and without a second thought doctors ripped out their healthy reproductive organs, striving for placid, postsurgical women in a sort of bizarre reproductive spin on the lobotomy.'[28]

Although the diagnosis of hysteria was finally officially discounted in 1952,[29] the practice of hysterectomy (surgical removal of the uterus) has continued as a kind of 'cure-all' for menstrual and menopausal maladies into contemporary times. The number of hysterectomies is inordinately high in developed countries like Australia, the USA, Canada, the UK and New Zealand.[30]

Well known women's health expert and OB/GYN physician, Christiane Northrup, M.D., claims that even though the overall rate of hysterectomies has gone down since it peaked in the 1980s (when about 60 % of women

---

26 Ibid., pp.49–63, in which the authors give a fascinating overview of the prevalence of hysteria throughout history, particularly during the Victorian era.

27 Ibid., p.49

28 Ibid., pp.57–58

29 Ibid., p.50

30 As cited by Charmaine Saunders in her illuminating paper, 'Hysterectomy and Female Castration: Popular Choices for Women in Affluent Societies'. Saunders writes: '..in Australia around 35,000 hysterectomies are performed each year. Around one in four New Zealand women will have had a hysterectomy by the age of 50. In Canada, nearly 40% of women over 60 have had a hysterectomy. In the UK, around 100,000 hysterectomies are performed every year. In France there are 60,000 every year.' See: http://www.feministagenda.org.au/IFS%20Papers/Charmaine2.pdf

in the US had their uterus removed by age 65) they are still performed too often when other options are available.[31] Ernst Bartsich, M.D., a gynecological surgeon at Weill-Cornell Medical Center in New York, agrees and says that while it may be an 'acceptable procedure' it doesn't make it 'necessary in so many cases.' He asserts that of the 617,000 hysterectomies performed annually in the United States, 76–85% could be unnecessary.[32]

Rich woman, poor woman: the classist divide

Let's wind back to the late 1800s when middle and upper-class women were still languishing on divans in well-to-do drawing rooms with this mysterious 'hysteria'.

These Victorian women were advised to rest during their menses, which was perhaps one of the few benefits of being considered 'sensitive'. Lara Owen, menstrual educator and author, quotes from a medical book of the time:

> We cannot too emphatically urge the importance of regarding these monthly returns as periods of ill-health, as days when the ordinary occupations are to be suspended or modified.[33]

Although this recommendation for menstrual rest may have been coming from a condescending and outdated perspective that was tied up with the strange and repressive ideas around 'hysteria', there is validity to this idea. There are many benefits women can gain from giving themselves the time to rest during their monthly period and these will be explored in chapter four.

The working class women of Victorian times, however, were not afforded this luxury of resting when they bled. In fact, things had become a lot worse for these women due to the shift from farming to factory life, which meant they no longer enjoyed the natural rest periods due to the fluctuation of

---

31 Christiane Northrup, M.D., in *Women's Bodies, Women's Wisdom: Creating Physical and Emotional Health and Healing* (p.166) writes: 'More than one-fourth of American women will have this procedure by age sixty.' And, 'The undervaluing of the uterus by doctors and public alike has contributed to the fact that, after caesarean section, hysterectomy is the second most commonly performed major surgical operation in the United States' (p.65).

32 See: http://edition.cnn.com/2007/HEALTH/07/27/healthmag.surgery/

33 Quoted by Lara Owen in *Her Blood is Gold: Awakening to the Wisdom of Menstruation*, p.12

the seasons and rhythm of farm life. Lara Owen explains, 'In a matter of decades, workers in Europe and America shifted from living in a culture which responded to the rhythm of the moon and sun to one in which work was determined by the clock and by machines.'[34]

The sacred power of menstruation

In the House of the Moon, women of all ages gathered together to celebrate the life-giving, life-sustaining powers of their blood and to strengthen their connections with the natural rhythms and cycles of life.

—JASON ELIAS AND KATHERINE KETCHAM
—REFERRING TO NATIVE AMERICAN PRACTICES[35]

In some ancient, pre-Christian, goddess-worshipping, or generally more matriarchal societies, the positive power of menstruation was recognised.

In ancient rituals and ceremonies, menstrual blood was considered a valuable ingredient. According to Barbara Walker, in the *Encyclopaedia of Myths and Secrets*, menstrual blood appears both in mythology as well as real-world practices as a powerful substance that could afford immortality to Egyptian pharaohs, Celtic kings, and even early Taoist practitioners. It was 'used for everything from an ingredient in wine given to Greek gods, to both a beverage and bath for fellow deities of the Hindu Great Mother.'[36] Interestingly, the root of the word 'ritual' comes from the Sanskrit word 'r'tu' which means menstruation.[37]

In Indian Vedic culture as well as Native American Indian tribes, it has always been the practice for menstruating women to be separated from the rest of the tribe or village in menstrual huts or lodges, or even just in a separate room of the house. The women are expected to rest from their usual duties, avoiding cooking and caring for the family and the rest of the tribe.

This practice of separation could be viewed as another example of entrenched fear and mistrust of a woman's monthly bodily process, which certainly has been the case in many cultures. But it can also be viewed as an

---

34   Ibid., p.11

35   Jason Elias and Katherine Ketcham, *In the House of the Moon: Reclaiming the Feminine Spirit Healing*, p.156.

36   As quoted by Stein and Kim in *Flow*, pp.38–39

37   Joy F. Reichard, M.A. in *Celebrate the Divine Feminine: Reclaim your power with Ancient Goddess Wisdom*, p.239

acknowledgment of the sacredness of a woman's bleeding time, along with a recognition of the necessity for her to rest and renew her energy during this time. Jessica H. Simmons, anthropological researcher and founder of Sacha Mama Creations, claims, 'much misunderstanding is birthed from the view of Western mentality when peering into such customs.' Simmons goes on to say:

> It seems, to a society attached to feminist ideas, that because a woman is removed and there are traditions that are exclusively for women, that it was somehow a forced concept by male power. Yet, this is farther from the truth than some would realise. In fact, in all that I have witnessed and experienced, such customs are in reverence to the power of the woman, not the inferiority. I believe we are the ones who invoke inferiority concepts to our women because we DON'T respect or recognize this power, and instead choose to replace ritual and ceremony with fast-paced lifestyles that do not allow us to remove ourselves and feel our own power.[38]

Thomas Buckley and Alma Gottlieb in *Blood Magic: The Anthropology of Menstruation* concur, suggesting that menstrual taboos can be interpreted on many different levels and were most definitely not always repressive towards the female:

> Many menstrual taboos, rather than protecting society from a universally ascribed feminine evil, explicitly protect the perceived creative spirituality of menstruous women from the influence of others in a more neutral state, as well as protecting the latter in turn from the potent, positive spiritual force ascribed to such women. In other cultures menstrual customs, rather than subordinating women to men fearful of them, provide women with means of ensuring their own autonomy, influence, and social control.[39]

Lara Owen suggests the red dot Hindu women put between their eyebrows was originally menstrual blood and was done to invoke the 'visionary aspect of menstruation'. She explains:

38   Jessica H. Simmons in an online blog: https://earthmedicine2015.wordpress.com/2015/10/19/the-ceremony-of-bleeding/

39   Buckley and Gottlieb, *Blood Magic: The Anthropology of Menstruation*, p.7

The blood carries in it the cells of the body, and therefore it contains the knowledge of the DNA. The genetic code, the lineage, is contained within the bloodstream. Every cell in the body is a microcosm of the whole. By painting the third eye with our blood we open ourselves to the knowledge hidden in the genetic code. This knowledge includes deep ancestral awareness and can bring understanding of our own family patterns and also of the human family. [40]

A woman from the American Indian Yurok people in contemporary California, who carries on the tradition of her foremothers of separating herself during her menstruation, explains why she continues to honour this tradition:

A menstruating woman should isolate herself because this is the time when she is at the height of her powers. Thus the time should not be wasted in mundane tasks and social distractions, nor should one's concentration be broken by concerns with the opposite sex. Rather, all of one's energies should be applied in concentrated meditation 'to find out the purpose of your life', and towards the 'accumulation' of spiritual energy. The menstrual shelter, or room, is 'like the men's sweathouse', a place where you 'go into yourself and make yourself stronger.[41]

The practice of menstrual separation has been prevalent in many ancient cultures and it is perhaps Anita Diamant in her novel, *The Red Tent*, who first disseminated this idea widely amongst modern, Western women. Diamant's seminal book offers a feminist re-telling of the life of the biblical character, Dinah. The author describes how Dinah's people lived in tents that were used for various purposes, including the 'red tent'. The red tent was a sacred space where the women of the tribe would gather when they would all menstruate in synchrony with one other and in alignment with the dark moon each month.[42] These women would take their monthly rest in the

---

40 Owen, *Her Blood is Gold*, pp.119-120. Independent midwife Jane Hardwick Collings adds: 'The third eye area is also the place of the pineal gland, referred to in ancient knowledge as the, 'seat of the soul,' so this practice could well increase connection and communication with one's "higher self"'—http://www.moonsong.com.au/the-spiritual-practice-of-menstruation/

41 Buckley and Gottlieb, *Blood Magic*, p.190

42 This echoes what Buckley and Gottlieb, in *Blood Magic*, concluded about the Yurok American Indian women—that they menstruated in synchrony 'utilizing the light of the moon to regularize their menstrual cycles...', p.207

red tent; tell each other stories, eat delicacies, and massage each other's feet as they bled upon the hay.

The whole tribe acknowledged that this was an important practice for its women to support their strength and fertility. There was no hiding or shame around this practice that revered a woman's fertility and was a true embodiment of a positive monthly ritual around menstruation.

> *In the red tent, the truth is known. In the red tent, where days pass like a gentle stream, as the gift of Innana courses through us, cleansing the body of last month's death, preparing the body to receive the new month's life, women give thanks—for repose and restoration, for the knowledge that life comes from between our legs, and that life costs blood.*
>
> —ANITA DIAMANT[43]

The first bleed: an important rite of passage

> *It is said in Native ways that this first blood is the richest and the most powerful a woman will ever have. On this day, she is very special and honoured, for she is becoming like her Mother the Earth: able to renew and nurture life.*
>
> —BROOKE MEDICINE EAGLE[44]

In addition to the monthly ritual of separation that allowed women to rest and renew their energy during their period, many traditional societies also had practices to celebrate and honour a young girl when she first reached puberty and began to bleed.

A girl's first menstrual period is called her 'menarche' and Diamant writes of how the red tent was also a sacred space for menarche rituals, echoing practices that have existed across the world, particularly in cultures like that of the native American Indians. The Navaho people carried out an elaborate menarche ritual for their young girls that included 'seclusion, instruction of the girl in the taboos she must observe as a menstruating woman, and a large tribal celebration when the seclusion and instruction was complete.'[45]

---

43   Anita Diamant, *The Red Tent*, p.193

44   Quoted by Elias and Ketcham in *In the House of the Moon*, p.159

45   Delaney, Lupton and Toth, *The Curse*, p.33

In India, the menarche has traditionally been celebrated as an important and positive transformation for young girls into women, and their rituals have also involved a period of seclusion, instruction, and then public rejoicing. Authors of *The Curse: A Cultural History of Menstruation*, Delaney, Lupton, and Toth, explain how the Deshast Brahmins, after the obligatory period of seclusion, placed the girl 'on a little throne' and she was 'visited by neighbours and relatives, given presents, and washed in ceremonial oil.'[46]

Among the Dagara people of West Africa, the initiation of girls is performed each year for all the girls who have started to menstruate in the preceding year. Christiane Northrup M.D. writes, 'this ceremony is the beginning of a long period of mentoring that includes information about sex, intimacy, and the special healing powers of the menstruating woman.'[47]

The common theme for the various menarche rituals across cultures is one of preparing a young girl for womanhood, 'an emphasis on the entrance to a sexual life and on the importance of the procreative function to the life and welfare of the society,' write Delaney, Lupton and Toth.[48]

MENSTRUATION TODAY

The more rigid, linear and out of touch with the feminine,
with soul life and natural rhythms a culture becomes,
the more severe will be the disturbance a woman
experiences within her cycle. The menstrual cycle is both
a monitor for her own wellbeing, and the world's.

—ALEXANDRA POPE[49]

This little meandering through the human history of menstruation helps explain today's current attitudes. Our modern society still labours under a sense of shame and taboo around the subject of menstruation that has

---

46 Ibid., p.34

47 Northrup in an online article, 'Celebrating a girls first period'. http://www. drnorthrup.com/celebrating-a-girls-first-period/#sthash.tWBtQo5x.dpuf This is footnoted by Northrup as coming from Lara Owen, *Honoring menstruation: a time of self-renewal*. (Freedom, CA: Crossing Press), p.35.

48 Delaney, Lupton and Toth, *The Curse*, p.25

49 Alexandra Pope, *The Wild Genie: The Healing Power of Menstruation*, p.220

characterised many patriarchal cultures of the past. This taboo is evident when simply considering the embarrassment that accompanies a blood stain on a women's skirt, or a tampon accidentally falling out of her handbag, or her whispered request to a female colleague for a spare tampon because she just got her *period*.

Although women are no longer the unwarranted victims of the irrational fear and ostracism that has occurred throughout history, there is currently an entrenched, cultural denial of menstruation that is harming women in its own insidious way. Women are living in a culture that negates the bloody realities of menstruation with sanitised versions that are depicted on television commercials with the images of blue liquid on a dazzling white (dioxide-dyed) sanitary pads. This denial extends to the practice of 'menstrual suppression' in which doctors press women to take advantage of modern contraceptive options that 'liberate' them from the 'inconvenience' of their body having to undergo its monthly bleed.

Denying the imperative of women's cyclical bodies is the result of a hangover from the Victorian attitude towards working-class women's bodies that I touched on in my wrap-up of the 'her-story' of menstruation. Women are expected to function optimally within the inexorable rhythm of the five day working week (for mothers it's more like a seven day working week!) allowing no space for recognition of their own internal womb rhythms, which are in turn connected to that of the moon's.

Through relinquishing the Victorian notion of the upper middle class woman as a passive, sensitive creature who should most definitely rest during her monthly period, society has essentially 'thrown the baby out with the bathwater'—pardon the pun! Lara Owen writes, 'there is usually at least a glimmer of truth in any ideology, and the physicians of the Victorian era were not completely wrong when they emphasised the importance of menstruation in women's overall health, the relationship between the womb and the psyche, and the wisdom of rest during the period.'[50]

Consequently, these days women are trapped in a linear paradigm that doesn't support their feminine bodies and psyches. Modern society tends to view menstruation as a 'curse' (a long-standing nickname in the West), or at best, as an inconvenience. Women basically try to ignore it all—they stick a tampon in, take a painkiller if necessary, and forge on as normal.

---

50   Owen, *Her Blood is Gold*, p14

If symptoms like period cramps, tiredness, and pre-menstrual headaches do demand their attention, they suffer in silence, considering this their inevitable 'feminine lot'.

Perhaps some of the blame for this 'grimace and bear it' attitude can be attributed to the first and second waves of feminism—the suffragettes in the early 1900s, followed by the 'Women's Liberation Movement' of the 1960–80s.[51] While these earlier manifestations of feminism were critical in granting women many invaluable freedoms and equalities, they also generated an unrealistic expectation that women needed to be viewed as just the same as men. It was believed that if women were viewed as 'weaker' in any way this would hamper their progress towards gender equality. This is where the third wave of feminism (spanning the 1980–90s) with its branches of 'difference feminism' and 'spiritual feminism'[52] offers a more refined understanding that we are in fact *equal but different*. It's this difference that needs to be honoured to support our ongoing mental and emotional health and wellbeing as women.

A recognition of this 'difference', of women's true, inherent feminine natures, needs to be honoured with monthly rest, and this takes courage, as Lara Owen describes:

> When I discuss ancient ideas about the spiritual power of menstrua-
> tion with successful aspiring women, one of the biggest fears is that
> this will in some way affect their myth of being 'just as good as a
> man, and sometimes better'. Many women don't want to go deeper
> into menstruation; they are scared of what they will discover. It suits
> them to suppress their feelings with tranquilisers, to spray with vagi-
> nal deodorants to disguise the smell of the blood, to numb their pain
> through painkillers, and to absorb their blood with tampons so they
> never have to actually see it. It's easier to be a successful woman in a
> man's world if you hardly recognise that you menstruate at all.[53]

---

51 A good overview of the three waves of feminism can be found in this online article: http://www.gender.cawater-info.net/knowledge_base/rubricator/feminism_e.htm and also this here: https://www.progressivewomensleadership.com/a-brief-history-the-three-waves-of-feminism

52 Chris Bobel in *New Blood: Third-Wave Feminism and the Politics of Menstruation*, (p.66) describes 'feminist-spiritualists' as 'menstrual activists who work to reclaim menstruation as a healthy, spiritual, empowering, and even pleasurable experience.'

53 Owen, *Her Blood is Gold*, pp.14–15

Promoting a modern menarche

In addition to lacking a tradition that acknowledges the importance of sacred rest during our periods, we are also without any established rituals to celebrate our entrance into womanhood—the menarche.

Think back to your first period. It's likely there was little, if any, fuss made by your family and friends. If you're lucky, it was a neutral event, but for many women it may have be played out as a negative memory that can colour their attitudes towards their bodies for the rest of their lives. My mother was sent home in disgrace from her Catholic girls' school when she bled onto her school uniform. Without any education and support, as well as the public shaming, the whole event was bewildering and embarrassing.

Things are a little less dire these days; compared to when my mother was growing up. Young girls are now more educated around the medical process of menstruation. However, we still don't tend to honour or celebrate this event in a teenage girl's life.

It is time we come full circle and for women to create their own modern menarche rituals to support their daughters, their friends' daughters, their granddaughters, or their nieces in beginning their relationships with their monthly cycles in a positive and empowering way.

The importance of menarche rituals

A symbolic act at the time of first bleeding recognises,
emphasises, and accepts the change which has occurred in
the child and becomes for that child the start of learning
from her own experience as she grows into maturity.

—MIRANDA GRAY[54]

Miranda Gray, author and menstrual-positive workshop facilitator, says that menarche is an important point in a young girl's life as it signals her transition from 'the linear nature of childhood to the cyclic nature of womanhood.'[55]

Many other menstrual-positive educators agree and suggest if women can take the time and conscious intention to honour the onset of menstruation for a young girl this will have positive flow-on effects for her experience of

---

54 Miranda Gray, *Red Moon: Understanding and Using the Creative, Sexual and Spiritual Gifts of the Menstrual Cycle*, p.159

55 Ibid

those other significant transition periods—birth and menopause. A colleague of mine, Moana Pearl, who has been involved in sacred women's business and women's spirituality for 25 years says:

> If a young woman learns to honour her body as sacred, to self-care and self-respect, then she will make healthy choices for her body, her sexuality, her birthing and her children. She will stay connected to her body's wisdom and learn from its changes, and her healthy entry into menstruation will support her through her menopause. She will be empowered and strengthened by knowing she carries (and is carried by) something of value, deeply connected to the cycles of the universe, something of mystery itself, the red thread connecting women throughout time, and all humans…as every human has been birthed through a woman's body. She will recognise her menstrual cycle as a resource, a friend, a wise mentor, a sanctuary.[56]

Independent midwife Jane Hardwicke Collings makes the particular point that a woman's disconnection with her menstrual cycle can begin with an uncelebrated menarche, and this can have deep repercussions in how she births:

> To my mind, a major contributing factor to where we are at as a culture, why home birth and vaginal birth are threatened, is because the majority of women come to the birth altar unprepared, unknowing and unconvinced of the power and point of natural birth, and why is this so? Because they have been led to believe through their experiences of being a woman so far through their menarche and their menstruation, that the female body is essentially flawed, that medical science and technology will enable them to control the wayward unpredictable processes they must endure in the female body and that the fertility cycle of a woman is fraught with danger, blood, mess, pain, mood swings and inconvenience, which will interfere with a woman's productivity and contribution on a day to day basis.[57]

---

56   From Moana Pearl's online blog: https://moanapearl.wordpress.com/2017/05/

57   Hardwick Collings in her online blog: http://www.moonsong.com.au/the-connection -between-menarche-and-childbirth-from-one-rite-to-the-next/

Creating a menarche ritual

If you are the mother of a girl, you have the opportunity to help your daughter foster a positive connection with her femininity through co-creating a menarche ritual she can recall into her adulthood as beautiful and honouring.

So what does a menarche ritual look like? This is entirely limited by your own imagination but there are some terrific resources you may want to draw on for ideas and inspiration.[58]

Miranda Gray in her book, *Red Moon*, offers some helpful guidelines and symbols for your menarche ritual with your daughter, 'try to make the whole day of the rite of passage special for your daughter; do something together which is normally considered a treat and make it a family occasion if you feel that is appropriate,' recommends Gray.[59]

Dr Christiane Northrup shares some inspiring, modern-day menarche stories in her online article 'Celebrating a Girl's First Period', like this one which illustrates a simple way that you can include your daughter's 'elders':

> I wrote to my circle of female friends and family, asking them each to help me celebrate Molly from afar by sending a card, note, or reading that they would want to share with her whenever the day came. I planned to keep them all in a special envelope or booklet and wait for the time to share them.
>
> These women, including my college roommate, sisters-in-law, and childhood friend, all seized the opportunity to do something very special. What came back over the next few months were boxes filled with gifts, books, writings. I found a beautiful storage box covered in a floral fabric in which I would present these gifts, rather than the planned envelope or scrapbook. The box was filled with a series of butterfly objects—a butterfly necklace, trinket box, and hairclips to signify her transformation; a Celtic plaque depicting the maiden, mother, and crone to educate her about the cycles of life; photos of one of her aunts in 'stylish' cat-eye glasses at the age she first menstruated; a book of teen wisdom; a big box of gourmet chocolates from a grown cousin who said this would

---

58 Lucy H. Pearce, in her book *Moon Time: A Guide to Celebrating your Menstrual Cycle*, in a section entitled, 'Activities to celebrate your daughter's menarche', offers some simple and practical ideas—location 2273 (Kindle edition)

59 Gray, *Red Moon: Understanding and using the creative, sexual and spiritual gifts of the menstrual cycle*, pp.159–167

always make her feel better at 'that time of the month.' And there were many, many written words of wisdom and memory from these wonderful women, including an awkward note from her grandmother (my mom), who simply didn't know what to say to acknowledge an event that was so very private when she was a girl.

The day Molly got her period, she was very matter-of-fact, as she often is about life. Before she got into bed, I took her into our guest room and pulled out the celebration box. She first read the card from me, which explained what she was about to receive, and then together we opened the large fabric box and all the beautifully wrapped gifts from her 'sisters' inside. For that hour, it was as if all of the women we knew were right there in the room with us, a circle of women drawn together across distance and time. Together we shared what women are all about—memories, advice, and deeply held feelings.[60]

Moana Pearl, who has shepherded young girls and their mothers through the sacred passage of menarche for almost twenty years, offers these words of caution to those designing a menarche ritual:

If we overlay a shallow, plastic, contemporary version of a ritual celebration on menarche it could become like a birthday party with red balloons. Menarche rituals and ceremonies carry powerful symbolism. Have clear intention. Dig deep inside. Go gently. Get support from others who have held these ceremonies before. Be sure it's not only about her as a person, it's bigger than that. Remember, it's not what we say that will imprint our girls most, it's how we live, moon by moon, breath by breath.[61]

As these ancient menstrual-positive ideas around honouring and celebrating a women's menstrual period and the menarche take root in our modern consciousness, women have the unique opportunity to embrace and adapt these ideas as their own and to share them with their daughters and their community. Gradually, we can change the culture that has long perpetuated an unhelpful and even harmful attitude around this most natural of bodily processes. After all, the fact that we bleed every month represents the very heart of what it means to be a woman and it's time that this was no longer devalued in contemporary society.

---

60 Northrup, online blog: http://www.drnorthrup.com/celebrating-a-girls-first-period/

61 Pearl in her online blog: https://moanapearl.wordpress.com/2017/05/

Healing your own menarche

If your memory of your own experience of menarche is less than re-splendent, you can always do some healing work around this to help you move forward in a way that positively reframes your attitudes around your cycle. This can support you in your current life-phase and may also heal any physical or emotional imbalances or blockages that are impeding your optimal health and connection with your femininity.

One healing method is the quintessentially feminine therapy of talking and sharing. Get together with a close girlfriend or female family member to consciously discuss your respective experiences around your first-bleed. Take turns really listening to each other's story—'holding space' for each other. This means that you are totally present in a caring, non-judgemental way for the other woman that allows her to freely express and move through all her feelings around her experience of menarche.

Perhaps you can finish your sharing-time with your 'soul sister' by each setting a positive intention for how you would like to now honour your menstrual cycle each month (see p.80 for some ideas on honouring your menses). Or if you are no longer menstruating, you could set a positive intention for including more self-care into your life as a post-menopausal woman.

Another way you can support yourself in processing your menarche experiences is to journal. For example, write a letter to your younger, teenage self from your now more mature self, offering your younger self-loving words of advice and support.

If you feel that you have any significant trauma around your teenage experiences of menstruation and early sexuality it may also be necessary to seek professional counselling support.

Regardless of what method you use to process any dishonouring experiences around your menarche it's always important to give yourself the gift of *gentle acceptance*. Yoga lends itself so beautifully to this intention, especially a Feminine Yoga practice that embodies the concept of *ahimsa* or self-compassion (read more about this important Feminine Yoga principle in chapter three), which can support you so gracefully through the physical and emotional challenges that may arise throughout your womb-cycles.

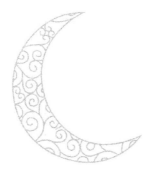

Part Two
Getting Started

CHAPTER TWO
THE EBB AND FLOW OF THE WOMB

When I teach a session explaining the physiology of the menstrual cycle on yoga teacher training courses and workshops, I am constantly surprised to discover how few women are well acquainted with the inner workings of their wombs.

Developing a sound understanding of how your menstrual cycle works, as well as its four 'energetic' phases, is the first step to building a healthier relationship with your body and its cycles. This understanding will also help you gain the most from the Moving with the Moon practices detailed in this book.

THE MONTHLY CYCLE: WHAT'S ACTUALLY GOING ON?

A woman's monthly cycle averages 29.5 days, just like that of the moon. This is only the *average* as many women have shorter or longer cycles that can range from 21 to 35 days. Your reproductive cycle responds to a rise and fall in hormones and is commonly divided into two phases.

The first phase, known as the 'follicular' or 'proliferative phase', begins on day 1 of your cycle when you start to bleed. Women usually bleed for anywhere between 3 to 5 days. When you menstruate, the hormones, oestrogen and progesterone are at their lowest levels. During or just after your period, the pituitary gland responds to a signal from the hypothalamus to stimulate the growth of 10 to 20 eggs that develop in their shells, called 'follicles', within the ovaries.

The follicles produce an increasing amount of oestrogen, which is responsible for creating a new, bloody lining to the uterus called the 'endometrium'. This thickening of the womb is the body's way of preparing for a potential pregnancy—a thick and juicy endometrium creates a receptive home for a fertilised egg to burrow into and therefore establish pregnancy. Oestrogen also converts the mucus around the cervix (entrance to the womb) into copious slippery like 'egg-white' or 'fertile mucous', which facilitates the passage of sperm as well as lengthening its life span (sperm can live for approximately five days in fertile mucus).

Around day 14 (again, this is just the average), ovulation occurs. This is when the most mature egg ripens and bursts out of its follicle, and from the ovary, and into the fallopian tube that connects down to the uterus. The egg can live in the fallopian tube for anywhere between 12 to 24 hours. If you have well-timed sex around ovulation, you can potentially fall pregnant. In this instance, sperm travels up through the vagina, through the cervix, into the uterus and then continues to swim up the fallopian tube to merge with the ripe egg. If fertilisation occurs, the fertilised egg, now called an embryo, will travel down the fallopian tube and implant into the endometrium (lining of the womb), about six days later. The body will then continue to produce increasing levels of progesterone and oestrogen to sustain the pregnancy.

After ovulation, the second phase called the 'luteul' or 'premenstrual phase' commences. During this phase of the menstrual cycle, the empty shell around the egg, now called the 'corpus luteum', produces high levels of progesterone. Progesterone continues to thicken and nourish the endometrium (lining of the womb) which dries up the cervical mucus and vaginal sensation, and raises the body temperature.

If pregnancy does not occur, the corpus luteum will shrivel and die and cease its production of hormones about 14 days after ovulation. The lining of the womb (endometrium) breaks down and is shed as menstrual blood, and so begins day 1 of the cycle again, your body having completed a full circle.[62]

TRACKING YOUR CYCLE

If I asked you where you are right now in your menstrual cycle, would you know?

For many women the only time they know for sure where they are positioned in their cycle is when they are bleeding (menstruation).

However if you're trying to get pregnant, or manage your fertility naturally, or become more attuned with your body and your emotions by embarking on a Moving with the Moon yoga practice, you'll need to know how to track your cycle. This means ideally learning to recognise when you ovulate.

Simple ways you can tell you are ovulating include observing changes in your vaginal mucus and the position of your cervix. When you're ovulating, the vaginal mucus will become copious, clear, and slippery, like egg white. You should be able to stretch it between two fingers, just like

---

62   These are the references I used for this little overview of the menstrual cycle:
      Honoring our Cycles, Katie Singer, *Women, Hormones and the Menstrual Cycle*,
      Ruth Trickey, and, *Natural Fertility: The Complete Guide to Avoiding or Achieving
      Conception*, Francesca Naish.

egg-white. When you put your finger inside your vagina and feel for your cervix (the entrance to your womb) it will be higher than normal. For me, it feels like my vaginal canal becomes longer, bigger, softer, and more open when I am ovulating and therefore fertile.

During ovulation, supporting your body's natural biological urge to procreate, you are also likely to feel sexier than at other times of the month. Although many women also report their libido peaks again just before they menstruate.

Keeping a record of how many days your cycle lasts every month, over a number of months, can also help give you a picture of when you ovulate. I have mentioned that the *average* point in the cycle for ovulation to occur is around day 14, which would be true for you if you have a 28 or 29 day cycle. However, if your cycle is much shorter, you will ovulate earlier. Some women ovulate very early—sometimes just after their period—and therefore produce fertile mucus along with menstrual blood. This means these women can actually get pregnant when they have sex during their menses. You can reliably use this calculation method, known as the 'calendar method', of ascertaining when you are ovulating, if you have regular cycles (over at least the last six months). Simply subtract 14 days from your shortest cycle length, so if it's 26 days, subtract 14, and you will know that your ovulation phase is *around* day 12.[63]

I've offered a very brief introduction to working out when you're ovulating. I urge you to do your research if you're not sure and especially if you're trying to achieve or avoid pregnancy. There are many excellent books[64] that go into detail about the various 'natural fertility' techniques you can use to track your cycle. Additionally, there are 'apps' you can download onto your mobile device into which you can enter your personal cycle data that then indicates when you might be ovulating.

---

63   Reference: Christiane Northrup M.D., *Women's Bodies, Women's Wisdom*, p.423.
     A more precise version of this 'calendar method' calculation for determining your
     approximate date of ovulation is explained on a Queensland Women's Health Fact
     Sheet (http://womhealth.org.au/conditions-and-treatments/understanding-your-
     menstrual-cycle-fact-sheet), as follows: 'For women with regular cycles, an easy way
     to approximate the time of ovulation is to subtract 16 from the number of days in
     the cycle and then add 4. This will calculate the span of days in which ovulation
     is most likely to occur. For instance, a woman with a 22-day cycle is most likely to
     ovulate between days 6 and 10 of her cycle (22-16 = 6 (+4 =10).'

64   I recommend these two books to give you a comprehensive 'how to' guide for
     tracking your cycle in order to achieve or avoid pregnancy, or, just understand
     your cycle better: *Natural Fertility: The Complete Guide to Avoiding or Achieving
     Conception*, by Francesca Naish, and, *Honoring Our Cycles: A Natural Family
     Planning Workbook* by Katie Singer.

THE LUNAR CONNECTION

Our bodies know about change, rhythm, and cycles. This is
women's eternal, universal secret. Nature is rhythm, and our
bodies are part of nature—not only the immediate earth
environment but the exquisite vast movement of the cosmos.

—CAMILLE MAURINE AND LORIN ROCHE[65]

So far, I have explained that the average length of the menstrual cycle (29.5 days) is actually the same as the lunar cycle (the time that it takes the moon to orbit the earth). It's fascinating to explore this connection between the moon and a woman's body a little further. Just as the moon affects the oceanic tides it also impacts on the inner tides of a woman's womb. It appears that ovulation can be triggered by the light of the full moon due to its interaction with a woman's melatonin levels and her hormonal system.

Fertility naturopath Francesca Naish writes that the pineal gland (which interacts with our governing hormonal glands of the hypothalamus and pituitary) responds to changes in light and darkness, indicating that a woman's hormonal system can be influenced by lunar-light.[66] Christiane Northrup M.D. refers to studies that show higher rates of conception (and therefore ovulation) occur around the full moon, whereas there is a decrease in conception (and therefore ovulation) around the new moon.[67]

Lara Owen makes the compelling point about the connection between the relatively unchangeable length of women's luteal phase and how this can potentially relate to the unchangeable cycle of the moon:

> The endometrium is shed fourteen days after ovulation; out of the whole menstrual cycle, this time period of bleeding fourteen days after ovulation is the most regular and widely experienced by women everywhere. This means that if the full moon triggers ovulation, then women will bleed fourteen days later, on the new moon.[68]

---

65 Camille Maurine and Lorin Roche, *Meditation Secrets for Women: Discovering your passion, pleasure, and inner peace,* p.147

66 Naish, in *Natural Fertility* (p.89) writes: '.. it has been shown that the light of the full moon increases levels of the follicle stimulating hormone (FSH), via the hypothalamus and pituitary glands. We also know that light is absorbed, via the optic nerve, and used as a 'nutrient' for the endocrine system, and that the pineal gland ('the third eye') is also light-sensitive.'

67 See Northrup, *Women's Bodies, Women's Wisdom,* p.104

68 Owen, *Her Blood is Gold,* p.23

According to Francesca Naish, in the Zambezi valley in Africa, women have known for a very long time that the moon influences women's monthly cycles and they 'expect to ovulate at the full moon and menstruate when the moon is new.' This is aided by an architectural adaption in which the roofs of their houses have a special opening for the full moon to shine through.[69] Another example is the Yurok American Indian women who menstruated in synchrony 'utilising the light of the moon to regularise their menstrual cycles.'[70]

The white moon cycle

In modern urban settings, the moon's light is diluted by artificial lights, and women's cycles can also be thrown out by other factors like diet, pollutants, stress[71], and spontaneously synchronising with women close by. This means that there is no guarantee that women's bodies will be so easily influenced by the moon.

These days, women tend to menstruate at all different times of the lunar month, although studies show that more women do still bleed with the new or dark moon.[72] Dr Christiane Northrup says that when women live together in natural settings their 'ovulations tend to occur at the time of the full moon, with menses and self-reflection at the dark of the moon.'[73]

This predominant pattern of ovulating with the full moon and therefore bleeding with the new or dark moon is known as a 'white moon cycle'. According to the ancient healing-science of Ayurveda, the 'white moon cycle' is optimal for strengthening a woman's menstrual health and fertility. Dr Robert E. Svoboda, an American Ayurvedic physician, writes that when a woman ovulates with the full moon, 'the heavens encourage her body and mind to be plump and juicy,' and menstruating with the new moon helps her body, 'to expel unused fertility juices.'[74]

---

69 Naish, *Natural Fertility*, p.105

70 Buckley and Gottleib, *Blood Magic: The Anthropology of Menstruation*, p.207

71 See chapter eight, 'Menstrual Medicine', for more information on the connection between stress and an imbalance in the menstrual cycle.

72 Penelope Shuttle and Peter Redgrove in their pioneering book, *The Wise Wound*, which is heavy with research, cite a study by Walter and Abraham Menaker of 250, 000 hospital births that came up with the following conclusion: 'The evidence presented here shows a small but statistically significant lunar (or sun-moon) influence on the human birth-rate, and presumably on the conception rate and, perhaps, on the ovulation rate... The peak of conception and probably ovulation appears to occur at full moon or a day before it,' (p. 150).

73 Northrup, *Women's Bodies, Women's Wisdom*, p.106

74 Dr. Robert E. Svoboda , *Ayurveda for Women: A Guide to Vitality and Health*, p.29

Lucy Pearce, author of *Moon Time: A Guide to Celebrating Your Menstruation*, writes that women who have charted their cycles and find they are menstruating with the dark moon report feeling more 'in flow' and 'attuned to themselves'.[75]

There are many possible ways to encourage your cycle to sync to the moon and to follow this 'white moon cycle'. These include meditation and intention-setting, mudra (hand gestures),[76] and, exposing yourself to the light of the full moon—sleeping with the curtains open to let the full moon flood in. There is even a field of practice called 'lunaception'[77] in which you can mimic the light of the moon and sleep with a night light on for three nights in the middle of the month to precipitate ovulation.

Personally, I experience the extraordinary phenomenon in which every few months my body seems to spontaneously adjust the length of my cycle, so I have an unusually long or short cycle to bring me back in line with a 'white moon cycle'.

The red moon cycle

Some women notice they actually bleed with the full moon, which is the opposite to the 'white moon cycle'. This pattern, known as a 'red moon cycle', occurs when women ovulate with the *new* moon and bleed with a *full* moon.

---

75 Lucy H. Pearce, *Moon Time*, location 1064 (Kindle edition)

76 Ayurvedic women's health expert, Maya Tiwari, in *Women's Power to Heal through Inner Medicine*, says practising Yoni Mudra (see p.327 in this book for illustration and instructions) can help strengthen our Shakti energy and 'redirects the menstrual blood back in accordance with the new moon' (p.155). Tiwari also advocates 'Uttara Vasta', a Wise Earth Ayurvedic herbal douche practice as an effective way of aligning you to the moon (ie: a 'white moon cycle').

77 The idea of 'Lunaception' was first popularised by Louise Lacey in her groundbreaking book, *Lunaception: A Feminine Odyssey into Fertility and Contraception*—see: http://lunaception.net. I first came across a description of this practice in *The Garden of Fertility* by Katie Singer, (pp.159-163) which cites some interesting research on the practice and benefits of night lighting on the female menstrual cycle. Dr Christiane Northrup in her book, *Women's Bodies, Women's Wisdom* (p 104), refers to a study in which two thousand women with irregular menstrual cycles managed to regulate their cycles by sleeping with night lighting (citing F.A. Brown, 1972. 'The clocks: Timing biological rhythms,' American Scientist).

Miranda Gray assures women, 'both cycles are expressions of the feminine energies and neither is more powerful or more correct than the other.'[78]

Whether your body is following a 'red moon' or 'white moon' cycle may depend upon your particular focus in your life at the time, as Jane Hardwicke Collings clarifies:

> It has felt to be the case over and over that a full moon ovulation is when you are in the baby-making phase of your life, and dark moon ovulation is when you are not and you are birthing deep parts and aspects of yourself rather than babies. Bleeding at the dark moon aligns with the energy of the moon at this part of her cycle and supports retreat, enables release, purification, cleansing, renewal and rebirth. Bleeding always lures us inward, into our cave, for a time of contemplation, release and renewal, when the moon is full and we are bleeding, it is as if the lights are on in our 'cave' and we cannot hide from the parts of us that we 'need' to face and let go of.[79]

Miranda Gray agrees and says, 'the red moon cycle' shows an orientation away from the expression of the energies in procreation and the material world and towards inner development and its expression.'[80]

The dance between white and red moon cycles

Throughout your fertile life cycle, you may find that you experience both 'red moon' and 'white moon' cycles, or that your cycle is in transition from one to the other. Becoming more sensitive to the subtle differences in your cycle and how it parallels with the moon in its various phases, allows you to recognise your changing needs—physical, emotional, and mental—that you can address in how you work, love, play, and practise your yoga. Jane Hardwicke Collings sums this up beautifully:

> Our menstrual cycle is our barometer of our being, it is directly affected by our lifestyle, health and stresses. It will get us to the right place at the right time. The journey to know this uncovers the women's mysteries and takes a woman forward on her path of personal awareness and

---

78 Miranda Gray, *Red Moon*, p.77

79 Jane Hardwicke Collings, from her online blog titled, 'Menstrual Lunar Asynchrony', Spring 2011: http://www.moonsong.com.au/menstrual-lunar-asynchrony-2/

80 Miranda Gray, *Red Moon*, pp.76-77

shows her the interconnectedness of everything. Through exploring her menstrual cycle she is invited into the realm of feminine wisdom, power and strength. She comes to realise that she needs to take responsibility for her life.[81]

The moon as metaphor

Just as the moon sheds her shadow to be born again, so do women shed their blood in an ongoing process of renewal and regeneration. Filling with light and emptying into darkness, the moon has come to symbolise the dynamic, eternal nature of life, and women, because their bodies are privileged to follow these natural cycles, carry within their hearts and souls the moon's gentle wisdom.

—Jason Elias and Katherine Ketcham[82]

Let me emphasise that there is no right or wrong as to how your menstrual cycle should relate to the lunar cycle. This overview of 'red' and 'white moon' cycles is not intended to make you feel inadequate if your body does not neatly match with one of these cycles and you are therefore not bleeding regularly with the new or full moon. I certainly don't want you to feel that this is yet another thing for you to be good at, to succeed at, to 'conquer'—these are all out-dated attitudes stemming from the masculine paradigm that only serve to hinder the much-needed quality of feminine self-acceptance.

If you find that your menstruation and ovulation coincide with the waxing moon or waning moon this is totally valid too! You can still look to the moon as a reference or gauge for where you are at in your cycle no matter how uniquely your body correlates to its phases.

My main point is that developing your awareness of how your bodily cycles mirror the phases of the moon deepens your connection with your body and the changes you experience internally and externally, which results in a positive flow-on effect for your health and your enjoyment of your menstrual cycle.

---

81 Jane Hardwicke Collings, from her online blog titled, 'Menstrual Lunar Asynchrony', Spring 2011: http://www.moonsong.com.au/menstrual-lunar-asynchrony-2/

82 Elias and Ketcham, *In the House of the Moon*, location 283 (Kindle version)

Referencing the moon will make you aware that the changes in your monthly cycle are what keep you constantly connected to those of nature. Simply look out at the moon each night to feel that connection. Regardless of how your body uniquely syncs with the lunar cycle, you will develop an appreciation of the mirroring energies of your body and the moon. You will understand that with the build-up and then release of the uterine endometrial cells, along with the ripening and disintegration of a potentially fertile egg, and your rise and fall in physical energy, your feminine body is essentially 'waxing' and 'waning' every month, reflecting the journey of the moon into fullness and then emptiness again.

Tami Lynn Kent in *The Wild Feminine* suggests that the energy of menstruation is 'a physical reflection of the uterine capacity to hold or release.' She says that just as women's bodies (wombs) know when to hold and release during the monthly cycle, so too can they take this innate ability into all of life's major transitions: 'Changing jobs, reinventing or dissolving a marriage, creating a new partnership, sending a child off to college, completing a major project, losing a parent, facing a serious illness, making a new home: all major life events require that we choose what to hold or release in order to make a complete transition.'[83]

THE FOUR ENERGETIC PHASES OF YOUR CYCLE

The earth has her seasons when autumn leaves fall, while vital sap is withdrawn before its vigorous resurgence in spring time. By adopting a positive attitude to this most natural of womanly processes, we can use full awareness of menstruation and its implications to experience our bond with Mother Earth and join in the rhythms of the cosmos.

—SWAMI MUKTANANDA[84]

From a purely physiological perspective, as previously detailed, a woman's monthly menstrual cycle consists of two phases: the follicular/proliferative

---

83 Tami Lynn Kent, *The Wild Feminine: Finding Power, Spirit and Joy in the Female Body*, pp.212-213

84 Swami Muktananda, *Nawa Yogini Tantra: Yoga for Women*, p.41

phase and the luteal/premenstrual phase. However, if you track the array of physical and emotional changes that you can experience during your cycle, it becomes clear that the menstrual cycle can also be viewed in terms of four 'energetic' phases.

Various menstrual-positive educators posit the four phases of the menstrual cycle as a way to more deeply appreciate fluctuations of a woman's cycle. I particularly resonate with Miranda Gray's exploration of these four phases in her inspiring book, *The Optimized Woman: Using Your Menstrual Cycle To Achieve Success and Fulfillment*. Gray puts forward a kind of cyclical, 'life-coaching' model which suggests that if women can tune into their changing physical energy, moods and mental states that become evident throughout the four phases of their cycle, they can adjust their workload and their self-expectations accordingly to maximise their wellbeing and productivity.

Moving with the Moon

In this book, I've added the lunar metaphor as a way of deepening our awareness of these four phases. And I have broadened this idea into a yoga context, as I endeavour to answer this question: *how can we adjust our yoga practice to reflect the changing needs of the four phases of our menstrual cycle and therefore support ourselves on a holistic level?*

So what are these four phases and what do they mean for your life and your yoga practice?

The Dark Moon (menstrual) phase

This phase correlates with your menses. When there is no moon, or a 'dark moon', your natural inclination is to stay indoors. In the same way, the energy of menstruation encourages you to retreat inwards.

As your uterus works hard to shed its menstrual blood, there is usually a natural dip in your energy. This is the most sensitive time in your cycle— your immune system is at its lowest point and you actually need more sleep at this time of the month![85] It represents the dormant 'winter' phase of your cycle.

---

85   See p.71 in chapter four of this book for more details on the physical sensitivity of this phase, i.e., lower immunity and need for rest and sleep.

Miranda Gray calls this the 'reflective' phase.[86] It's when you can reflect on the events and feelings of the past month, and let go of anything that no longer serves you. It not only involves a physical cleansing of the body as the endometrial lining is released, but also an emotional cleansing. To do this you need to take some time and space for yourself, as much as possible, and separate from your duties as mother, wife, girlfriend, worker, and nourish your energy with deep, inner reflective practices.

A Dark Moon yoga practice

This is your time to 'lush it up' with gentle Restorative Yoga that encompasses only those postures that are safe and appropriate for menstruation (see chapter four for details).

During this phase you are more receptive to deep states of relaxation and meditation than at any other point in your cycle, so this can be harnessed with a quiet, interior practice that will include time to breathe and just 'be'. Create a sacred space for yourself—light some candles, play some soothing music, and turn off the mobile phone!

The Waxing Moon (pre-ovulation) phase

This phase occurs from post-menstruation until just before you ovulate—what is typically called the follicular of proliferative phase in the medical model. Miranda Gray calls this the 'dynamic' phase.[87]

In the same way that your energy is building, your uterine lining is also proliferating, and your hormone levels are escalating. This phase equates seasonally to spring, or to the waxing phase of the moon.

After the heaviness and often lower energy of your menstrual period, in this Waxing Moon phase you emerge like a butterfly from its chrysalis, with renewed vigour. The more challenging hormonal symptoms that accompany the Waning and Dark Moon phases of your cycle no longer encumber you.

---

86 Miranda Gray in *The Optimized Woman: Using your menstrual cycle to achieve success and fulfilment*, writes: 'The *Reflective* phase is probably the most profound catalytic tool we have for changing actions and goals and our relationship to ourselves, and also for deepening our level of connection, experience and understanding of the universe and our place in it. To actively use this tool we need to slow down. We need to accept that we can't match the pace of the world for a few days and make room for the *Reflective* phase abilities', p.59

87 Gray writes in *The Optimized Woman*: 'The joy of the *Dynamic* phase is the feeling it brings of self-confidence, independence and the increased physical energy and mental clarity which empowers us to take action. This is the time to take steps and start those groundbreaking, life-changing exploits,' p.78

This is when you exhibit the most 'yang', or 'masculine' qualities of your cycle. You are driven and full of energy. Your focus is outward, and you may find it's when you are most productive and outcome-oriented.

A Waxing Moon yoga practice

In the first few days after bleeding has completed, you'll need to ease back into your regular yoga practice to allow time for your uterus to recover and your energy to rejuvenate.

After that, you can go for it! This is your time to shine in your yoga practice! Tackle those more challenging and dynamic postures during this phase of your cycle. However, don't forget to also take time to ground and balance your energy so that you don't overstimulate the nervous system and burn out.

The Full Moon (ovulation) phase

Around the time that you ovulate and are potentially fertile every month, you can usually notice a subtle shift into this phase, which is like the summer of your cycle. When the moon is full, your natural inclination is to be outside and revel in its light and beauty. It is the same for your Full Moon phase. This is the time when your energy is extroverted, reflecting this full moon energy.

Just like the Waxing Moon phase, you continue to feel energetic and outwardly focused. However, rather than the achievement-oriented, ego-driven energy that gets things done, you move into more of the nurturing, mother energy.

Miranda Gray calls this the 'expressive' phase[88] because it's when you become more relationship-focused and you naturally reconnect with those who are close to you—most particularly your lover. Now you sparkle in your femininity and you are generally at the peak of your sexual appetite and openness towards others, which reflects the womb's biological imperative to receive and 'hold'.

---

88 Gray describes the 'Expressive Phase' as a 'feeling-oriented phase' (*The Optimised Woman*, p.94) and writes: 'The *Expressive* phase abilities and skills develop around the time of ovulation and are usually experienced a few days before and a few days afterwards. Like the *Reflective* phase, the *Expressive* phase is the pivot time in our cycle, characterized by a weakening of the driving force of the ego,' and 'During the *Expressive* phase, work colleagues' and customers' needs and feelings have a higher priority than our own project. We are also more willing to 'go with the flow' and to allow things to develop in their own time.' (p.95).

A Full Moon yoga practice

This is when you are at your most feminine and your yoga practice becomes playful and flirtatious with 'womb dances' and hip-opening fertility sequences. You can also embody the loving, open, 'feeling-energy' of this phase with heart-opening yoga postures.

However, be careful not to get carried away and overstretch during this time; you need to make sure you balance your practice with stabilising postures as the surge and then drop in oestrogen in the body at this time can cause instability in the sacrum and lower back.[89]

The Waning Moon (premenstrual) phase

In your Waning Moon phase, your physical and emotional energy and fortitude begin to wane. Your focus moves inwards, which reflects the moon moving towards darkness and emptiness. This phase spans the time after ovulation up until you start to bleed again. It epitomises autumnal energy in which your body is preparing to retreat (for the Dark Moon phase to come).

In modern society this is the much-maligned aspect of a woman's cycle—it's when we often experience premenstrual symptoms (PMS). Women commiserate with each other about the numerous annoying and sometimes distressing PMS symptoms, ranging from bloating, to headaches, to moodiness. However, if you can learn to honour and embrace all of the changing faces of your cycle, even this more challenging phase, you may in fact find that your overall experience of this phase becomes much more positive.

Miranda Gray calls this the 'creative' phase,[90] which has helped me immeasurably in reframing my own experience of this time. I have learnt to value my heightened intuition and creative abilities that become obvious during this phase, and to cut myself some slack in terms of limiting my expectations for tackling left-brain, rational, detail-orientated tasks during this time.

---

89 See chapter six, p.207 in this book for more details (and yoga contraindications) on how the sudden withdrawal of oestrogen that occurs post-ovulation can potentially cause lower back injury.

90 Gray writes of the 'Creative Phase': '..it offers talents and opportunities that I don't have at any other time, such as flashes of brilliant insight and awareness, and the opportunity to clear out my emotional baggage and find out what really matters to me', *The Optimized Woman*, p.39.

A Waning Moon yoga practice

Very often your temper and your nerves are frayed during this premenstrual phase. This is the time to practise grounding, soothing sequences and enjoy long relaxation (Yoga Nidra[91]) practices. And, Inversions, Inversions, Inversions![92] Inversions not only calm the nervous system, but also help balance the hormonal system, which can be more necessary at this time of the month than any other!

With the arrival of the dark moon (either real or metaphorical) and the shedding of the uterine lining, the cycle begins anew, symbolising your interconnection with the universal rhythms of death and re-birth.

Understanding and harnessing your unique four-phase-cycle

As we have seen, the length of women's cycles can vary considerably, so this will mean the duration and timing of each of your four phases will be unique to you. For example, if you have a longer cycle, you will find that your Waxing Moon phase is longer than a woman who has a shorter cycle. To ascertain your own unique, Moving with the Moon, four phases pattern, I recommend that in addition to familiarising yourself with the general principles of tracking your cycle (see chapter two), you chart out your own 'menstrual dial'[93] over several months.

A menstrual dial looks like a kind of 'pie chart'—a circle with wedges within it representing each day of your cycle—and is a visual way to very quickly discern a pattern, from month-to-month, of certain physical, mental or emotional characteristics that tend to arise for you within each of the four phases, or even more precisely, on a particular day of your cycle each month.

When I started to keep a menstrual dial, I noticed that without fail, every month, on day 18, I would shift abruptly from my sanguine Full Moon (ovulation) phase to my more challenging Waning Moon (premenstrual) phase with sudden 'symptoms' of anger and irritability. My

---

91   See p.268 for a Waning Moon Yoga Nidra (deep relaxation) practice.

92   See Appendix 2 for examples of some Supported Inversion postures.

93   You can download a free, menstrual dial template from Miranda Gray's website here: http://www.optimizedwoman.com/womens-lifecoaching-articles.html
Or, purchase a beautiful moon dial by Lucy Pearce (author of *Moon Time*) here: http://shop.womancraftpublishing.com/category-s/1822.htm

newfound understanding of this particular pattern made it easier for me to have forewarning that allowed me to take care of myself (and those around me!). This meant that I ramped up my cooling, calming stress-management techniques and tried to avoid stressful, confrontational situations on this, the most emotionally volatile day of my cycle.

Understanding the subtle patterns, like this, that threaded through my cycle, allowed me a compassionate space that may have otherwise been unavailable to me. I was able to realise that the emotions I tended to experience on those days were hormonally induced, which somehow helped me not to take myself (or others) too seriously!

As you make daily notes of the physical, emotional and energetic changes that you experience throughout your menstrual month, you'll start to recognise an obvious pattern that can become your own Moving with the Moon template. This will then serve as a useful guide, indicating when you need to adapt your yoga practice to the various phases of your cycle. As you get to know your own body better, you'll be surprised and delighted with the results of this deeper understanding, which is beneficial not just for your yoga practice but for your daily life 'off the mat'.

CHAPTER THREE
PRINCIPLES AND GUIDELINES FOR A MOVING WITH THE MOON PRACTICE

KEY PRINCIPLES OF A FEMININE YOGA PRACTICE

*The body has its own way of knowing, a knowing that has
little to do with logic, and much to do with truth, little to
do with control, and much to do with acceptance, little to
do with division and analysis and much to do with union.*

—MARILYN SEWELL[94]

While this book offers an extensive library of postures and practices that you
can use for specific guidance throughout your monthly cycle and into menopause, you may also find it lastingly useful to gain an understanding of the key,
Feminine Yoga principles underlying a Moving with the Moon practice. Once
you are able appreciate and integrate these principles, along with a practical
understanding of the changing requirements of your cycle or life-stage, you
will find that you can be more intuitive in your daily practice. You will have
the tools to sensitively listen and respond to your body-mind's changing needs,
allowing you to creatively craft your very own Feminine Yoga practice.

---

94 Found on: http://www.livinglifefully.com/body.htm

Feminine Yoga principle one: *ahimsa*

When we refuse to take the time to treat our bodies, emotions,
and minds with reverence and love, they will often remind
us—not so kindly—by failing to respond when we need
them. Our ability to think clearly recedes. We may experience
sadness and depression. After a time our lack of ease may
allow disease to creep into our life. Then we are obliged to
take care of ourselves... It is much more pleasant and fun to
do it willingly, before any dis-ease invites itself to your life.
Love for yourself is love for all.

—NISCHALA JOY DEVI[95]

Ahimsa is a foundational moral precept that appears in the ancient yogic text, *The Yoga Sutras of Patanjali*.[96] It is derived from two words—'a', meaning 'not', and 'himsa', meaning 'harm'. It therefore means 'non-harming', or 'non-violence'.

From an early age we are inculcated with the idea that hurting others is not socially or morally sanctioned; however we don't necessarily learn about the importance of also being gentle with themselves. For women this is perhaps even more true. Women are the nurturers of society and they are often too busy taking care of others to consider that they also need to take care of themselves. Sometimes they only realise the importance of self-care when they become sick or injured and receive a 'wake-up' call from their body's intelligence.

This concept of self-compassion is the overarching principle of Feminine Yoga, no matter where you are in your monthly cycle or life-stage. Ideally, once you have truly embodied this idea of self-care and self-love you can proactively implement it in your life so that it becomes a daily habit and not

---

95 Nischala Joy Devi, *The Secret Power of Yoga: A Woman's Guide to the Heart and Spirit of the Yoga Sutras*, p.181

96 There are many translations of *The Yoga Sutras of Patanjali* that delineate the '8 Limbs of Yoga'. One of my favourites is an interpretation by Nischala Joy Devi, *The Secret Power of Yoga*, because it looks at the sutras with fresh eyes, from a feminine perspective, and serves as a wonderful reference to support a feminine, Moving with the Moon approach to our yoga practice.

just something you do to try to fix yourself when something goes wrong. As Liz Koch, somatic educator and author, suggests:

> What we need is more capacity to build our ability to endure pleasure. What is it to feel good? What is it to allow the system to become more intelligent, more resilient? Most of us don't have that. We have the idea that we only do something to get us out of pain. We don't do it because it brings us pleasure; because it brings us a sense of calm, a sense of nourishment. We don't know how to nourish ourselves, through movement as well as through food. So you're learning to take care of yourself.. to continue this exploration of nourishment.[97]

Yogic tools that can help you embody *ahimsa* within your practice include the relaxation and meditation practices that are sprinkled throughout this book, as well as Restorative Yoga (see Appendix 3). These tools all teach us to be gentle with ourselves.

The very concept of Moving with the Moon is *ahimsa* in action, because it involves skilfully tuning in to the changing daily needs of your body so that you only practise to an intensity that is appropriate for what is going on for you at that particular point in your monthly cycle, on all levels—physically, mentally and emotionally. Cultivating your own Moving with the Moon home practice, rather than attending one-size-fits-all group classes can be so beneficial. An evolving personalised practice helps you avoid the pitfalls of a gung-ho group class energy, which can tempt you to override your individual needs.

Another way to embody *ahimsa* is to examine how you treat yourself, and others, *off* the yoga mat. *Ahimsa* comprises one of the ten ethical guidelines (five *yamas* and five *niyamas*) for living that are described in the ancient *Yoga Sutras*. These guidelines were created to inspire people to lead an authentic yogic life that extended way beyond the practice of just the Asanas (postures). If you are to truly practise *ahimsa*, you need to ask yourself these big questions: *Can I deepen my mindfulness around my intentions, thoughts and actions towards others—are they kind, are my words necessary? Can I learn to forgive myself implicitly when I invariably 'fall down' and act unkindly or inappropriately towards myself or others?*

---

97 This quote is from my transcript from an audio lecture Liz Koch delivered as part of an online course I attended. See Koch's website for more information on her courses and publications: http://www.coreawareness.com

Ultimately, your yoga 'off the mat' practice in which you set the intention to live as mindfully and gently as possible is very similar to your 'on the mat' practice. It is a *practice*. And that's the key thing to remember when you fail. Which you will! Just get back on your mat (either your real yoga mat or your metaphorical one) and begin again. The relentless challenges of motherhood have taught me that one on a very profound level! Forgiveness, letting go of judgement (of self and of others), and an active gratitude-practice, are all ways you can bring more of the nectar of *ahimsa* into your daily life.

Feminine Yoga principle two: womb centring

When the womb is ungrounded, we can be scattered, inefficient, moody, and exhausted. It can seem like we never have enough time to get what we want done, and the things we want always seem just out of reach. We can be reactive, unable to step back from people, events and relationship experiences to allow appropriate action. We feel like life is too fast, that it is passing by too quickly, and we cannot quite catch up to it.

—PADMA AND ANIYA AON PRAKASHA[98]

In our hectic lives we are prone to 'living in our heads', as we worry, stress and fuss our way through our days, weeks, months and even years. Many people do not know how to ground their awareness in their body, particularly their lower-body. As a yoga teacher I see this so often reflected in how people breathe. A 'heady' person will very often have a shallow, upper-chest way of breathing that can exacerbate the stress response. In their yoga practice, these people have great difficulty sensing into their body and tuning into it to make subtle adjustments or softenings where needed. They will intellectualise everything, rather than *feel*. In essence, this is an example of an over-masculinisation that buries women's innate femininity.

It's vital for your health and wellbeing as a woman that you form a healthy relationship with the lower two energy centres—your root, or *muladhara chakra*, located at the perineum and vagina, as well as your 'womb-space', or *svadistana chakra*, located within the pelvis, specifically, the uterus.

---

98 Padma and Anaiya Aon Prakasha, *Womb Wisdom: Awakening the Creative and Forgotten Powers of the Feminine*, location 893 (Kindle Version)

Back in the 1970s, Aviva Steiner, a physical education teacher, developed a series of womb-stimulating and nourishing movements to regulate women's cycles. She claimed that if women don't move the energy within their pelvic region they are at risk of creating menstrual and menopausal imbalances and lowering their fertility.[99]

Dr Christiane Northrup agrees that the free flow of pelvic energy is vital to a woman's health: 'Fibroids, endometriosis, diseases of the ovaries, and other pelvic disorders are manifestations of blocked energy in the pelvis,' she writes.[100]

> *The quality of energy flow in the female pelvis, including the flow of each ovary, the uterus, and the vagina, impacts on a woman's overall vibrancy. Like nutrients drawn from the soil that are essential for a plant's growth, the flow of pelvic energy through a woman's root determines the vitality of her womanhood.*
>
> —TAMI LYNN KENT[101]

Defining the womb-space and your root

The womb is a woman's creative centre. It's literally the space in which she can create new life when she nurtures a baby for nine months. However, even if a woman never carries a child in her womb, it is still the energetic centre for creative energy in her life. The womb-space can correlate with the *dantien* or *hara* from Eastern traditions such as Taoism, Chi Kung and

---

99   Adelheid Ohlig in her book, *Luna Yoga: Vital Fertility and Sexuality*, writes of her teacher and mentor, Aviva Steiner: 'Aviva discovered that a woman's energy source is in her pelvis, in her sexual organs. If a woman's energy is allowed to flow freely into the rest of her body, the woman will live a healthy, long life and have tremendous energy and vitality. If the energy is locked in the pelvis, reproductive problems and a variety of diseases from PMS to cancer are promoted,' p.35.

100   Northrup, *Women's Bodies, Women's Wisdom*, p.87

101   Tami Lynn Kent, *Wild Feminine*, p.14. Also from Kent: 'When a woman knows how to access her root place, she finds the energy for building her creative dreams, nurturing her creations, and changing the core patterns that diminish her radiance,' p. xxiii

martial arts. The *dantien* or *hara* is said to be located about four finger widths below the navel and is considered to be the 'power centre' in which vital *chi* or energy is stored—for both women and men.[102]

Another way to locate your womb-space is to place your thumbs at the navel and extend your index fingers down to form a diamond shape (see Figure 1).

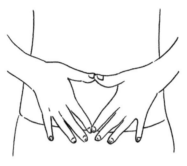

Figure 1

Deep into your body behind your index fingers is the rough location of your womb. In reality, you don't need to be too specific about the physical location; what you're aiming to do is to build your feeling, awareness and ultimately energy in the *general* lower belly and pelvic region.

It's very easy to start to build a tangible connection with your root-centre. Just squeeze your pelvic floor or vagina in the same way you do when you are doing 'kegels' (pelvic floor exercises). If you're not familiar with exercising the pelvic floor, think of the muscles you use to stop the flow of urine when you are on the toilet, or, imagine you are squeezing a pencil in your vagina. To get concrete feedback, you can try putting your index or middle finger in your vagina and then squeezing your finger.

---

102   Rachael Jayne Groover in her book *Powerful and Feminine: How to Increase your Magnetic Presence and Attract the Attention You Want*, suggests that the *dantien* (also called the '*lower dantian*') or *hara* correlates with the feminine womb-space (p.63). Christiane Northrup M.D. says that 'the hara, this low-belly body center (which also includes the ovaries) is associated with power, passion and creativity'—*Women's Bodies, Women's Wisdom*, p.163. Christopher J. Makhert, author of *Dantien: Your Secret Energy Centre* (York Beach ME, Samual Weiser Inc., 1998) defines the 'Dan-Tien Personality' as somebody who is 'collected, responsible, helpful' and with a 'modest attitude'. He goes on to say, 'They are self confident but do not seek the limelight, and they are not interested in impressing or dominating others. Yet they radiate quiet power and attract admirers and follows'. These could be described as the more feminine characteristics!

Squeezing and toning this vaginal and perineal area will help foster a healthy connection with the root of your body as well as achieving many benefits such as healing or preventing prolapse and incontinence, and boosting your enjoyment of sex.

At the same time, it's also important to learn how to relax your pelvic floor and vaginal muscles, particularly when you are menstruating, as I point out in chapter four.[103] If these muscles are permanently switched on, tension can accrue. It's all about creating *elasticity* of these muscles. From an energetic perspective, it's about generating energy-flow around the perineum and up into the pelvis. The first step to doing this is fostering a subtle awareness and sensitivity of this part of your body.

Shakti Prana

In Feminine Yoga, we talk about encouraging the flow of *shakti prana* within the pelvic bowl. *Prana* is the energy or life-force that moves around the body and *shakti prana* is the sacred, feminine energy that is present in these lowest two chakras—the root and womb-space. Maya Tiwari (Mother Maya) explains, 'shakti prana is the body's inherent reproductive life force; when in a state of balance, it protects the health of the reproductive organs, genitals, womb, belly and breasts.'[104]

On a purely physical level it also makes sense to promote blood flow to the pelvic region. The health of the pelvic organs (ovaries, uterus, fallopian tubes) is greatly improved when they receive unimpeded blood flow. Tight pelvic muscles can restrict the natural, healthy circulation within the pelvis. The Classical Women's postures (see Appendix 2) work to promote pelvic circulation—both physical and energetic—by opening the hips, stretching the pelvic floor and bringing space and softness to the belly.

Ways of connecting with your womb-space and the root-chakra

Yoga postures

As mentioned, the Classical Women's postures promote energy and blood flow to the pelvic area. The pelvic tilting movements involved in the Cat-Cow Pose (see Figure 47 and Figure 48, p.129) and Supine Pelvic Tilts, (see Figure 105 and Figure 106, p.171) also move and generate energy in this area.

---

103   On p.87 I explain how engaging the pelvic floor (mulha bandha) is contraindicated during menstruation.

104   Maya Tiwari, *Women's Power to Heal through Inner Medicine*, p.155

Breath

In yoga we say that the breath represents, and is a way to move and activate *prana* (the essential life force or energy) throughout the body. This book will later explore various breathing techniques, most significantly the Soft Belly Breath (see p.100). You can use this practice to breathe more deeply into your deep, lower belly and pelvic floor area, therefore activating and nourishing your *shakti prana*.

Meditation and visualisation

One of the important and characterising features of a Moving with the Moon approach is beautiful, feminine meditation practices that help you inhabit your womb-space. You will enjoy plenty of these meditations throughout this book.

Touch

I often rub my hands over my belly in an instinctive, nurturing gesture. This instantly helps me drop my awareness down and out of my busy mind. It reminds me to relax and soften my belly, which helps with alleviating stress and tension, and nourishes my abdominal and pelvic organs.

Movement

Circling and swaying your hips is an instinctively feminine way to nurture and strengthen your *shakti prana*. You can incorporate these movements within your Feminine Yoga practice (see Figure 187 in the Classical Feminine Flow Full Moon Sequence, p.230), or you can simply put on some inspiring music and enjoy some juicy, sexy free-dance movements.

Pelvic floor activation

As previously detailed, engaging the pelvic floor, known in yoga as 'Muladhara Bandha', is a simple way to not only bring awareness into your root, but also to tone the all-important pelvic floor muscles. In addition, pelvic floor work helps you to subtly tone the deep, abdominal muscles (specifically, the transversus abdominus). There will be instructions throughout the sequences indicating when to activate your pelvic floor during the posture practice.

Fostering your creativity

As I have mentioned, the womb-space is a woman's creative, power centre. Finding ways to express your creativity can nourish the energy there.

Take up or reconnect with a creative pursuit that fills you up—whether it be writing, painting, dancing, gardening, craft or music, to name just a few! There is so much joy to be found in indulging in something creative, just for the sake of it; to express yourself—your deepest soul energies—not because there is any specific purpose, for instance to make money, but just for the love of it.

Beginning or renewing your commitment to your creativity can bring profound benefits to the health and vitality of your reproductive organs as well as your nervous system as you learn to relax more and 'find your flow'.

Ana's story: reconnecting with the womb-space

At the age of 42, I experienced a health crisis which shook my assumptions and by association, my life, to the very core. I suffered total burnout due to an overload of stress and ultimately an excess of the 'masculine' in my life. I had been single parenting for almost a decade as well as running my busy yoga teacher training business in which I was responsible for many administration and teaching staff.

Even in my relationship with my partner at the time, I felt that I was the main one who was responsible for holding things together. I was accountable, too accountable. If you're familiar with the work of Alison A Armstrong[105] you'll know that she suggests that accountability is a defining masculine characteristic. Men, with their predominance of testosterone thrive on being accountable, on being responsible—on the 'single focus' of getting the job done, on being 'outcome focused'. Women don't have the same levels of testosterone (just one small peak around ovulation) to sustain this 'hunter instinct' and they burn out if they feel compelled to be accountable for too long.

My healing crisis revealed to me a clear irony: I always thought with all the work in women's health and yoga that I'd been doing that I was very connected with my womb-space—no problems there! However, as I sat with my friend and spiritual healer Anna Watts[106] and meditated on my chakras, I realised that when she prompted me to feel into and visualise my Sacral Chakra, my womb-centre, my 'female creative space', I saw only a

---

105   Alison A. Armstrong author of *The Queen's Code* and personal growth facilitator is renowned for her work around understanding the differences between men and women in relationships.

106   Find out more about Anna Watts's work here: https://www.spiritwayhealing.com.au

barren, dark, inhospitable place—a dark cave. This was no surprise when you consider one of my most distressing burnout symptoms was constant heart arrhythmia (ectopic heartbeat) and breathlessness which left me feeling like my energy was all up in my chest (the home of the masculine).

In time, as I began to heal, I furnished this space, in my mind's eye, so that I feminised it. I added a day-bed with colourful cushions, rich velvet drapes, a warm fire in the centre. My womb-space gradually became somewhere I felt more comfortable to spend some time 'hanging out'.

At my third session with Anna I finally experienced my womb-space as filled with light and clear energy, breezes and pastel-coloured drapes, and I could feel myself dropping down into this space. My weeks of meditations, visualisations, womb-dances and breath-work dedicated to embodying this space had paid off and my energy had finally dropped, or 'earthed' down to where it should be. Wow! What a relief!

I was then able to access a new way to soften into my natural femininity that had been there all the time, but had been suppressed and ignored. It's not just about 'thinking' your way to connect with your womb-space, you have to *feel*, and to do that, use whatever tool works for you whether it be breath, meditation, yoga postures, chanting, dance—or a combination of all!

The womb-heart connection

Not only is it important for women to connect with their womb-space, but it's also beneficial to form a positive connection with another key feminine-centre, the heart-space, or in yogic terms, the 'Heart Chakra'.

The heart-centre is our energetic home for love, unconditional love, and by softening into this space in conjunction with, and in alignment with the womb-space, you can support yourself in healing your connection to the feminine.

Here's a beautiful Womb-Heart Meditation that will support this softening into the feminine and feeling the connection (feedback-loop) between the womb-space and heart-space, which is integral in supporting your fertility.

Womb-heart Meditation

Begin by placing both palms on your lower belly, your womb-centre and take some lovely, full Soft Belly Breaths (see p.100). Allow your deep, lower belly to open to the breath; to receive the breath; to receive this moment.

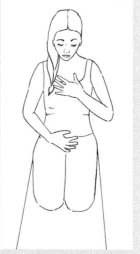

Now, place your left hand on your heart-centre (in the centre of the chest) and keep your right hand on your lower belly, your womb-space, or 'womb-heart' (see Figure 2).

Your womb-space, behind your right palm, is your centre for nurturing new life. Deep within your uterus is where the seed of love grows into a fully formed baby or idea.

Figure 2

Your womb-space is also your 'womb-heart' because it is so closely connected to the energy of your heart-centre, and it has its own energetic, beating heart.[107]

Your heart-centre, behind your left palm, is your epicentre for love—deep, abiding, unconditional love. It has the capacity to keep opening and opening like a lotus flower unfurling its petals in the sun—feeding yourself and others with love.

There is a free flow of energy between these two energy centres. Traumas that affect your heart can affect the uterus and the free flow of blood and energy between these two physical and energetic points in our body.

So as you rest now, deeply into yourself, feel the sensations, the subtle permutations of energy beneath your left and right palms. Feel the flow of energy between these points—up and down your soft solar plexus.

Know that this simple practice helps you come home to yourself and allows you to embrace the divine in everyday life.

Namaste

107　I owe the idea of the 'womb-heart' to Nischala Joy Devi who writes: 'Women are graced with what is often referred to as the 'womb heart.' It relates to the 'beating heart' through intuition and feelings. This legacy of love is so powerful that it is able to sustain a new life. The beating heart and the womb heart each hold the sacred essence of consciousness,'—*The Secret Power of Yoga*, p.60

Feminine Yoga principle three: *apana*

Work with apana, and apana will work with you.

—ROBERT SVOBODA[108]

The third principle of a Feminine Yoga practice is *apana*. According to ancient yogic subtle physiology and Ayurveda, the sister-science to yoga, there are five *vayus*[109] or 'energies' that govern different bodily functions and aspects of your being and they all need to be in balance for your optimal health and vitality. *Prana vayu*, residing in the chest and head, is the energy that governs your inspiration and taking things. It also nourishes the brain and the eyes. The force behind *prana vayu* is upward and propulsive and is generally considered more 'masculine' in its essence. *Apana vayu* is the opposite, more 'feminine' quality of energy flow that is represented by a downward movement, residing in the pelvis, and nourishing the pelvic organs.

Healthy *apana* (the downward movement of energy) is essential in supporting elimination of your bodily wastes to avoid imbalances like constipation or diarrhoea. Additionally, *apana vayu* is responsible for eliminating mental and emotional toxins from your bodies, which can support your whole, mind-body health. Specifically, for women, the processes of menstruation and birth are also governed by the energy of *apana* and it is therefore an important principle when working with a more feminine-based yoga practice.

Because *apana* is a grounding energy it can help balance your *vata* levels. *Vata* is one of the three main Ayurvedic constitutions (of which everyone has a predominance of one or several) that is related to the air-element— see Appendix 1 for more information on these three constitutions or *doshas*. When you have an excess of this *vata* energy in your body, you can feel anxious, 'spacy' and ungrounded. It is therefore useful to focus on cultivating *apana vayu* at times of high *vata* such as during perimenopause, as well as during your premenstrual (Waning Moon) and menstruation (Dark Moon) phases of your monthly cycle.

---

108 Dr Svoboda, *Ayurveda for Women: A Guide to Vitality and Health*, p.79

109 Ibid., p.60. Dr Svoboda provides an overview of these five *vayus* which are also aspects of the Ayurvedic *dosha* (or constitution) of *vata*: *Prana* (extends from the diaphragm to the throat), *Udana* (extends from the throat to the top of the head), *Samana* (extends from diaphragm to the navel), *Vyana* (permeates the entire body from its seat in the heart), *Apana* (extends from the navel to the anus).

Yogic tools for harnessing the power of *apana*—which will deepen the therapeutic value of a feminine-focused yoga practice—include breathing techniques such as the Apana Breath (see p. 102) as well as various meditation and visualisation practices described in this book. Grounding, floor-based postures such as the Classical Women's postures (see p. 441) and sequences like the classical joint-freeing and digestive toning sequence, known as Pawanmuktasana (see p. 407) also encourage the energy of *apana*. Some Standing poses, like the Standing Goddess (see Figure 394, p. 447), are also wonderful for sending the breath (and therefore energy) down through the legs into the earth, channelling *apana*.

GUIDELINES FOR YOUR MOVING WITH THE MOON HOME PRACTICE

Create a sacred space

Find a dedicated practice space in your house, whether it's a corner of a room, or a separate room. Mark this space as your sacred, feminine space with items and images that are beautiful and significant for you. You can create a feminine altar with flowers, candles, statues, crystals, feathers, or other items from nature. You might include a photograph of your guru if you have one, or of a person or people who are special to you, who inspire you. I have an uplifting affirmation pasted on the wall near my practice space, and I sometimes place my favourite, inspiring book on my altar.

Make your Moving with the Moon home practice space entirely your own; you may find over time you add special things to it as they come into your life, building upon your sacred space and therefore the intention for your feminine practice.

If you are including Hindu or Buddhist statues on your altar you might want to opt for one or several of the more feminine icons like Tara (Mother Goddess of peace and protection), Kuan Yin (Mother Goddess of compassion, mercy and kindness), Durga (Mother of the Universe Goddess), Lakshmi (Goddess of wealth, prosperity and fertility), or, Saraswati (Goddess of knowledge, wisdom and the arts).

With the devotion and energy you have imbued in the choice and placement of your beautiful, sacred items—as well as setting aside a dedicated practice space—you're creating a fertile space for a regular home practice. This will nourish and support you throughout the fluctuations within each month and throughout your feminine life transitions.

Ultimately, creating a sacred, dedicated space will allow you to be more inspired to get on your mat—which is often the key 'stumbling block' for beginning and experienced practitioners alike.

Prop yourself up

Restorative Yoga is an invaluable tool in your 'feminine tool box' (see Appendix 3 for some sample Restorative Yoga postures). Integral to this specialised, therapeutic practice are several yoga props. Invest in a yoga mat, yoga bolster, one or two yoga-blankets (thick beach towels can substitute if necessary), a yoga block, a yoga strap and an eye bag, and you'll have everything you need to do most Restorative postures. A couple of the postures require two bolsters, however, you could always roll a few blankets up into a cylinder to replicate a second bolster if you prefer not to purchase a second bolster.

If you haven't done Restorative Yoga before, you won't regret the investment in these yoga props. You will discover these supported postures are wonderful, especially for those days when you are tired, exhausted, and depleted (for example when you are bleeding), or when you just need a more gentle, supportive practice that nourishes your nervous system and provides deep rest for your body and mind.

Initiate from the left

In a Moving with the Moon, feminine approach to the yoga, I advocate that you initiate from the *left* side. This means that when you are doing a Salute to the Sun, or in the Moving with the Moon vernacular, a 'Lunar or Womb Salute'[110], you always initiate from the left side by stepping back first on the left leg (into the lunge) and always stepping forward first on the left leg (into the lunge again), before doing it all on the right side.

Likewise, when you are practising an asymmetrical posture, do the left side first.

Why? Because there are two hemispheres or sides to the brain—the left hemisphere that generally controls the more rational, factual, and therefore more typically, 'masculine' thought processes; and the right hemisphere, which is responsible for the more creative, intuitive and

---

110 This book includes a Full Moon Salute on p.225 and a Waning Moon Salute on p.278.

therefore more typically 'feminine' thought processes.[111] Therefore the connection can be made that because the left side of the brain controls the right side of the body and the right hemisphere of the brain controls the left side of the body, we must emphasise the left side of the body in our yoga practice to foster feminine essence.

Consider how society is built on right-sided dominance, with nine out of ten people being right-handed.[112] So often in yoga and other forms of physical exercise, people are traditionally encouraged to initiate from the right side of the body.

It's time to break this paradigm!

Yoga teacher and 'eco-feminist' Moana Pearl recommends a 'simple but catalytic action towards reclaiming a truly feminine inner authority as women' is to extend this habit of initiating from the left side into your daily life—making your morning juice with your left hand, or using your left foot first when entering or exiting a building. She goes on to elucidate that in many Native American Indian traditions, the left side of the body is related to 'feminine nature and maternal lineage', whereas the right side of the body connects 'our paternal lineage, and our masculine aspects.'[113]

The same left-side emphasis also applies when you perform the classical Pranayama (yoga breathing) practice called Nadi Shodhana (the Alternate Nostril Breath—see p.105). We appropriate this practice for Feminine Yoga by always starting and ending a round through the left nostril. In addition to the reasons listed above this is also because in yogic physiology, the left nostril relates to the lunar, receptive, feminine, subtle energy channel, or *ida nadi* (which runs from the perineum to the 'third eye'), whereas the right nostril relates to the solar, active, masculine channel or *pingala nadi*.

---

111 Reference: https://www.livescience.com/32935-whats-the-difference-between-the-right-brain-and-left-brain.html

112 Reference: https://www.livescience.com/17009-left-handedness-ambidexterity.html

113 Moana Pearl: https://moanapearl.wordpress.com/page/4/ Pearl also writes: 'Because Western culture is so left brain dominant in our approach to language and thought process, as women we can benefit from putting our attention to the use of the left side of the body in our yoga practice to encourage our shakti, our feminine nature, and our intuition, on and off the mat.'

Other tips and considerations

- Always practise yoga on an empty stomach, allowing at least 1.5-2 hours after eating beforehand.

- If you're having trouble keeping up the discipline for a regular practice, it can help if you practise at the same time every day. This way it becomes a habit, something like a 'Pavlov's dog' scenario. Find the best time in your day when you know you won't be disturbed, distracted or tempted to put off your yoga practice. A good time can be the early mornings, before you have breakfast, your children are awake, and your day begins; or evenings, just before bed for a gentle, wind-down practice.

- Another way to support your practice is to begin and end it with a ritual. This may be as simple as lighting a candle and incense or burning your favourite essential oils before you begin, and finishing by chanting the sacred mantra 'om' three times to complete your practice, with your hands in the Heart-Womb Mudra (see Figure 2, p.59).

- Don't set yourself up for failure. Short, regular practices are better than longer, less frequent practices. Even as little as 10-20 minutes can be so beneficial to help you recalibrate, refresh your energy and sprinkle a little bit of magic into your day.

- If you can't seem to motivate yourself to get on to your mat, try 'tricking' yourself into it. Simply tell yourself that you'll just go lie on your mat for a little while. Just rest in a supine position like Constructive Rest Position (see Figure 19, p.95)—no expectations. After some time, you may find that instinctively, your body starts to move and stretch into other positions that feel good—stretching, opening, releasing, energising. Before you know it, you may find that you are moving from one posture to the next and you have completed a full yoga practice, despite yourself!

- Always finish with Savasana. Savasana, or the Corpse Pose, is the final, resting position that is performed at the end of a yoga practice. It is is a potently relaxing practice that calms the nervous system and allows you time to integrate all the postures and practices that you've just done within your body-mind. I once heard another yoga teacher describe this practice as like the 'recovery room' that you transition in to, after surgery. You don't just get up and leave after you've had an operation, healing is only complete after you've taken time to rest in 'recovery'. It is usually done lying on your back, but you will also find other Restorative options for Savasana in this book that involve resting in a prone position, on your front (see Appendix 3). Either way, it is important to spend at least five minutes in Savasana before you re-assimilate into the rest of your day.

- Set up an atmosphere of playful experimentation in your yoga practice. Let your body be your laboratory. Explore how each posture and sequence of postures and practices makes you feel in your body, mind and emotions. Tweak your practice accordingly. If something feels really good and shifts you into a more positive physical and emotional space, then that's a good sign. However, if something that you're doing doesn't feel good—leaves you feeling uncomfortable, in any pain, or just doesn't feel 'right'—don't ignore this feedback. Make your Moving with the Moon practice your very own so that it serves your unique needs each day, month and year that you get onto your mat.

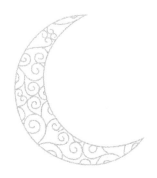

Part Three
Exploring the Four Phases

Chapter Four
THE DARK MOON: BEING WITH THE FLOW

*Each month I am sensitive to the first twinges of my womb.
I am waiting and listening for her signal that my
'bleeding time' is here. If my cycle is in tune with
the moon, I watch as the world draws into darkness,
moving towards no moon, dark moon.*

*Sometimes, in the days before I actually bleed,
my womb teases me and offers me clusters of
deep inner sensations—'pre-cramps'.*

*But then finally my time is come! I sense deep
inside me: my cervix opens as my womb begins
its work of shedding and letting go.*

*Usually the sensations build gradually and consistently in
intensity until I feel the full grip of my Dark Moon time
upon my belly, upon my centre, upon my very consciousness.
My belly becomes very soft, my pelvic floor heavy, my legs
weary, very weary. With these visceral sensations, the sharp
edges of my mind and emotions soften too, and I let go of
actively trying to will myself and others to be 'this way'.*

*I welcome these sensations and the feelings that
accompany the 'big exhale' in my month. I have
prepared for the arrival of my Dark Moon time. Where
possible, I have cleared the way in my work and home
life so that I can allow my body to bleed and rest.*

Then, it's just about surrender. The same as for birth.

—ANA'S MENSTRUAL DIARY

The onset of bleeding, as your uterus sheds its lining, indicates the start of the Dark Moon phase—the hibernating, winter phase of your cycle. This phase carries through until your body stops bleeding, but from a Moving with the Moon perspective, the first 1-2 days of bleeding is regarded as the deepest time of retreat. This is when your energy is usually at its lowest point and your focus is very internal.

To fully appreciate how to use yoga to support you when you are menstruating, it's helpful first to understand the fundamental need for rest and reflection that characterises this phase.

CHANGING THE PARADIGM

The fact that so many women in our society call menses 'the curse' is sufficient indication of how far away from a naturally healthy life we strayed when we took women out of their menstrual huts and told them to work through the month no matter what.

—DR ROBERT E. SVOBODA[114]

As explored in chapter one, modern women are forced to operate within the dominant, linear, masculine paradigm that refuses to honour the natural fluctuations of the menstrual cycle and views menstruation itself as something to be ignored or even suppressed. How different might women's experiences of their menses be if they viewed it in a more positive light? How would it be if we welcomed our monthly bleed as a precious opportunity to rest and nourish ourselves—rather than resisting and resenting it, and seeing it as something to 'push on through'?

The philosophy behind a Moving with the Moon, feminine approach to yoga suggests that the key to enjoying your period and even falling in love with your cycle is to reframe this time as your 'monthly holiday'. This represents a resurgence of those time-honoured practices celebrating the arrival of a woman's bleeding each month as a gift that signified her fertility and the potency of her womanhood.

---

114   Dr. Robert E. Svoboda, *Ayurveda for Women: A Guide to Vitality and Health*, p.72

As we have seen, in Native American cultures there was no question that their women be given the time and space to rest and retreat during their 'moon-time'. 'Most if not all traditions of Native American spirituality hold the moon-time as a sacred time of purification during which women do not go into ceremony or use sacred objects such as pipes and feathers,' writes Native American Shaman, Nicholas Noble Wolf. 'Often people from the Western culture see this as a disrespectful and negative stereotyping of a woman's menstrual cycle. We traditional people do not see it this way, as moon-time is a place of honor and beauty.'[115]

Like those women of indigenous, pre-industrial cultures who bled with the dark of the moon and took time out in their 'moon lodges', 'menstrual huts' and 'red tents', the modern woman can learn to treasure her own 'moontime' as her special, monthly mini-retreat. We have much to gain by adopting this new (or rather, old) practice. Simply by making the time and space for monthly rest and contemplation, you will find that you re-emerge from your menstrual cocoon each month with renewed vigour. You'll start to notice the difference compared with those times when you don't afford yourself a menstrual retreat; if you *don't* take your 'moontime', you may notice a toll on your available energy levels for the rest of the month.

A DELICATE PHASE

*Women have a tremendous fear of feeling our tiredness. We are
afraid that if we let ourselves feel it we will never get up again.
My tiredness is mine. I have earned it.*

—ANNE WILSON SCHAEF[116]

Reflecting the quiet energy of the dark moon, women generally experience their menstrual period as a time when they are lower in energy, and they tend to feel more sensitive and introverted. In addition to the common menstrual complaints of cramping, headaches and bloating, many women report feeling more tired as their uterus works hard to expel its lining (endometrium). With the drop in hormones—oestrogen and progesterone—that

---

115 Nicholas Noble Wolf, 'The Gift from the Moon—how moontime came to women and how it might be honoured', www.nicholasnoblewolf.com

116 Anne Wilson Schaef, *Meditations for Women Who do Too Much*, 'February 5' (no page numbers).

presages your menstrual period, there is also a decline in your immune system that can make you more susceptible to catching colds and flus and leave you feeling more fragile than at other times in the month.[117]

During the menstrual phase, women need to take extra care of their health. Dr Elizabeth Lyster, MD, an American board-certified OB/GYN physician recommends that women reduce external stress while their bodies are coping with the process of menstrual bleeding.[118] And, it's no surprise to learn that menstruating women, along with new mothers and babies, actually need more sleep![119]

Furthermore, as we approach our menses, the cervix drops lower in the vagina and opens and softens to allow the blood to pass through, and this can subtly add to a woman's feeling of vulnerability at this time.

---

117 'The body can be particularly receptive to outside factors during the menstrual cycle, such as stress and immune system cell changes', notes the United States National Library of Medicine. 'The body goes through its cyclic repair during menses, as the many molecular and cellular interactions that are part of menstruation take place. Keeping your body healthy and your immune system at its strongest is especially important at "that time of the month"' (See: www.livestrong.com.) The research paper, 'Impact of Stress, Gender and Menstrual Cycle on Immune System: Possible Role of Nitric Oxide' by scientists from the Department of Physiology, Hacettepe University Medical Faculty, Turkey, concludes, 'The luteal phase differed from the other groups due to the presence of suppressed immune response to acute stress.'
(See: https://cyclesresearchinstitute.wordpress.com/2010/06/26/impact-of-stress-gender-and-menstrual-cycle-on-immune-system-possible-role-of-nitric-oxide/.) Alexandra Pope, in *The Wild Genie* writes, 'The immune system, our physical boundary, which is more vulnerable premenstrually, appears to mirror the thinning of psychological boundaries. I've encountered a number of women who get flu symptoms before they bleed as well as sometimes before ovulation. Women with chronic health problems, such as allergies and inflammatory conditions often find their symptoms increase at these times.' (p.81).

118 From an interview with Elizabeth Lyster, MD, as quoted in this online article: http://simplystated.realsimple.com/2012/09/21/how-to-avoid-colds-and-flu-this-fall-really/

119 Lucy H. Pearce writes in *Moon Time: A guide to celebrating your menstruation* (location 1078, Kindle edition), 'New mothers and babies require higher levels of sleep and rest. And so do menstruating women'. This could be partly due to the fact that women are more likely to suffer sleep disturbances premenstrually as well as in early menstruation'. (See: Monica Mallampalli PhD, MSc., SWHR director of scientific programs, *Why we need to pay more attention to women's sleep*, at: http://www.huffingtonpost.com/michael-keaton/women-sleep_b_5399748.html)

Maya Tiwari, an Ayurvedic women's health expert, counsels that women should 'go at a slower pace' during their period, to allow the body to cleanse itself. She writes, 'you are [also] advised to pare down your activities to the bare essentials so that body, mind and spirit may experience the least degree of intrusion'.[120]

THE IMPERATIVE FOR REST

Retreating from the normal routine and everyday intrusions is necessary so that you can remain mindful of the great transformational experience of shedding the lining of the uterus (endometrium) so that it can be renewed once more.

—MAYA TIWARI[121]

The integrative health modalities of both Ayurveda and Traditional Chinese Medicine (TCM) agree that resting during menstruation can enhance a woman's overall health. Maya Tiwari says that if you pamper yourself on the first day of your period—no work, no worries, no cooking, no cleaning—your reproductive health will benefit enormously.[122]

Acupuncturist and TCM practitioner Chi Fung Lee says that a woman should rest and be quiet when she is menstruating, and that people around her should be more thoughtful so that her nervous system is not triggered. 'For some women, they need more sleep because they are losing blood—losing chi, leaking out their essence. Their energy is depleted,' says Lee.[123] Lara Owen, author of *Her Blood is Gold: Awakening the Wisdom of Menstruation*, adds that the Chinese believe that the cause of many gynaecological complaints is 'faulty behaviour during menstruation', that includes, 'getting cold, lifting heavy objects, overworking, and eating inappropriate food'.[124]

120   Maya Tiwari, at: http://www.mypeacevow.org/womenpower.php

121   Maya Tiwari, *Women's Power to Heal through Inner Medicine*, p.66

122   Maya Tiwari, *Ayurveda: A life of Balance: The Complete Guide to Ayurvedic Nutrition and Body Types with Recipes* (as paraphrased by Linda Sparrowe in *Yoga for a Healthy Menstrual Cycle*, p.43)

123   From a skype interview with Chi Fung Lee (Amsterdam), July, 2014.

124   Lara Owen, *Her Blood is Gold: Awakening the Wisdom of Menstruation*, p.31

According to Ayurveda, the *dosha* (constitution) of *vata*[125] predominates during the menses. The *vata dosha* regulates the nervous system, and when this *dosha* is out of balance (in excess), we tend to experience stress-related symptoms such as anxiety and insomnia that may also have a flow-on effect of inducing menstrual imbalances. This means that to take care of your menstrual health, you need to pacify your *vata* by controlling your stress levels, particularly during this more delicate phase of your cycle.

Modern Western medicine also recognises the connection between stress and our menstrual cycle. American obstetrician Christiane Northrup, M.D., even goes so far as to claim, 'I have come to see that all kinds of stress-related diseases, ranging from PMS to osteoporosis, could be lessened a great deal if we simply followed our body's wisdom once per month.'[126]. Alexandra Pope, author and pioneering menstrual health educator, aptly describes the menstrual cycle as a woman's 'stress sensitive system'.[127] In other words, an imbalance in the menstrual cycle can reflect a larger imbalance within a woman's body (and psyche!), particularly within her nervous system. The hypothalamus is a gland in the brain that controls and integrates the overlapping functions of the endocrine (hormonal) system and the autonomic nervous system. Within the female hormonal system, the hypothalamus sends messages to the pituitary gland, signalling it to produce hormones essential to a woman's menstrual cycle. Because the hypothalamus links the brain to the hormonal system, and is positioned close to the emotional centre of our brain,[128] it can be adversely affected by

---

125 See Appendix 1 in this book for a definition of the constitution of *vata* and the three Ayurvedic *doshas*.

126 Christiane Northrup M.D., in her article, 'The Wisdom of the Menstrual Cycle', http://www.drnorthrup.com/wisdom-of-menstrual-cycle/

127 Alexandra Pope, *The Wild Genie—The Healing Power of Menstruation*, p.23

128 Linda Sparrowe in *Yoga for a Healthy Menstrual Cycle* (p.5) makes an assertion about the susceptibility of the hypothalamus to stress. The idea that the female hormonal system can be adversely affected by stress, causing menstrual imbalances (such as strong menstrual cramping, endometriosis, amenorrhea and infertility) is also reinforced by extensive scientific and medical literature, too numerous to mention here. See Dr Christiane Northrup in her book, *Women's Bodies, Women's Wisdom* (throughout chapter five) where she explains the connection between stress and various menstrual imbalances. And this online article—http://www.mayoclinic.org/diseases-conditions/amenorrhea/basics/causes/con-20031561—explains how stress can be a cause of the menstrual irregularity, amenorrhea. Additionally, a press release from the *UC Berkley News*—http://berkeley.edu/news/media/releases/2009/06/15_stress.shtml—explains how stress can have a negative impact on a woman's fertility. Finally, also see chapter eight, p.306 in this book.

stress, which can cause it to send faulty messages to the pituitary gland and result in an imbalance in your hormones—ultimately an excess or deficiency of oestrogen or progesterone.

Moreover, when you become stressed, your autonomic nervous system moves into 'fight or flight' response (emanating from the sympathetic nervous system)[129] and your body produces stress hormones including cortisol, to provide an appropriate response to the perceived 'threat'. If you are chronically stressed, your body doesn't have an off-switch for the production of cortisol and it continues to flood your bloodstream. This can result in a kind of 'hypervigilance',[130] in which your stress tolerance becomes very low and your body maintains an almost constant state of alarm precipitated by even minor, inconsequential events. Eventually, the body runs out of enough cortisol to deal with these perceived stressors and starts to steal from sex hormones, like progesterone, and a pre-hormone called pregnenolone, which can then tip the balance of your reproductive system.[131]

It's clear then that the basis for a healthy menstrual cycle can be found in how well you manage your stress levels. Keeping your stress to a minimum is important throughout the whole month, but even more so when your energy is already compromised during your more delicate bleeding time. Therefore, one very simple and effective way to nourish your nervous system and benefit your hormonal health is to make sure you create the time for rest and retreat away from life's daily challenges—even if just for a short time.

---

129   The Autonomic Nervous System controls the 'automatic' functions of our body, like breathing and heart-rate. It consists of two 'branches'—the 'sympathetic' and 'parasympathetic nervous systems'. 'The parasympathetic nervous system (PNS) controls homeostasis and the body at rest and is responsible for the body's 'rest and digest' function. The sympathetic nervous system (SNS) controls the body's responses to a perceived threat and is responsible for the "fight or flight" response.'—reference: http://www.diffen.com/difference/Parasympathetic_nervous_system_vs_Sympathetic_nervous_system

130   A useful definition of 'hypervigilance' can be found here: https://en.wikipedia.org/wiki/Hypervigilance

131   I first encountered the concept of 'Pregnenolone Steal' in *The Hormone Cure* by Sara Gottfried, M.D., pp.45-46. A variety of references to this phenomenon can be found online, on various medical and scientific websites.

A TIME FOR REFLECTION

Women naturally seek their rebirth at every new moon by releasing their profound life-making material back to the earth.

—MAYA TIWARI[132]

Not only does slowing down and resting during your menstrual period enhance your physical wellbeing, but it will also provide the opportunity for emotional healing and growth. You can take advantage of the lower ebb in your energy that typifies menstruation to take pause in your busy life and reflect on where you've been and where you are now headed. In this way, every month you can enjoy a 'rebirth'—as you create the space to let go of aspects of yourself that are no longer serving you and set intentions for what you want to manifest in the following month.

Alexandra Pope captures the cathartic opportunity offered by our monthly-bleed when she writes:

> Giving yourself the permission to do absolutely nothing at your bleeding is a ritual. This is particularly powerful if you are generally a "driven" person. Be tender and sweet, take the phone off the hook, switch off the mobile for 24 hours (I mean it!) and surrender. Feel all the cells of your body release tension, tiredness, toxins. Let your being empty of all the stuff of the past month... everything. Cry, ache, dream and dream some more. Bliss out.[133]

Taking time to rest and reflect also offers you the potential opportunity of gaining fresh insights into current challenges or dilemmas in your life, so that when you emerge from your Dark Moon, 'reflective' phase,[134] you may find you can move forward in a more positive way with these new understandings gleaned from your retreat time.

As a yogini, I can't help but view my Dark Moon time using the metaphor of the breath. This quieter time in my month reflects the 'big exhale' followed by a natural 'pause'. After the release of the 'exhale' when your body empties, you can simply just allow yourself to 'be' during the 'pause'

---

132   Maya Tiwari, *Women's Power to Heal Through Inner Medicine*, p.65

133   Alexandra Pope, *The Wild Genie: The Healing Power of Menstruation*, p.136

134   Miranda Gray in *The Optimized Woman*, calls the menstrual period the 'reflective' phase.

that naturally follows—your bleeding time. You can surrender all need for rational thought and structure, which feels completely in alignment with your natural right-brain inclination during this phase.[135]

Shining One,
Breathing out, let go
And fall into knowing all of creation
As existing within space,
And you are absorbed in that
Vibrant empty fullness.
In this moment your body is intimate
With space, exchanging essence for essence.
Balancing in the midst of vast emptiness,
Know utter freedom.

—RADIANCE SUTRA:: 35, LORIN ROCHE[136]

Native American cultures have long considered that women are naturally more attuned to their intuitive side during the menses and they have traditionally revered a woman's 'moontime' as a powerfully psychic time in which her dreams and visions could provide deep wisdom and guidance for the whole tribe. 'In the Dark of the Moon as we begin our bleeding, is the time when the veil between us and the Great Mystery is the thinnest,' writes Native American author, healer and visionary Brooke Medicine Eagle. 'It is the most feminine, receptive time for women, and its function is exactly that to be receptive. The Moon time then becomes a

---

135 Christiane Northrup, M.D., says that research shows that the right side of the brain becomes more active during our premenstrual phase—see *Women's Bodies, Women's Wisdom*, p.108. I also found a study (http://onlinelibrary.wiley.com/wol1/doi/10.1002/hbm.21126/abstract) entitled 'Dynamic Changes in Functional Cerebral Connectivity of Special Cognition during the Menstrual Cycle', which concluded, 'The behavioral data confirmed the right hemisphere advantage for the figure comparison task as well as changes of the right hemisphere advantage during the menstrual cycle.'

136 Lorin Roche, PhD in his interpretive translation, *The Radiance Sutras* (the ancient Tantric text known as the 'Vijnana Bhairava Tantra'), p.70

time of retreat and calling for vision.'[137] You may have noticed yourself that your dreams are more vivid during the lead up to and during your period, reflecting this heightened connection with your subconscious.[138]

It follows that meditation comes most easily for women at this point in their cycle. Given the right preconditions—rest and retreat—a woman can slip into deep states of meditation and embrace the beauty of contemplation that is so regenerating for her body and spirit. 'Rather than fight this experience,' Miranda Gray writes, 'we can instead simply enjoy our natural ability to let go and leave aside our ego self and gain the benefits of stress relief and well-being that meditation can bring.'[139]

> *Surrender to rest. Turn the mind gently inward and allow the tensions to leave. Then you can hear what is most deeply true. This is pratyahara, choosing freely to accept or leave the external situation and direct your attention inside. It is as the psalm says, "Be still, and know."*
>
> —BIJA BENNETT[140]

When next you menstruate, instead of going against this more quiet energy, are you able to withdraw from social, family and work commitments (where possible) and schedule some 'me-time', some dreaming, reflective time? In my own family matrix, I announce to my husband when I am in my 'red tent' and he supports me by appreciating that I am naturally more tired at this time of the month and he often cooks and cares for me on the first day of my bleed so that I can surrender to total rest. I even try to educate my 13-year-old son by letting him know that I am on my period and that 'mum is tired today and needs to rest'.

---

137   Brooke Medicine Eagle from *Buffalo Woman Comes Singing*, as cited by Jason Elias and Katherine Ketcham in *Feminine Healing* (p.165). Alexandra Pope in *The Wild Genie*, also explains how the Native Americans regarded a woman's menstruation as equivalent to the man's 'vision quest', when a man would venture into the wilderness. 'It would come to a woman unbidden as she menstruated. All she need do was to be still,' writes Pope, p.66.

138   Dr Northrup in *Women's Bodies, Women's Wisdom* (p.107) cites studies that 'have shown that women's dreams are more frequent and often more vivid during the premenstrual and menstrual phases of their cycles', and this is footnoted with the references: Harman, 'Dreaming Sleep (the D State) and the Menstrual Cycle', *Journal of Nervous and Mental Disease*, and Swanson and Foulkes, 'Dream Content and the Menstrual Cycle', *Journal of Nervous and Mental Disease*.

139   Miranda Gray, *The Optimized Woman*, p.61

140   Bija Bennett, *Emotional Yoga: How the Body can Heal the Mind*, p.140

*I have learnt to be gentle with my exquisitely sensitive and
vulnerable self at this time of the 'moon-th'. Safe in my Dark
Moon, menstrual cocoon, I withdraw from the outside world and
I tune inwards to the pulse, the internal rhythm of my womb.*

—ANA'S MENSTRUAL DIARY

A REALITY CHECK

At this point you're probably thinking, 'I'm a busy woman with many conflicting demands upon my time and energy. It's unrealistic to expect that I can drop everything!' I agree! You may not be in the position where you can take the whole day off from your work or family responsibilities to retreat into your 'red tent', but are there small ways you can lighten your load and steal even just a little time for yourself to honour your Dark Moon time?

Herbalist and author of *105 Ways to Celebrate Menstruation*, Kami McBride offers a slew of juicy menstrual honouring ideas and says that it's important that we give ourselves at least two full hours of solitude when we bleed.[141] I tend to concur, and try to take a few hours off to rest on my bed on the first and heaviest day of my period. I retreat there to doze, to read, to daydream. I know that this small investment in my own rest-time pays off for me later in the month by returning enhanced energy when I move into my Waxing Moon (post-menstruation) and Full Moon (ovulation) phases, and most importantly, flows on to make my most challenging phase, the Waning Moon (premenstrual) phase, easier to manage.

Even when I can't take time off, I lower my expectation of how productive I can and should be on the first day or so of my bleeding. I cut myself some slack! If I've had a hard day teaching or in the office running my business, I make sure that I create space for a gentle, wind-down evening. I try to avoid cooking—I organise take-out, or pull a pre-prepared meal from my freezer—or if he has time, my husband takes on the cooking. At the very least, at some point in my day, I try to make time for a nurturing Dark Moon yoga practice. Even twenty minutes or so of gentle, Restorative Yoga gives me the pause that I need to honour my Dark Moon time and withdraw from the outside world.

---

141   Kami McBride, *105 Ways to Celebrate Menstruation*, p.27

Giving yourself the time to rest and retreat during your monthly period takes discipline, even courage. It is so easy to fill our days with 'must dos' and our heads with worries. In our linear-based reality that is suited to the more constant masculine energy, as women, we need to deliberately carve out our cyclical rest-time, which may feel against the grain of social expectations. 'We live in a culture which demands that we are "turned on" all the time. Always bright and happy. Always available for intercourse—both sexual and otherwise with people,' writes Lucy Pearce.[142]

Once you start taking mindful pause in your menstrual month, you'll be spurred along by the positive results you will observe; you will realise how this simple practice enhances your connection with your body and your menstrual cycle, and has positive flow-on effects for your overall health.

PRACTICAL WAYS TO HONOUR YOUR DARK MOON BLEEDING TIME

There are so many wonderful ways you can honour this natural time of stillness during your menstrual month and build positive habits around taking care of your health and wellbeing. Here are some starting suggestions for you to try when you bleed. They may also inspire you to come up with your own Dark Moon rituals.

- Go to bed early or sleep in (or both!).
- Take a nap.
- Read your favourite book.
- Sip your favourite herbal tea.[143]
- Eat nourishing, warming foods like soups or stews.
- Decline social invitations and stay quiet at home.
- Write in your journal—reflecting on the month that's been and setting intentions for the future. Or, use your journal like a

---

142 *Lucy H. Pearce, Moon Time: A Guide to Celebrating your Menstrual Cycle*, location 1094 (Kindle edition)

143 Relaxing, soothing teas for menstruation recommended by herbalist Kami McBride include chamomile, lemonbalm and passion flower (*105 Ways to Celebrate Menstruation*, p.40). I enjoy sipping on 'red' or 'pink' herb teas like rose and rosehip tea. Lucy Pearce, author of *Moontime: A Guide to Celebrating your Menstrual Cycle*, also recommends red raspberry leaf tea, to tone the uterus and relieve nausea, and nettle tea to boost your iron levels (Kindle version: location 1876).

beloved friend to work through any feelings that have bubbled to the surface at this deeply intuitive time of your month.
- Take a gentle walk in nature.
- Practise some nurturing Dark Moon yoga to relax and soothe your body and soul. Your Dark Moon yoga practice may consist of one posture, or a sequence of postures (see the Dark Moon sequences at the end of this chapter) or it may just be your favourite breathing, relaxation or meditation practice (sprinkled throughout this chapter)—whatever you intuitively feel will nurture your energy.

YOGA FOR THE DARK MOON PHASE

The yogic 'red tent'

Often I've stepped from a world where I've been working too hard, my mind in overdrive, my commitments overwhelming, and I feel beyond tired during my Dark Moon time. So soothing then to unroll my yoga mat and let my body soften and yield upon my bolsters. As my body lets go into the gentle shapes that I offer it, my mind and emotions too can pull back from their inner attack, and instead the inner-smile returns. All balance and equanimity returns as things drop back into the simplicity of breath and sensation. When I emerge, I feel connected. My body feels whole and feminine again. Peace reigns within and without.

—ANA'S MENSTRUAL DIARY

I was enjoying a post-class cup of tea with a yoga teacher friend and his female student one day, when the student shared with me that she regularly suffered from severe menstrual distress. Every month she bled heavily and suffered strong menstrual cramps. I asked her if she still attended my friend's yoga class—a strong, dynamic Asana (posture) class—when she was menstruating. The woman looked at me blankly and replied that, yes, of course she did; she simply took some painkillers and threw herself into the practice. After all, she loved my friend's yoga class! I then asked her how she felt after doing his class. 'Awful!' she said unequivocally. I gently suggested that perhaps there might be another way for her to support herself during her period—either resting or doing her own gentle yoga practice.

A Dark Moon menstrual yoga practice is one of the best ways I know to support myself at this sensitive point in my cycle. Even if it's just for 20 or 30 minutes, I close the door on my many commitments and create my own metaphorical 'red tent', softening into a soothing, restorative, lushly Feminine Yoga practice.

As I say to my yoga students, if you are feeling tired, 'crampy' and low, you have a few critical choices: you can ignore these feelings and push on through and end up feeling worse; you can sprawl on the sofa, watching day-time television, binging on potato chips and chocolate, feeling sorry for yourself; or you can get out your bolster, breathe and relax, and enjoy a rejuvenating yoga-rest.

To create your own yogic 'red tent', set up a space for yourself where you will not be disturbed (if possible!), whether it be a separate room, or part of a room. Light some candles, burn essential oils or incense, listen to feminine music, or simply savour silence, and allow the alchemy of Feminine Yoga to work its magic on your body and soul.[144] Enjoy the sequences at the end of this chapter, or make up your own. But before you do, read on to gain an understanding of the important principles and guidelines for your Dark Moon yoga practice.

Principles of a Dark Moon yoga practice

The dark moon provides a cosy climate for a woman's
sadhana or rest, reprieve and replenishment.
Mother Moon takes to recharging her Shakti during
this time. Likewise, a woman is advised to create a
gentle space to conserve her feminine powers and
inculcate her creative potential during this time.

—MAYA TIWARI [145]

To get the most enjoyment and benefit from your Dark Moon menstrual practice, it's important that you have a good understanding of how to adapt the yoga postures appropriately for this more sensitive time of the month. Not just any yoga will do! Remember, we are no longer practising yoga like a man. We now understand that yoga needs to be adapted for the unique needs of our feminine cycle.

---

144   For more tips on establishing and maintaining a home yoga practice see p.61 in chapter three.

145   Maya Tiwari, *Women's Power to Heal Through Inner Medicine*, p.78

Let's look as some fundamental principles behind a feminine approach to yoga for your Dark Moon time.

Make space for the 'mini-birth'

The smooth muscle (myometrial) layer of the uterus contracts with a strong downward force during childbirth and is one of the strongest muscles in the body.[146] A woman can feel the effects of this powerful muscle in action as it pushes the baby out of the body during labour and also when she experiences menstrual cramps. Prostaglandin F2 alpha is the hormone responsible for triggering uterine contractions for *both* menstruation and labour. If you've given birth and your labour started gradually, you may recall the early part of labour felt just like period cramps.

Effectively, when you menstruate you may experience the same sensations and process as early labour. And if you suffer from menstrual anomalies, such as endometriosis or fibroids,[147] which can manifest as painful cramping (thought to be caused by an excess of these prostaglandins[148]), the sensations may even be ramped-up to approximate those felt during more established labour.

Therefore, your menstruation is like a 'mini birth', and you need to consider this when choosing the type and qualities of your movements during your period. Just as when you are in labour, you will want to be gentle with yourself during your monthly-bleed. It's best to practise movements that create softness and space in the belly to support your hard working uterus. You will want to avoid twisting, compressing and wrenching the belly (uterus), and you will be focused on conserving your energy as much as possible.

---

146   The uterus is considered to be the strongest muscle in the body by weight 'based on the ability of the uterus that weighs only 1.1 kg (40 oz) to deliver an infant. This 1.1 kg uterus can exert a force of 100 to 400 N of downward force with each contraction.' Reference: https://www.buzzle.com/articles/strongest-muscle-in-the-human-body.html

147   See chapter eight in this book for more information on various menstrual irregularities including endometriosis and fibroids.

148   Jason Elias and Katherine Ketcham in *Feminine Healing* (p.184) write, 'Recent research indicates that high levels of the hormone prostaglandin F2 alpha create uterine spasms and cramping sensations'. Christiane Northrup, M.D., in *Women's Bodies, Women's Wisdom* also mentions this connection between Prostaglandin F2A and menstrual cramps and how this hormone (and other inflammatory chemicals) can be propagated by stress.

Support *apana*

> *Menstruation has an inward and downward movement in the body. Part of accessing the deep wisdom of the feminine involves moving from the yang experience of outward expression and achievement to the yin experience of going inside and listening to the deep recesses of the soul.*

—KAMI MCBRIDE[149]

As women we are fortunate because our bodies offer us the valuable opportunity for monthly cleansing and 'purification'. The Ayurvedic belief is that every month a woman's body cleanses itself of any accumulated *ama* or toxins. These can be toxins caused by improper diet, intake of drugs, as well as mental and emotional stress. Dr Robert E. Svoboda suggests that this in-built purification system is a 'second chance' to purify our blood and is perhaps even one reason why women live longer than men![150]

To facilitate this removal of toxins, a woman's body needs to harness the power of *apana*. As mentioned in chapter three, *apana* is a concept in yoga and Ayurveda referring to the downward movement of energy that operates from the navel to the anus. *Apana vayu* is the flow of energy or *prana* that is responsible for eliminating substances from the body; urination, defecation, ejaculation, birth and menstruation are all governed by the energy of *apana*. Therefore, all the movements and even Pranayama (breathing practices) and meditation practices[151] that you adopt during menstruation need to facilitate this downward flow of energy. In concrete terms, supporting *apana* means that you will want to exclude any movements that invert the body. This will then assist in the effective removal of *ama* and help you achieve and maintain maximum health and wellbeing as a woman.

This idea of supporting the process of *apana* also extends to how a woman manages her menstruation. It is recommended from the Ayurvedic and Feminine Yoga perspective that you avoid or minimise the use of tampons as these interfere with this natural downward flow of energy. Instead, try reusable cloth pads or moon cups because they do not prevent *apana*. Cloth pads or moon cups are environmentally friendly and help you

---

149   Kami McBride, *105 Ways to Celebrate Menstruation*, p.13

150   Dr. Robert E. Svoboda, *Ayurveda for Women*, p.71

151   '...you can eliminate some of your mental wastes by meditation', says Dr. Robert E. Svoboda in *Ayurveda for Women*, p.63

stay connected to the process and ritual of menstruation, especially if you water your garden with your nutrient-rich blood either directly from the moon-cup or from the water in which you've soaked your cloth pads.[152]

Foster cooling and grounding energy

According to yoga teacher and author of *The Women's Yoga Book*, Bobby Clennell, heat is discharged from the body during menstruation.[153] This makes sense when you consider how hard the uterus is working to discharge the thickened endometrium (uterine lining), particularly if you're experiencing a lot of cramping. To balance and minimise this heating, *yang* energy, you need to ensure the quality of your yoga practice is *yin* or cooling in essence. This means avoiding the over-stimulation of a more 'solar' practice and instead working with a 'lunar' focus that is cooling, soothing and calming.

As we have seen, menstruation is a woman's monthly time of *vata*, which is the Ayurvedic constitution (*dosha*) associated with the element of air.[154] When you have too much *vata* you are likely to become over-sensitive, overwhelmed, anxious, scattered and ungrounded. A Dark Moon menstrual yoga practice should therefore aim to calm and ground your energy by incorporating slow, meditative movements that include longer holds of gentle, supportive variations of the postures, and lots of floor-based work.

---

152 Sex coach and journalist, Laura Anne Rowell gives some compelling reasons for switching to either a moon cup or cloth pads. She points out the potential toxic and carcinogenic effects of the synthetic materials that commercial pads and tampons are made of, not to mention the detrimental environmental effects. She also gives some handy advice on diluting your menstrual blood to apply as a garden fertilizer because of its high nitrogen and protein content. See: https://www.honeycolony.com/article/the-power-of-menses/

153 Bobby Clennell, *The Women's Yoga Book: Asana and Pranayama for all Phases of the Menstrual Cycle*, p.18. Also, this article—https://www.avogel.co.uk/health/periods/symptoms/sweating/—suggests that we may feel hotter (temperature-wise) when we menstruate, due to hormonal imbalances.

154 See Appendix 1 For more information on the three Ayurvedic *doshas*.

Contraindications and cautions for your Dark Moon yoga practice

So far, we've discussed how a sensitive Dark Moon yoga practice should include movements that keep the belly soft and open, facilitate the downward movement of energy, and that are grounding, cooling and ultimately restful. Bearing these principles in mind, here are some more specific guidelines for what to avoid or modify during your menstruation.

Modify or avoid: Twists

Avoid Closed Twists that involve a strong action on the abdominal area, such as Marichyasana III (Seated One Leg Twist—see Figure 3); and Ardha Matsyendrasana (Half Lord of the Fish Pose Twist—see Figure 4), as these postures constrict the uterus and also compress the other reproductive organs, and may cause flooding or clotting of the menstrual blood. Instead, do their open versions (see Figure 5 and Figure 6).

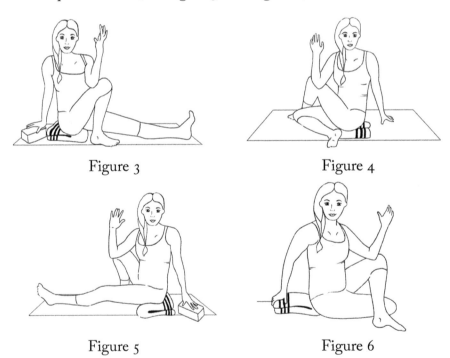

Figure 3   Figure 4

Figure 5   Figure 6

Other safe, gentle twists that are appropriate for menstruation include the simple Cross-legged Twist (see Figure 7) and Bharadvajasana (Sage Twist—see Figure 8.)

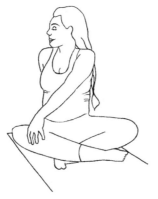
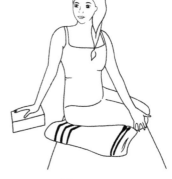

Figure 7   Figure 8

Avoid: abdominal and pelvic floor exercises

Strong activation of the abdominal muscles in postures like Paripurna Navasana (The Boat Pose—see Figure 9) should be avoided while you are bleeding. As previously mentioned, the reason for this is that we want to allow for space and softness in the belly during menstruation—facilitating the 'mini-birth'—plus, our strength and energy is naturally di-

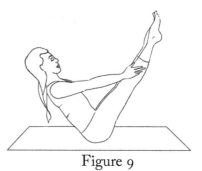

Figure 9

minished. Trial if for yourself—practise a strong posture like the Boat Pose that requires a great deal of core strength while you are menstruating; it's likely to feel counter-intuitive and it can deplete your energy reserves further.

In order to hold yourself stable in postures that require strong abdominal engagement, you may end up overly relying on the back muscles because the abdominals naturally don't support the body as they would during the rest of the month. You may also be more likely to overuse the deep core, psoas muscle (connecting the trunk to legs), which is undesirable, as a tight psoas, according to Liz Koch, a somatic therapist and expert on the psoas, can be a contributing factor in menstrual cramping.[155]

---

155   Liz Koch explains how this can occur in her article, 'How Does the Psoas Influence Menstrual Cycles', at, www.coreawareness.com as well as in her book, *The Psoas Book*. On p.61, Koch writes, 'The experience of menstrual cramping has been successfully relieved by releasing the psoas muscle.'

The lower energy locks or Bandhas—Uddiyana Bandha (Upward Abdominal Lock) and Mula Bandha (Pelvic Floor Lock)—should also be avoided when you are menstruating. Uddiyana Bandha involves a strong action of lifting and scooping the abdominals, which is counter to our intention of keeping this area soft. In addition, both Bandhas involve a drawing up of the energy into the body that goes against the natural downward movement of energy (*apana*).

Avoid: Inversions

You've probably heard before that you should avoid practising Inversions during your period, but you may not know *why*. There are several good reasons for avoiding what I call the full, 'Active Inversions' like Headstand, Shoulderstand, Handstand, as well as Viparita Karani (Legs up the Wall Pose—see Figure 410, p.453), with the hips raised on a bolster.

Firstly and most obviously, if women turn their bodies upside down when they are menstruating, they are going against the flow—both the literal, physical flow of the blood as well as the energetic downward flow or *apana*. If you block the natural *apana* of your menses, you also prevent the proper release of *ama* (toxins) from the body. Dr Svoboda says that the potential back-flow of the blood and the reversal of *apana* can be responsible for menstrual anomalies like endometriosis and it can also cause vaginitis, ovarian cysts and uterine fibroids.[156] As Bobby Clennel says, it's 'common sense' to avoid Inversions during your period since 'the menstrual process is one of discharge'.[157]

---

156   Dr. Robert E. Svoboda, in *Ayurveda for Women*, p.70, says, 'When *apana* moves upward it can create endometriosis, which can produce severe pain during menses. This condition occurs when fragments of endometrium (the uterine lining) travel upward from the uterus into the abdominal cavity instead of down and out through the vagina as normally happens each month. This tissue can only move upward when *apana* makes it do so, which *apana* will only do when its own flow has been reversed'. It should be noted, however, that the theory of 'retrograde menstruation' as being a cause for endometriosis has been called into question (see *Clinical Gynecology*, Bieber, Sanfillipo, Horowitz, Shafi p.205) but is yet to be categorically disproved. For example, the Mayo Clinic still lists retrograde menstruation as one of the potential causes—http://www.mayoclinic.org/diseases-conditions/endometriosis/symptoms-causes/dxc-20236425). Either way, if there is any risk of retrograde menstruation (and therefore reversal of *apana*) causing endometriosis, then it makes sense to avoid Inversions, just in case!

157   Bobby Clennell, *The Women's Yoga Book: Asana and Pranayama for All Phases of the Menstrual Cycle*, p.19

Secondly, when viewed from a Western physiological perspective, we discover that Inversions are also problematic. According to yoga teacher and doctor, Mary P. Schatz, M.D., Inversions can cause vascular congestion.[158] Schatz says that when we invert, the effect of gravity on blood vessels that are embedded into the broad ligaments of the uterus that take away blood from the uterus (veins), can become blocked and can cause a pooling of blood in the uterus. If Inversions cause us to bleed more than usual the result may be that we feel 'weak and emotionally vulnerable'.[159]

A third reason to avoid Inversions when you are bleeding is related to the potential for injury in the lower back or sacrum. When practising the stronger Inversions like Handstand or Headstand, it's essential to recruit the abdominals to create stability and support for the spine. However, as already noted, a woman's overall strength, and therefore her abdominals are weaker than normal during this time of the month, and she should avoid activating them to support the natural process of the monthly 'mini-birth'. Without the full use of your abdominals to support you in these Inversions you risk injuring your lower back that is already vulnerable and more unstable than normal due to the presence of the hormone 'relaxin'. This hormone, as the name implies, relaxes and softens the ligaments and joints in the body, specifically in the lower back and pelvis, and is produced

---

158   See: Mary P. Schatz, M.D. online article, 'A Woman's balance: Inversions and Menstruation' (http://yoga4leongal.blogspot.com.au/2009/05/womans-balance-inversions-and.html_—'During inversions, the uterus is pulled toward the head by gravity, causing the broad ligaments to be stretched. This can cause stretch and partial collapse or occlusion of the thin-walled veins, while allowing the uncollapsed arteries to continue to pump in blood. Thus, more blood enters the uterus via the arteries than can be carried away by the veins. The vascular congestion that results can lead to increased menstrual bleeding,' writes Schatz.

159   "… weak and emotionally vulnerable"—so writes Yuko Yoshikawa in a *Yoga Journal* (Sep/Oct 2000, p.101) article, 'Everybody Upsidedown'. Interestingly well known yoga teacher and physical therapist, Judith Hanson Lasater says Inversions may cause the vessels *supplying* blood to the uterus to be partially blocked by the weight of the uterus as it's pulled by gravity (opposite to Dr Schatz's theory—see previous footnote). Lasater says that Inversions can therefore cause a temporary decrease or even cessation of the menstrual flow followed by a sometimes heavier flow. See Judith Lasater PhD., *Relax and Renew: Restful Yoga for Stressful Times*, p.158. Either way, whether you subscribe to Schatz's or Lasater's view, they both agree the result is heavier bleeding, which suggests it's best to avoid Inversions when we bleed.

late in your cycle to allow the cervix (entrance to the womb) to open to facilitate menstruation. This explains why you may often have an achy-back just before or at the start of your menses, and research shows that women are more vulnerable to injury at this time of the month.[160]

Avoid or minimise: strong Standing poses and dynamic Vinyasa

As we've seen, the engagement of the abdominal and pelvic floor muscles is counter to the *apana*-energy of menstruation, which means that Standing postures are also not ideal during your period. This is because you are less able to call on the support of your core muscles to provide stability for your back in the Standing postures. Additionally, the strength and stamina required to execute these poses—especially the Warrior postures (see Figure 10 and Figure 11)—is not necessarily available to you at this monthly time of natural, low ebb in your energy.

A final reason for avoiding or, at the very least, minimising your stay in the more dynamic Standing postures is that they can be heat-building and, as mentioned above, during menstruation you should be working to cool the body and mind, rather than continuing to activate heating, *yang* energy.

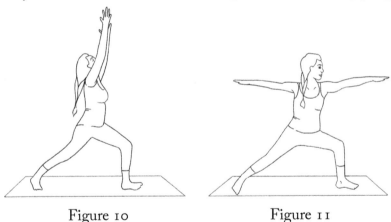

Figure 10   Figure 11

In the same vein, you should avoid a dynamic Vinyasa practice (flowing, linked postures), particularly sequences that involve 'jumpings' (jumping from one posture to the next) and lots of strong poses during your period. In addition to the Warrior poses, other examples of overly strong and

160 See BBC News article, 'Menstrual Cycle Injury Risk Link'— (www.news.bbc. co.uk/2/hi/health/6354303.stm), which cites research undertaken by London's Portland Hospital, concluding that women are more likely to injure them-selves at specific times in their menstrual cycle: 'At the end of the cycle, levels of [another hormone], relaxin rises. This is to allow the cervix to open so that menstruation can occur, but it also means the ligaments in general are softened'.

heating postures, which also require a lot of core activation, are the Plank Pose (see Figure 12) and Chaturanga Dandasana (Push-up Pose—see Figure 13)

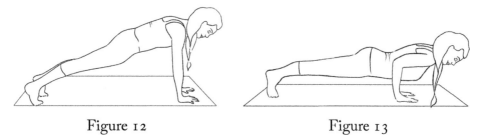

Figure 12   Figure 13

If you do feel an urge to perform these more dynamic postures and Vinyasa, it's preferable that you leave them for the latter part of your menses when your flow is light, and your energy tends to be on the increase again.

Avoid: strong Backbends

It is generally recommended that you avoid the strong, active Backbends like Urdvha Dhanurasana (Wheel Pose—see Figure 14) and Urdhva Mukha Svanasana (Upward Facing Dog—see Figure 15) during your Dark Moon menstrual time. These postures are essentially *yang* in their nature and they require a lot of energy to perform and, as we've learnt, this is a time to indulge and rest your body, rather than push your limits.

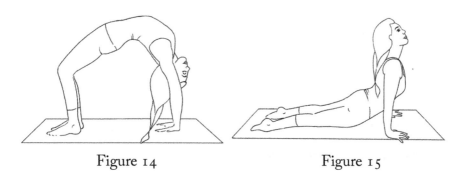

Figure 14   Figure 15

A further reason to refrain from practising these kind of Dynamic Backbends is due to the potential lower back and sacral vulnerability caused by the luteal and early menses surge in relaxin. Just as with the Active Inversions, without the proper engagement of the abdominals— which we've already discovered are best kept soft— you can risk injuring the lower back.

While simple Backbends like Setu Bandhasana (the Bridge Pose— see Figure 16) are fine to practise during the menses, they can be quite heating, and when performed in succession or held for too long, can be too strenuous. It is therefore best to focus on the supported version of Bridge Pose—with a block (on its lowest edge—see Figure 17) or bolster under the sacrum/torso (see Figure 399, p.450).

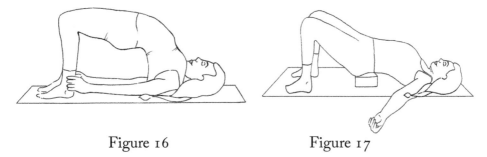

Figure 16   Figure 17

Avoid: *yang* Pranayama

During your menstrual period I recommend you avoid the more *yang* breathing practices that involve rapid, strong breaths, like Kapalabhati (Skull Shining Breath—see p.268 for instructions) and Bhastrika (Bellows Breath/ Breath of Fire). Both these Pranayama involve short, rapid breaths, whilst pumping the belly in and out, and are overly stimulating and heat inducing and involve too strong an action on the abdomen.

Now that you know what to avoid, the next question is: what postures and practices *can* you do to support yourself during your Dark Moon time?

What is a Dark Moon menstrual yoga practice?

As you have probably gathered by now, the overall tone of a therapeutic practice for menstruation is gentle so that you can work *with*, not against, the energy low that generally occurs at this time of the month. Therefore, one of the best ingredients for a nurturing Dark Moon practice is Restorative Yoga.

Restorative Yoga: active relaxation

Restorative Yoga involves the practice of many of the common yoga postures in supported, graduated variations. By propping yourself up with bolsters and folded blankets (and sometimes chairs and yoga blocks), you are able to comfortably stay in a posture for longer periods—sometimes up to 10 minutes—which enhances its therapeutic benefits. These benefits are wide ranging, depending on the posture, but it's safe to say that all Restorative postures[161] work on calming the nervous system and quieting

---

161   See Appendix 3 for an overview of the types of Restorative postures we employ in a Feminine Yoga practice.

the mind, countering the stress response. This makes Restorative Yoga an invaluable tool for all phases of your menstrual cycle, but most especially during your more vulnerable Dark Moon phase.

The magic of Restorative Yoga is that you don't have to expend energy to gain energy! If you are feeling tired, sluggish and heavy in your body and mind, you will find that a Restorative practice—even as short as 15-20 minutes—can make a real difference to how you are feeling both mentally and physically.

Judith Hanson Lasater, the doyenne of Restorative Yoga in the West,[162] describes it as 'active relaxation' and says that this unique practice balances the masculine energy of *prana* (that powers the upper body from the diaphragm upwards), with the feminine energy of *apana* (that powers the lower body, from the diaphragm downwards—most specifically, the abdominal area). 'Restorative yoga balances these two aspects of energy so that the practitioner is neither overstimulated nor depleted,' writes Lasater.[163] In summary, it's an alchemical practice that lends itself perfectly to the mood of this time of the month, providing deep rest and healing.

Beneficial postures and practices

A Dark Moon practice is largely floor based, consisting of Supine and Sitting postures.

Grounding Seated Postures

Sitting postures are very appropriate for your Dark Moon time due to their non-strenuous nature and grounding effects. Two such Seated postures are Baddha Konasana (Bound Angle Pose—see Figure 383, p.441) and Upavista Konasana (Wide Angle Pose—see Figure 384, p.442), which are both what I like to call 'Classical Women's' postures.[164] These are the postures that are universally recommended by yoga therapists as being helpful for promoting a healthy reproductive system.

On a physical level, the Classical Women's postures release muscular tension in the pelvic area, creating space there for the uterus to work most

---

162 Judith Lasater's book, *Relax and Renew: Restful Yoga for Stressful Times* is a veritable Restorative Yoga 'bible'. It includes sequences for women's cycles—for menstruation, pregnancy and menopause—as well as for various ailments like back pain, headache, insomnia and even jet lag!

163 Lasater, *Relax and Renew*, pp.7-8

164 See Appendix 2 in this book for more some examples (and their benefits) of these beneficial poses for women.

efficiently during the menses, and they help to boost blood circulation in the pelvic and abdominal areas, which promotes easeful menstruation. Geeta Iyengar, well known Iyengar teacher and specialist in yoga for women's health, says of Baddha Konasana: 'This pose is a boon to women as it tones the kidneys, alleviates urinary and uterine disorders, prevents sciatica and hernia. It also strengthens the bladder and the uterus'.[165]

On an energetic level, these Classical Women's postures release stagnation and boost the flow of *prana*, or *shakti prana*[166] around the reproductive organs. In particular, Baddha Konasana harnesses the beneficial, grounding energy of *apana* that relates to the inner thighs, pelvic region (including pelvic floor) and lower back. Sandra Anderson, yoga teacher and author from the Himalayan Institute, suggests that this posture is one of the most 'powerful postures for awakening and directing *apana*.'[167]

In addition to the seated variations already mentioned, the Classical Women's postures can be adapted as Restorative postures—using bolsters, blankets, blocks, straps and a chair—either as supported, Supine Heart-Openers or Supported Forward Bends.[168]

Restful Supine postures

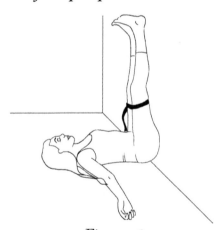

When you're tired, or even exhausted at this time of your cycle, any posture that involves lying on the back feels exquisite! Whether it be a static, hip-opening Classical Women's posture like supported Supta Padangusthasana II (Reclining Big Toe Pose—see Figure 387, p.444), which opens and softens the pelvic area, or gently rocking or circling the knees in Apanasana (Knee to Chest Pose—Posture 2, p.124), which massages the lower back and eases menstrual cramps, Supine postures provide an opportunity

Figure 18

for the body to rest while gently targeting key areas of the body.

---

165   Geeta S. Iyengar, *Yoga, A Gem for Women*, p.141

166   See p.55 in chapter three for a definition of *shakti prana*.

167   Sandra Anderson, *Yoga International*, 'The Five Prana Vayus in Yoga: Apana', May, 2013 https://yogainternational.com/article/view/the-5-prana-vayus-in-yoga-apana

168   See Appendix 2 for examples of some Classical Women's Heart-Opener and Forward Bending Restorative postures.

Supine postures to begin or end your menstrual Dark Moon practice include menstrual-friendly Inversions like Chair Savasana (see Figure 414, p.455), or Viparita Karani (Legs up the Wall Pose—Figure 18), both of which can be very soothing for the common menstrual symptoms of tired, aching legs and lower back. Note, it's important that these postures are practised *without* the hips raised on a folded blanket or bolster so that the pelvis is not inverted.

Constructive Rest Position: better than a coffee!

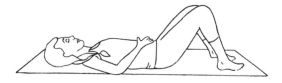

Figure 19

I often like to begin my Dark Moon practice with the Constructive Rest Position (CRP—see Figure 19). Originally conceived by somatic therapist, Mabel Todd,[169] this deceptively simple posture is beneficial for relieving menstrual backache and cramping, and is profoundly rejuvenating. Donna Farhi, an internationally renowned yoga teacher, says Constructive Rest Position is 'an alternative to a nap, cup of coffee or piece of chocolate!'[170]

To practise CRP lie on your back with the feet hip width apart and a comfortable distance away from the buttocks so that the pelvis is in neutral. When you have correctly positioned the feet in relation to the buttocks, there should be a feeling of the thigh bones and shin bones resting lightly against each other like two playing cards positioned in a delicately balanced triangular formation. This allows for a feeling of the head of the femur (thigh bone) to ground into the hip socket, which relaxes the hip flexors, quadriceps and abdominal muscles, and ultimately releases any holding in the psoas muscle.

Liz Koch says that resting on the floor in this particular fashion enables us to unravel patterns of tension from deep within our core outward, and

---

169   This is according to Donna Farhi in *Yoga for Women Therapeutic Practice Sequences* (e-book, 2009, p.3). However, Liz Koch in *The Psoas Book* writes that Lulu Swegard coined this name in the 1930s. Either way, it was a pioneering somatic therapist who first created and named this position, and it has now been widely touted by contemporary somatic therapists and yoga teachers like Liz Koch and Donna Farhi.

170   Donna Farhi, *Yoga for Women Therapeutic Practice Sequences*, p.3.

it 'frees the central nervous system from much of the stimuli that evokes habitual response patterns to gravity.'[171]

The iliopsoas complex of muscles are deep core muscles that connect the trunk to the legs, and run from the lower back through the core of the body, passing through the pelvis and finishing at the groin, inside each thigh bone. Branching off the psoas-major muscle at the pelvis is the iliacus, a fan-shaped muscle that lines the inside of the pelvic basin. Because the psoas runs through the pelvis, the nerves of the reproductive organs embed in this muscle. According to Liz Koch, if these psoas muscles are tight and constricted, this can cause or exacerbate menstrual cramping because the muscles can spasm around the nerves that innervate the reproductive organs. Therefore, Koch claims that by gently releasing the psoas in CRP, you can have a positive impact on your menstrual health.[172]

The Constructive Rest Position is also helpful in fostering the *apana-energy* that is beneficial for the Dark Moon phase as well as for your entire menstrual cycle. With the soles of the feet resting on the floor, CRP lends itself well to the practice of the grounding Apana Breath (see p.102). As you exhale, focus on sending any feelings of heaviness, tiredness and tension from your pelvis through your legs, into your feet, and into the earth. During your Dark Moon phase, it's so therapeutic to spend some time here in this restful, reclining posture, and really tune in, getting a sense of the yielding of the feet into the earth that then rebounds and sends energy (*prana*) from the feet, back up through the legs, into the pelvic bowl, and into your womb-space.

Supta Baddha Konasana: the mother of all postures

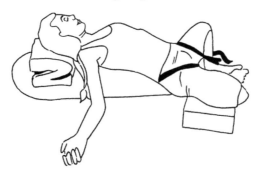

Figure 20

---

171   Read about the numerous benefits and applications of the Constructive Rest Position (CRP) in Liz Koch's books: *The Psoas Book* and *Core Awareness*, as well as in her many articles and videos at www.coreawareness.com

172   Liz Koch, in her article, 'How Does the Psoas Influence Menstrual Cycles', at www.coreawareness.com as well as in her book, *The Psoas Book*.

Included in this group of restful, Supine postures for healthy menstruation are the Restorative 'Heart-Opening' postures (see Appendix 3), in which you lie back over a bolster, blankets or yoga blocks.

Deserving special mention is the Classical Women's posture, Baddha Konasana in its Restorative variation—Supta Baddha Konasana (Reclining Bound Angle Posture— see Figure 20). Patricia Walden, a senior Iyengar-trained yoga teacher from the USA, describes this Restorative posture as the 'mother of all *asanas*'.[173] This blissful posture softens and creates space in the belly and pelvic area, can ease menstrual cramps and heaviness and congestion in the belly and pelvic floor. It is also particularly rewarding when your energy is quite low, as it opens the chest and lungs, facilitates deeper breathing and rebuilds your energy.

According to Judith Hanson Lasater, Supta Baddha Konasana supports the menstrual flow to move down and out and 'harmonizes the *apana*, or feminine, energy in the abdomen by creating a receptive vessel in the belly and pelvis.' She also says that psychologically, this posture creates a 'deep opening with safety and support'.[174]

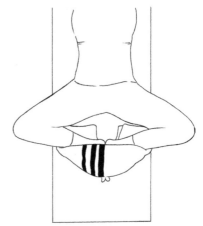

If you are practising this posture for any length of time, it's important that you support the knees to facilitate maximum softening and release in the belly and pelvic area. Do this by placing a block (see Figure 20), folded blanket or bolster under each knee, or wrap a long blanket roll (see Figure 21) around the front of the shins and ankles, and tuck it under the outer shins, near the knees.

Figure 21

173   Linda Sparrowe and Patricia Walden, *The Women's Book of Yoga and Health*, p.94

174   Judith Lasater, *Relax and Renew*, p.162.

Cooling Seated Forward Bends

The introspective nature of Forward Bends, particularly supported, Restorative Forward Bends, perfectly suits the tenor of your Dark Moon time of the month. These postures instil a sense of deep calm in the body-mind, relieving headaches, anxiety and irritability.

There is a natural internal focus that comes from folding ourselves inwards. From a physiological point of view, the act of resting the forehead on a support, such as a chair, bolster or brick, which characterises many Restorative Forward Bends, has a direct, balancing effect on the nervous system. In a posture like Supported Pascimottanasana (Seated Forward Bend—see p.451), the pressure on the forehead (from the chair or the soft props) helps relax the muscles around the eyes and forehead, and deeply soothes the nervous system because it engages your parasympathetic nervous system response ('relaxation response'[175]) by stimulating the vagus nerve.[176]

Pioneering yoga teacher BKS Iyengar says that Forward Bends are ideal for menstruation as they control the flow of blood and check excess discharge.[177]

---

175 Herbert Benson, founder of Harvard's Mind/Body Medical Institute, famously coined the term 'relaxation response'. This response is defined as your personal ability to encourage your body to release chemicals and brain signals that make your muscles and organs slow down and increase blood flow to the brain. Dr. Benson describes the scientific benefits of relaxation, explaining that regular practice of the relaxation response can be an effective treatment for a wide range of stress-related disorders,—from this article in *Psychology Today*, at https://www.psychologytoday.com/blog/heart-and-soul-healing/201303/dr-herbert-benson-s-relaxation-response

176 I have long been aware of the practice of supporting the forehead in Restorative postures in order to bring about a calming response to the body-mind. In searching for evidence as to why these forehead-supported postures work, I first came across an article about special needs children who instinctively press their foreheads into objects and people as a way of self-soothing. The article, 'Could your Special Needs Child's Forehead Stim be a Healing Mechanism?' (www.specialneedslove.net), led me to Mel Robin's, *A Physiological Handbook for Teachers of Yogasana* and this reference to the work of Cole (*Relaxation Physiology and Practice*, unpublished notes, 1994), '... when pressure is applied to the forehead of the orbits of the eyes, there is a parasympathetic vagal heart-slowing reflex that becomes operative.' Note, the vagus nerve is the largest cranial nerve that connects the brain to the parasympathetic nervous system as well as the digestive system, heart and lungs.

177 B.K.S Iyengar, *Yoga, The Path to Holistic Health*, p.356

My all-time favourite Dark Moon posture is the nurturing Forward Bend, the Supported Child Pose (see Figure 22). If I had to choose one posture for menstruation this would be it! It's as comforting as cuddling a big teddy bear, and offers many benefits including relief from menstrual pain, fatigue, and an aching, tight back. It's also an ideal position to place a hot-water bottle or heat pack on the sacrum, while you rest and breathe through the pain of period cramps.

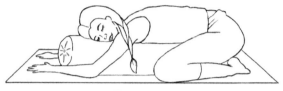

Figure 22

Gentle Standing poses

Your Dark Moon yoga practice is most restful and nurturing if it consists mostly of floor-based postures. However, you can also choose from some of the less active Standing poses. Good choices are the standing, Supported Forward Bends like Prasarita Padottanasana (Standing Wide-Legged Forward Bend—see Figure 404, p.452), or Uttanasana (Standing Forward Fold—see Figure 23), which offer the cooling, quieting effect on the body-mind of all Supported Forward Bends.

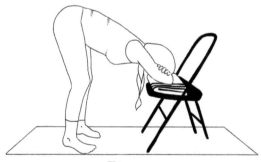

Figure 23

Two other Standing poses that can be helpful during your Dark Moon phase are the Classical Women's postures, Trikonasana (Triangle Pose—see Figure 24) and Ardha Chandrasana (Half-Moon Pose—see Figure 25). The hip and belly opening effects of these postures are beneficial in relieving abdominal congestion and cramping. They are best practised with support—have your back against the wall and one hand on a brick or chair (as pictured).

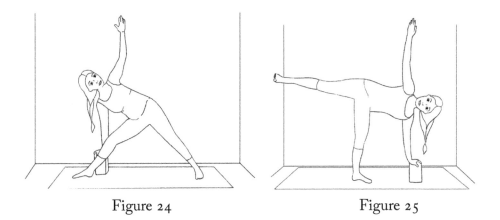

Figure 24   Figure 25

Dark Moon Pranayama

I have suggested that your monthly bleeding time is a metaphorical 'big exhale'—a time for letting go and surrendering to a gentler practice of self care and releasing of your obligations, even if for a short pocket of time. It therefore makes sense that your Pranayama (breath-work) focus will literally be on the exhale—the releasing and relinquishing of the breath into emptiness. When you emphasise a longer, deeper exhalation, you engage the relaxation response of the parasympathetic nervous system which counteracts the negative effects on your hormonal system of the 'fight or flight' or stress response of the sympathetic nervous system.

The Soft Belly Breath: letting it all go

Any regular-practising yoga practitioner will be aware of the calming benefits of breathing into the belly, sometimes called 'abdominal breathing', which is also the first stage in the full diaphragmatic or 'full yogic breath'. The Soft Belly Breath is essentially an abdominal breath with feminine intention: enhancing your awareness of, and connection with, your reproductive organs—your uterus and ovaries—or energetically speaking, your womb-space. It's a wonderful breathing practice for your menses as it facilitates receptiveness to the moment, which is such an integral aspect of the Dark Moon unravelling process.

After a few rounds of the Soft Belly Breath, you will automatically feel calmer and more connected with your body because this practice helps draw your energy out of the busy thoughts in your head and down into the more intuitive, feeling space of the belly.

This simple breathing technique also helps relax deep-held tension that can accumulate in the abdominal muscles. Stress can cause the abdominal muscles to become tense and hard which can contribute to menstrual cramps as well as reproductive imbalances.[178] Moreover, a vicious cycle can be perpetuated when a woman experiences strong, painful camps and the body's natural response is to tense up, which in turn, can cause more cramping!

As you breathe into your belly, focus on the feeling of the breath filling up the pelvic-belly that contains your womb and ovaries, enjoying the sensation of the breath softening this area and clearing congestion and heaviness in these organs and surrounding muscles. As you develop the practice, if you like, you can imagine the breath as white light, nourishing and healing your reproductive organs.

Drawing breath in and out of the body (and belly) is more than just a chemical exchange of gases, but also involves the movement of energy. In yoga, we call the breath *prana*—essential energy or 'life force'— and in Chinese medicine it is called *chi* or *qi*. It is understood in many complementary healing modalities that any blockages or congestion of the *prana* or *chi* in the body can cause imbalances, even illness. A simple breathing technique like the Soft Belly Breath can help first of all to bring your awareness to the subtle energy flow in your pelvic-belly (womb-space) and ultimately, with the intention and the energy behind the breath, move any stagnant energy in the pelvic area.

How to do it

Sit in a comfortable sitting position—kneeling, cross-legged, or in Diamond Posture (see Figure 26). You can also lie in Constructive Rest Position (see Figure 19, p.95), or a supported, Restorative position like Supta Baddha Konasana (see Figure 20, p.96)

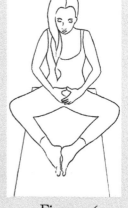

Once you're settled, begin by just allowing the breath to even and smooth out, and consciously relax any tension that you may perceive in your physical body.

Figure 26

---

178   The stress hormone epinephrine can cause the constriction of the blood vessels in the uterus which may, according to Dr Rahul Sachdev, specialist in Reproductive Endrocrinology and Infertility at the Robert Wood Johnson Medical School, impede a woman's fertility. Cited by Judith Hanson Lasater in her article in *Yoga Journal*, 'When you want to have a baby ... But Can't', at: http://www.yogajournal.com/article/lifestyle/when-you-want-to-have-a-baby-but-can-t/

Then, when you are ready, begin to direct the breath down into your belly—your womb-space. It can help to initially place one or both hands on your lower belly to get a sense of where you are sending the breath. With each inhalation feel the belly expand into the palms, and with each exhalation feel the belly soften back towards the spine, away from the palms. Progressively allow the belly to soften and open to the breath. Can you even begin to feel the breath touching right down into your pelvic floor as it too becomes elastic and receptive to the breath, doming down, ever so slightly, with each deep exhalation?

As you exhale, feel the breath empty completely out of the belly, releasing any tension and congestion. Take care not to harden or overly tighten the abdominal muscles as you fully exhale—just feel for a gentle drawing back of the navel towards the spine without accumulating any tension or force.

As you breathe this way, if you find that there is still a lot of tension and holding in the belly (or anywhere in the body), you can try combining the Soft Belly Breath with the Falling-Out Breath (see p.104), in which you employ a releasing, sounded-exhalation, through the mouth, to facilitate a deeper letting go.

The Apana Breath: detox your body-mind

Apana means 'air that moves away', and as we have explored, during menstruation, the body is governed by this quality of *apana*—the energy residing in the pelvis and lower abdomen that facilitates the movement of blood down and out of the body. In addition to correct choice of postures (i.e. choosing grounding postures and avoiding Inversions), we can also use the breath to facilitate this process of *apana*.

The Apana Breath is an energetic way that you can support your body's monthly detox as it releases *ama* (toxins), and it also has a balancing effect on your mind and emotions by helping ground you and connect with the earth.

The Apana Breath is a powerfully healing breath that supports the immune system, urinary and excretory systems, and strengthens your *ojas* or essential energy,[179] and, according to Sandra Anderson, helps keep the 'mind free of destructive forces'.[180] For women, it is a particularly beneficial practice because it can heal diseases of the reproductive system and help with menstrual problems.

---

179   David Frawley, *Yoga and Ayurveda*, p.254

180   Sandra Anderson, *Yoga International*, 'The Five Prana Vayus in Yoga: Apana', May, 2013, https://yogainternational.com/article/view/the-5-prana-vayus-in-yoga-apana

How to do it

The Apana Breath can be done in any Restorative posture that feels good for you, for example, Supta Badda Konasana (see Figure 20, p.96). This breathing practice also works well if you are in a position where the soles of your feet are in contact with the earth. So, it can be done in a standing position, like a basic Chi Kung Stance—feet shoulder-width apart (or wider), knees softly bent, tailbone heavy towards the earth (see Figure 27). Or for a very relaxing, grounding posture that supports the quieter energy of this time of the month, try doing it in the Constructive Rest Position (see Figure 19, p.95).

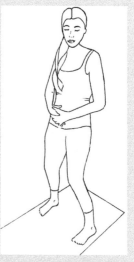

Figure 27

First, take a few gentle breaths as you settle into your chosen position. Then, take a deep breath down the entire length of your spine filling up into the back of the lungs, into the kidneys and adrenals (which sit on top of the kidneys in the mid-lower back, beneath the lowest ribs), into the belly, and down to the root of the spine at the perineum. Momentarily pause the breath there in the pelvic region. Then, as you exhale, imagine you are sending the breath out of your pelvis and down your legs into the earth.

As you work with this powerfully directed and grounding exhalation, visualise you are releasing any negative energy that is no longer serving you, into the earth. If you are feeling pain and congestion in your pelvis, lower back or uterus during your period, you can visualise that you are breathing this discomfort out and away with the long, releasing Apana Breaths.

Here's a visualisation, suggested by Ayurvedic practitioner David Frawley, which you may like to try as you work with the Apana Breath:

> View *apana* as a downward facing dark blue triangle in the region of the lower abdomen, from which the energy moves downward in lightning flashes, and grounds itself into the center of the earth below, where there dwells a special fire of strength and resistance.[181]

Another good pose to try the Apana Breath is the gentle Standing Pose, Prasarita Padottanasana (Standing Wide-Legged Forward Bend).

---

181   David Frawley, *Yoga and Ayurveda*, p.254

During your Dark Moon phase, practise this pose in its modified, supported version, with the forehead supported (see Figure 391, p.446), or with your hands on the floor or a prop and the spine at right-angles, your pelvis gently tipped forward (see Figure 28). These modifications allow for space and softness in the belly and offer an opportunity to circulate the flow of any stagnant energy in the pelvis.

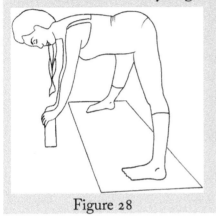

As you inhale, breathe into the pelvis, the sacrum and the pelvic floor. As you exhale, send the energy of the breath down the legs into the earth, pressing the soles of the feet into the mat, spreading the toes and lifting the insteps, so that there is a rebounding action of the descending energy of the breath down to the earth, which then feeds back into the vital organs of the pelvis.

Figure 28

The Falling-Out Breath: *Ahhh…*

The Falling-Out Breath is another breathing technique that harnesses the healing and relaxing power of the exhalation. Practised on its own, it's an effective Pranayama for releasing tension; combined with the Apana Breath, the cleansing and releasing effects are enhanced, which matches this phase of your cycle.

I first encountered this simple yet potent breathing practice when I trained in Phoenix Rising Yoga Therapy, the brainchild of Michael Lee, a yoga and stress management specialist.[182] Over the years, I have found this to be an invaluable tool to support the deepening of the letting-go process in Restorative postures—for both women and men.

How to do it

The practice is simple: take a deep breath in through the nose and then exhale deeply, sighing the breath out through an open mouth. Allow the lips, jaw and throat to be soft and feel free to make the sound of the breath audible as you release it out of the open mouth. Some people really enjoy making a deep, low 'ahhh' sound that emanates from the belly, from the sacrum, from the pelvic floor. It should feel like a deep, full-body sigh of relief that is totally delicious!

182   See more about Michael Lee's work here: http://pryt.com/

The Falling-Out Breath is particularly lovely used in Supported Forward Bending postures, like the Supported Child (see Figure 22, p.99). As you exhale through the mouth, you can accompany this with the visual imagery of the Apana Breath, so that you feel the exhale surrendered into the earth, letting go of anything that is no longer serving you in your month, and in your life.

The Feminine Alternate Nostril Breath

Nadi Shodhana or the Alternate Nostril Breath is a practice in which we alternate the flow of breath (ultimately—*prana)* between the left and right nostrils. Nadi Shodhana is used to cleanse the subtle channels or *nadis* of the body and will also help bring about balance between the right and left hemispheres of the brain. It is an especially beneficial way to calm nervous energy and relieve anxiety, and therefore an appropriate practice for your Dark Moon bleeding time when the *vata dosha*[183] can tend to dominate, which can make you feel delicate and easily overwhelmed.

When working with a feminine approach to yoga, I prefer to begin and end each round of Nadhi Shodhana with the left nostril. This is because the left nostril relates to the *ida nadi*, the lunar, feminine channel. The effect of activating this channel is calming and cooling. The right nostril relates to the *pingala nadi,* which is the solar, masculine channel, and when activated has a heating, stimulating effect on the body and mind.

Nadi Shodhana is a 'quick-fix' Pranayama. You only need to do a few rounds to feel instantly calm and grounded back into your body and into the present moment. It can be a practice that stands alone either at the beginning or end of your yoga practice, or it can work well to do a few rounds of Nadi Shodhana to prepare for meditation as it focuses the mind and draws your awareness to a subtler level.

How to do it

Sit in a comfortable position—cross-legged or kneeling—with the spine upright, chest open, shoulders relaxed and down.

Close the eyes and just settle into the seated position for a few breaths, breathing gently in and out of both nostrils and checking through the body that you are as relaxed and comfortable as possible.

When you're ready, prepare by bringing your right hand into Mrigi Mudra (Deer Mudra). Do this by tucking the middle and index finger into the palm at the mound of the thumb (see Figure 29) and bend your ring

---

183   See Appendix 1 for an explanation of the three Ayurvedic *doshas.*

finger slightly to sit on the little finger, so that the ring and little finger will kind of work as one.

Then, raise your hand, still in this Mudra, to the eyebrow-centre (see Figure 30) and prepare to begin a round by gently closing off the right nostril with your thumb and exhale through the open, left nostril. Then, inhale again through the left nostril, close off the left nostril with your ring finger (and little finger) and open the right nostril and exhale through the right nostril. Inhale again through the right nostril, then close off the right nostril, open the left nostril, and exhale through the left. This completes one round.

To go again, inhale through the open left nostril, exhale through the right nostril, inhale through the right nostril and exhale through the left nostril, completing another round.

Continue for another 5–10 rounds. As with all yoga Pranayama exercises, if you start to feel dizzy, breathless or uncomfortable in any way, cease the practice and breathe normally.

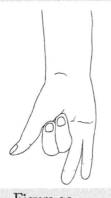

Figure 29

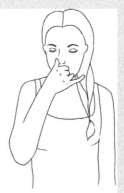

Figure 30

The Viloma Breath: creating space and energy

Viloma Pranayama is an interval breathing technique in which the breath is divided into three separate parts. It involves a very short hold of the breath that needs to be gentle and devoid of tension. Donna Farhi describes the subtlety of this momentary breath-hold: 'The pause should be a moment of suspension as when you say *'ah'*, rather than a feeling of contracting or holding the breath.'[184]

During menstruation, I like to do the Stage I version of this Pranayama that involves dividing the *inhalation* into three, and has the effect of deepening the *exhalation*.

---

184   Donna Farhi, *The Breathing Book*, p.157

As we have seen, any time that we focus on longer exhalations we ignite the rest, relaxation and repair response of our nervous system (parasympathetic), and we also harness the power of *apana*. This variation of Viloma Pranayama is also beneficial for when we are in a weakened state and need to gather energy, so it's ideal for the more vulnerable menstrual phase.

How to do it

The Viloma Pranayama is best done in a Supported Supine posture like the Reclining Goddess Posture (see Figure 398, p.450), or Supta Baddha Konasana on an inclined bolster (see Figure 388, p.444), because these positions open the chest and belly, and create freedom and space for the lungs and diaphragm.

Begin by allowing yourself to settle back into the support for the first few natural breaths. Relax your arms and shoulders so that the arms are hanging heavily from the shoulder sockets, and you feel loose at the elbows, wrists and finger joints. Soften the belly and swallow to relax the inner walls of the throat.

In this practice you divide the inhalation into thirds: begin by inhaling to a third of your lung capacity, then pause; then another third, then pause; then all the way, 100% capacity, and then pause there with your lungs full; then, exhale gently and fully. Take a normal, unbroken inhalation and exhalation in between before commencing your next 3-part inhalation.

Gradually you can add this additional visual image: imagine your torso is like a glass and as you inhale in thirds you are filling up your torso-glass with liquid from the base, all the way to the brim.

So, it goes like this: inhale a third of the way—visualise the breath filling from your pubic bone up to the line of your navel, and pause. Then, continue the inhalation from your navel to the mid-chest, up to the nipple-line, and pause. Finally, complete the inhalation all the way up to the top of the chest, to the line of the collarbones (over the very top lobes of the lungs), and pause momentarily, then exhale fully. Then take an unbroken inhalation and exhalation before commencing another round of the 3-part Viloma Inhalation.

Practise for as long as you feel comfortable. Initially this might only be for a few rounds of the 3-part inhalation, until you build up comfortably to 10–15 rounds.

Note, you can also try practising Viloma Stage II. Geeta Iyengar actually recommends this variation for menstruation. Simply, do the opposite of the above instructions. Instead of dividing the inhalation into three stages, practise a 3-part exhalation, with a long uninterrupted inhalation.

Dark Moon Meditations

The optimal time to meditate

Attuning to the metaphor of the moon, the menstrual phase can be likened to the quiet, reflective energy of the dark or new moon. It follows that your bleeding time is one of the best times in the month to meditate: when your energy draws inwards, you become more sensitive to subtle energies within and without. If you follow your body's cues when you bleed, you will respond by carving out some much-needed rest time to be in your 'red tent', which in turn provides an environment conducive to meditation.

Meditation helps you tap into your intuitive self, your inner teacher, and may therefore support the process of self-reflection that sits naturally at this point in your cycle—providing access to insights that may not ordinarily be available to you at other times in the month. Swami Muktanananda, author of *Nawa Yogini Tantra: Yoga for Women*, agrees that this is the time to give greater emphasis to meditation practices, and writes, 'Women are more sensitive and more psychically potent at this time, enhancing the possibility of a breakthrough in spiritual experience'.[185]

In the same way that menstruation affords an opportunity for the body to cleanse and renew, meditation, particularly at this point in your cycle, offers a cleansing of your mind. Meditation helps you empty all the thoughts and imperatives to 'do', to 'make things happen', and to be a certain way, either in a defined role for yourself or someone else.

Personally, I find that after the angst-ridden lead up to my period that characterises my Waning Moon, premenstrual phase, I really enjoy settling into an incredible feeling of peacefulness and 'okay-ness' once bleeding finally begins. I am instantly and gratefully transformed into a more *kapha* (connected with the earth element)[186] state of contentment and satisfaction with my lot in life. Meditation therefore is easy and aligns seamlessly with this natural, easeful space.

I will sit with this feeling of being enough

and let it be with me today

— ANNE WILSON SCHAEF[187]

---

185   Swami Muktananda, *Nawa Yogini Tantra: Yoga for Women*, p.148

186   See Appendix 1, explaining *kapha* and the two other Ayurvedic *doshas*.

187   Anne Wilson Schaef, *Meditations for Women who do too Much*, Alternate Meditation 5 (no page number)

Primordial Ooze Meditation

As I've pointed out, there is a strong downward pull of energy that connects women to the earth during their menses—the energy of *apana*. The Primordial Ooze Meditation is complementary to the Apana Breath Practice and can help transform any negative feelings or sensations that may arise during your Dark Moon phase. Meditation teachers and authors of *Meditation Secrets for Women* Camille Maurine and Lorin Roche write, 'When you relax into the downward ooze, the sensations often change to a balmy, sensuous connectedness.'[188]

This meditation involves cultivating the art of doing absolutely NOTHING! The aim is to simply feel—to tune into the subtle energies that are present for you at this time of the month.

How to do it

Sit with a cushion or folded blanket beneath your buttocks, and your legs folded into Siddhasana (see Figure 31). In this position, you can either have one foot placed in front of the other, in front of the groin, or tuck your right heel into the perineum and place the left foot in front or on top of the crease between the right thigh and calf.

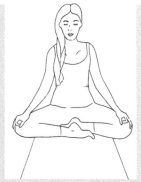

Figure 31

Allow your body to settle here, knees opening and down towards the floor, pelvis grounded. If your knees are a long way off the floor, it can help to support them by placing blocks, cushions or folded blankets underneath them to help give you a greater sense of connection with the ground and more support through the hips.

To begin this grounding meditation, tilt your spine slightly forwards from the hips and place your cupped hands onto the floor in front of you—fingers spread and connecting to the earth. In this gesture, the palms are concave, as you create a lift through the centre of the palms (see Figure 32). As you stay here for a minute or two, see if you can become aware of the energy of the earth channelling up through the centre of the palms of the

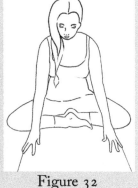

Figure 32

---

188   Camille Maurine and Lorin Roche, *Meditation Secrets for Women*, location 3418 (Kindle edition)

hands, up your arms and into your heart and down into your belly and womb-space. Holding this position a little longer, close your eyes and come into stillness, continuing to feel the energy from the earth coursing into the palms and up your arms, into your body. Concentrate very hard on this for just a little longer.

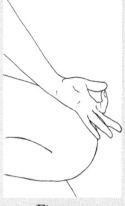

Figure 33

Then, release your hands away from the floor and rest the back of the hands on the knees, so that the palms are facing upwards, and you now have the fingers positioned into a relaxed, open Jnana Mudra (Wisdom Mudra), with the thumb and index fingers lightly touching (see Figure 33).

Now, just sit and let your awareness begin to draw further inwards. Notice the natural flow and rhythm of your breath, in and out of your nostrils. Soften the shoulders down away from the ears—feel them like ice melting into water. Soften the muscles around and behind the eyes. Soften the skin of the forehead and feel the skin of the temples slide back towards your ears. Relax the mouth and jaw, let the tip of your tongue rest lightly on the roof of your mouth. Swallow if necessary to *consciously relax the throat*. Move your awareness down your body to mindfully let go of any tension in the solar plexus and the belly.

After a little while, begin to deepen your breath and breathe down into your belly, your womb-space, and feel how this continues to release any tension or holding there. Just allow your soft belly to expand with the in-breath and soften gently back towards the spine with the out-breath. With this Soft Belly Breath, feel your awareness drop right down low into your body, into your womb-space, and out of your head.

Now, feel your connection to the earth again, this time through your base. Feel the pull of gravity down through your perineum, your sitting bones, heavy into the earth. Become aware of your Base Chakra. Imagine a beautiful deep, red lotus flower sitting at the base of your spine, at your perineum; admire the beauty and complexity of its dark, crimson petals. Underneath the lotus flower is the earth or rocks, whatever feels more solid and grounding for you. Visualise this flower as having deep roots or grounding cords that burrow deep down into the earth beneath you, right down into the bedrock. Feel how these roots, these grounding cords, support you in feeling grounded and solid, as you send some exhalations down into the earth beneath you.

Let go of directing your breath or awareness in any particular way at all. And let the breath be completely free. Just feel. Just feel into your whole body. Feel any sensations, pulsations of energy, anywhere, everywhere in your body. Feel your body shimmering with sensations, pulsating with energy.

Increasingly feel a sense of your body becoming liquid, smooth, oozing like honey, like chocolate melting in the sun. Feel the bliss of just allowing your body to *be*, yet at the same time, feeling so deeply into this state of being that you may begin to get a delicious sense of your body losing its boundaries; the boundaries of your body are merging with your surroundings.

There is no 'you', just this overriding sense of deliciousness, like you can taste the silence around you; it's like a sweet nectar. The air around you is thick and porous like your own body. Continue to feel into a sense of the honey-like, viscous fluidity of the body, as it flows beyond its boundaries. Be present to a complete feeling of bliss in every cell of your being.

Stay for as long as you wish, allowing any feelings or sensations to arise as you keep feeling into your body, your energy space, the spaciousness of your mind.

Then when you're ready, take a few deep inhalations to ground you in your body again and in this moment. Still with your eyes closed, rub your palms together vigorously to create heat and friction and then place the warm palms over the closed eyes. Take a few breaths here, breathing into the darkness of the palms over the eyes, feeling each breath energising you. Then, lower your hands and gently begin to open the eyes, but keep the focus of the eyes soft for a few extra moments just to allow the transition between your inner and outer worlds to be gradual and gentle.

Reflective Dark Moon Meditation

This meditation is inspired by the traditional Satyananda[189] meditation practice called Antar Mouna (Inner Silence). It's a simple mindfulness practice that involves inhabiting the *chidakasha* or 'mind space'—the mind consciousness that can be sensed as the area inside the forehead, or the space behind the closed eyes.

It is a wonderful practice for developing your 'witness consciousness' and the art of simply 'being', and there is no better time than your Dark

---

189   Satyananda Yoga is a system or style of yoga developed by Swami Satyananda Saraswati that incorporates practices 'derived from ancient and traditional sources', and is wholistic in its approach, including not just the postures but also meditation practices, pranayama and yoga philosophy. Read more here: http://www.biharyoga.net/yoga-vision/satyananda-yoga/

Moon or 'reflective' phase[190] in which to refine this practice. As discussed, a woman's bleeding time is her natural time of retreat, so this is the perfect time to do this inward-observing meditation that incorporates the yogic practice of *pratyahara* or 'withdrawal of the senses'.

Your heightened sensitivity during menstruation can make you more susceptible to becoming overwhelmed by perceived problems and issues within your life, says Satyananda yoga teacher and author Swami Muktananda.[191] She therefore suggests that if a woman takes the time for this kind of non-judgemental, witnessing meditation she can open up a space to create real solutions. 'Antar Mouna provides us with a psychological clear space, and allows us to get in touch with ourselves by acknowledging the parts of our being we often ignore,' explains Swami Muktananda. 'Just as our body is casting off substances it doesn't need anymore, so we too can throw off worn out ideas and self-images and make the most of this opportunity for self-renewal.'[192]

How to do it

Come into a comfortable sitting posture—cross-legged, Siddhasana (see Figure 31, p.109), or kneeling.

Close your eyes and allow yourself to settle into the position: centring your spine over your pelvis, sitting bones evenly grounding, heart-centre lifted, open and broad; shoulders relaxed and down, neck long, chin dropped slightly. Briefly scan your awareness through your body to check that you are as relaxed and quiet as possible in your body.

Now, bring your attention to your breath. Simply observe your natural breath, in and out of the nostrils, without trying to change or control your breath in any way.

Bring your attention to *chidakasha* (the 'mind-screen')—the space behind your closed eyes, just in inside your forehead. See if you can remain a witness of any images, thoughts, feelings that appear there in this black space behind the eyes. You are employing the same consciousness as if you were watching television—simply observing, with detachment, whatever appears on your psychic screen. You may see random pictures, you may notice a succession of thoughts or feelings, or there may be nothing.

---

190   Miranda Gray, *The Optimized Woman*, calls the menstrual phase, the 'reflective' phase.

191   Swami Muktananda, *Nawa Yogini Tantra—Yoga for Women*, p.40

192   Ibid., pp.40–41.

See if you can completely let go of all efforts, all impressions, all functions of the mind to do things, to make sense of things, but instead just remain aware of this space.

In time you may be aware that you are in the space, and yet the space is within you. You are the witness and the witnessed.

Stay here for up to 20 minutes.

You may find this practice challenging at first. Your mind may remain busy with mundane thoughts, the narrative of which may side-track you from witnessing-mind. Or, you may become sleepy and dull in the mind. That's fine. There is no need for judgement. The practice will develop and refine in time. The main thing is to let go of all effort and striving to be a particular way.

Dark Moon Relaxation Practices

The main theme for menstruation is all about rest and renewal of your energy during this delicate phase of your cycle. Deep relaxation practices can help rest your nervous system on a profound level by engaging the parasympathetic nervous system, precipitating your 'rest, digest and repair response'; this places you in a more receptive framework, balancing your stress response, and therefore brings your body-mind back into balance, allowing for deep healing and regeneration.

The following two deep relaxation practices can be done at any time, as self-contained practices to rejuvenate your energy, or to help you sleep. They can also be done at the end of your Asana (posture) practice to balance and centre you before you reintegrate into the rest of your day or evening.

Surrender to the Darkness Relaxation and Visualisation

This relaxation and visualisation practice is best done in a supine (Savasana) position and is good to do on the first or heaviest day of your bleeding, when your energy is at its lowest.

How to do it

Lie down in on your back on the floor or a bed. Have a bolster under your knees, if this feels more supportive for your lower back, and a small pillow or folded blanket under your head. You can cover your eyes with an eye-pillow, which will help relax the eyes, calm the mind, and tone the vagus nerve (connected with the parasympathetic, relaxation response). Use a blanket or shawl to cover yourself to make sure you'll be warm and comfortable for the duration of the practice.

Start by checking that you are lying in a straight line and rest your palms on your lower belly. Let your shoulders release back and down, feet falling out to the sides, as you loosen the hips, preparing for your deep, sacred rest. Remind yourself that this is *your* time; time to withdraw from the world to nourish your energy during your Dark Moon bleeding time. Soak up this intention of conscious rest into every cell of your body. Know that you've created this space just for yourself; you have nowhere to go, nothing to do, no one you need to be for anyone else. It's just your time to rest.

Feel your body becoming heavy and surrendered into the floor or bed beneath you, so that you have a sense of the earth embracing your weight, supporting you fully. It's as if the floor is pushing up into the weight of your body, allowing you to let go more fully.

Allow the breath to be quiet, natural, subtle, as you continue to enjoy the sensation of the entire body letting go.

Imagine now that your body is releasing back into a gigantic, deep, red, plush pillow. It's so soft, so supportive! Feel this softness all around you as you sink down more deeply.

Feel into your body now. Relax the facial features, the eyes sinking back in their sockets, like two pebbles sinking deep into a bottomless pond. Soften all the tiny muscles around the eyes, smooth out any furrows in the brow, and relax the upper and lower jaw. Swallow and consciously let go of any holding in the inner walls of the throat.

Move your awareness down through your body to relax the shoulders so that you feel the front shoulder-heads rolling back, and the chest broad and open. Relax the muscles at the bottom of the ribs, the floating ribs, and soften across the diaphragm; feel the back ribs spreading into the floor or bed beneath you. Feel the arms and legs heavy and loose.

Become aware of the entire back of your body and feel it very broad, very wide. Feel the body spreading into the floor, like chocolate melting in the hot sun.

Settle your awareness into the belly—relax there as you feel the gentle rise and fall of the natural breath in the belly, beneath your palms. Continue some deep Soft Belly Breaths here for a minute or two.

Now, become aware of the blackness behind the eyes: the infinite black space, the emptiness, the void, there behind the eyes. Feel into this blackness; go deeper and deeper into the blackness, so that it feels like you are being wrapped in blackness, in darkness. Feel the blackness go on extending so that your whole body is enveloped in darkness, soaking up the darkness. Feel the blackness so that it spreads in all directions—it's inside of you and all around you. There is no fear, no pain, no tension, just complete acceptance, complete surrender to the blackness, to the darkness.

Extend your awareness now to imagine that you can see the night sky above you—a mantle of utter blackness, studded with diamond constellations of stars. Gaze into this infinite blackness of space that has no end, no beginning.

Can you also imagine the outline of the new moon in this night sky before you? Feel the energy of the new moon; it's emerging from the darkness and there's a hesitant feeling of newness, new life, and growth.

Bring that image of the new moon into your womb-space now—the space beneath the palms. Breathe into your soft belly, your womb-space, as you visualise the new moon nestled in your womb.

Let go of the image of the new moon now, and imagine your womb is a room and you are inside it. Imagine this room as lush and darkly lit with soft, dark-red furnishings and curtains. It's warm and dark here. Picture yourself walking around this room, your womb-space, and you see a broom there. You begin sweeping with the broom. Sweeping up any debris in this beautiful, feminine room—sweeping away anything that you feel is unwanted, no longer needed. Keep sweeping until you feel that your womb-space-room is clean and new.

After a little while, come back into your whole body, and sense your whole body resting on the floor in this moment; resting your body as much as you can, supporting your hard-working body, your hard-working womb that is working to release your sacred Dark Moon blood.

Savour the last few moments of rest and rejuvenation, of this deep relaxation practice, just feeling, just resting within yourself.

When you're ready, roll on to your right side and rest there in a foetal position for a minute or two before coming up to a sitting position, rolling up through the spine as you do. Once you come to a comfortable sitting position, place your right hand on your womb-space, your left hand at the centre of your chest, at your heart-centre (Heart-Womb Mudra—see Figure 2, p.59).

Sit quietly for a few moments, or even minutes. Giving quiet thanks to your womb, the power-centre of your femininity. Giving thanks for the quietness and peacefulness of your sacred Dark Moon time: your special time to retreat and to rejuvenate your body and spirit.

Dark Moon Yoga Nidra

Yoga Nidra is a guided, deep relaxation practice that means 'yogic sleep'. The idea is that your body rests completely, but your mind remains quietly alert. It is a rejuvenating practice to support you when your energy is low, and it is said that one hour of Yoga Nidra is equivalent to 4 hours sleep![193]

Yoga Nidra is a powerfully healing practice that can help dispel anxiety, fatigue and depression. Yoga Nidra is more potent than many other relaxation practices because it helps us shift fully from the active, alert beta-brain-state to the more relaxing alpha-brain-state. In alpha, we are more open to positive suggestion (e.g. hypnosis) and this enhances the healing potential of Yoga Nidra.[194]

I have slightly adapted the traditional format of Yoga Nidra to suit the particular needs of women during their Dark Moon time.

How to do it

Lie down on to the floor—or on your bed—with a small cushion or folded blanket underneath the head and a bolster or pillow underneath the knees. Place an eye-bag on your eyes, and cover yourself with a blanket or shawl, if necessary, so you can be warm and comfortable for the duration of the practice. Make sure you have created a space for yourself where you will not be disturbed for the next 20 minutes or so.

Position the arms so that they are a little way out from the sides of the body and not touching the body. The palms are uppermost, fingers lightly curling. The feet are at least hip distance apart and allow them to fall out to the sides so that your hips are loose and relaxed.

Make any final adjustments to your posture so that you are as comfortable and supported as possible and that you will not need to move for the remainder of the relaxation practice.

---

193   This is a claim that I have come across frequently, touted by many proponents of Yoga Nidra, such as Swami Gurupremananda Saraswati in *Mother as First Guru*, p.43.

194   'During Yoga Nidra, the alpha waves covered the whole brain and were constant throughout the practice, while they occurred only partially and irregularly during the other relaxations. Furthermore, the level of alpha waves was constant throughout the entire Yoga Nidra, while it was irregular during the other relaxations,' writes Robert Nillson from the Scandinavian Yoga and Meditation School, referring to a research project at the Cologne University Clinic, Germany. See more at: https://www.yogameditation.com/reading-room/the-relaxed-state-and-science/

Now, feel your body settling in. Know that this is your time, just for you. Nowhere to go, nothing to do, nobody you have to be... Just *be*... Time to rest and honour yourself during this sacred time of your month, in your sacred 'red tent'. You can just let go here. You are completely safe and supported.

Take three slow, deep breaths: breathing in through the nose and breathing out through an open, relaxed mouth (Falling-Out Breaths). With each exhalation feel the weight of your body surrendering completely into the floor or bed beneath you. If you have been suffering menstrual pain, consciously use these Falling-Out exhalations to breathe out and away any tension that may have built up in the muscles in response to menstrual pain.

Then, allow your breath to become natural, there's no need to change the breath in any way, just let it be.

Now, bring your awareness to your *sankalpa*. This is your positive resolution for change, your deepest heartfelt desire. You may already have a *sankalpa* that you are working with, if so, bring this to mind now. Or, you can create a new *sankalpa*. It needs to be a short, positive affirmation in the present tense. If you like, you can cultivate one directly related to your 'moontime'. For example:

My bleeding time is easeful and joyful.
I honour myself during this sacred time and I am
completely connected to my body and my inner self.

Mentally repeat your *sankalpa* three times, with conviction. Planted deep into the fertile soil of your unconscious, your *sankalpa* is a potent agent for positive change in your life.

Now, let go of your *sankalpa* and become aware again of your breath—the natural rise and fall of your breath through the nostrils. Feel the breath subtle and easeful, without any force or strain. Simply allow the breath to find its own, natural rhythm. Feel the slight coolness of the breath on the inhalation as it draws in through the nostrils and the warmth of the breath, gently heated by the airways as you exhale.

We now begin the rotation of awareness around the body that is a key element of Yoga Nidra. As I name each part of the body, try to sense into that part of the body, picturing it, feeling it letting go. If you find that your mind wanders or becomes sleepy, bring yourself back to the practice, even if you must do this many times.

Begin by becoming aware of your left hand thumb, first finger, second finger, third finger, fourth finger. Palm of the hand, back of the hand, left wrist, forearm, elbow, upper arm, armpit, shoulder. Left waist, left hip, upper left leg, knee, lower leg, left ankle, top of the foot, sole of the foot, big toe, second toe, third toe, fourth toe, fifth toe.

Now, move your awareness to your right-hand thumb, first finger, second finger, third finger, fourth finger. Palm of the hand, back of the hand, right wrist, forearm, elbow, upper arm, armpit, shoulder. Right waist, right hip, upper right leg, knee, lower leg, right ankle, top of the foot, sole of the foot, big toe, second toe, third toe, fourth toe, fifth toe.

Now, moving up through the back of the body. Become aware of the left heel, right heel, back of the left knee, back of the right knee. Left buttock, right buttock. Sacrum, the bones of your sacrum. The lower back—left kidney and adrenal, right kidney and adrenal. The upper back—left shoulder blade, right shoulder blade. Back of the neck. Back of the head. Crown of the head.

Moving your attention now to the front of the body. Left side of the forehead, right side of the forehead. Left temple, right temple. Left eyebrow, right eyebrow, eyebrow-centre. Left eye, right eye. Left cheek, right cheek. The nose—left nostril, right nostril, bridge of the nose. The mouth—upper lip, lower lip. Inside of the mouth. Left side of the jaw, right side of the jaw. The tongue. The chin. The throat— swallow and relax the inner walls of the throat.

Become aware of the chest: left side of the chest, left breast, right side of the chest, right breast. Centre of the chest, heart-centre. Now become aware of your abdomen: upper-abdomen (solar plexus), mid-abdomen (navel-centre), lower abdomen (womb-space). Stay here for a few breaths, feeling each inhalation creating a sense of space and ease in your belly and womb-space; each exhalation releasing any tension or gripping in the belly.

Finally, become aware of your left hip, right hip, the pelvis—the bones of the pelvis. And now the vagina, the walls of the vagina. Feel the softness and openness of the walls of the vagina. And journey up through your vagina to the opening of the womb, the cervix. Sense your cervix—low and open as your womb releases its contents during this sacred time.

Now, bring your consciousness into your whole body. Your *whole body*, resting on the floor in this moment. *Whole body* awareness.

As you inhale, imagine warm, soothing water flowing up through your body from your feet up to your head. As you exhale, feel this beautiful, warm water cascading back down through your body all the way out through the soles of the feet. Continue this 'warm-water-breath' for a few rounds, allowing the soothing warmth to carry away any pain or muscle spasms that you may be experiencing during your Dark Moon time.

Now, I will take you through a series of mental images. Visualise each image as a picture in your mind's eye. Just watch these images in your mind-screen, as if you were watching them on a television screen.

The rising sun; ocean waves; a pink lotus; a fire burning bright; yellow clouds, smoky clouds; pink clouds; the setting sun; a smoky, blue sphere; the waves of the ocean—crashing to shore; a mountain range—silhouetted as the sun sets; a lush rainforest; a starlight night; a single candle flame; the infinite ocean, calm and quiet; a red lotus flower; the full moon shining bright on the ocean; a dark, starless sky; a scarlet-red lotus flower; a new, crescent moon.

Letting go of the visualisation practice now; become aware again of the breath at the belly, at the navel-centre. Simply watch as your navel rises, as you inhale, and sinks back down again, as you exhale. Stay here for several rounds of breath.

Now, letting go of navel-centre breathing, and bringing to mind again your *sankalpa*, your heartfelt prayer for positive transformation. Mentally repeat your *sankalpa* three times, with conviction, knowing, that in time, this will come to pass.

Bring your awareness now to your whole body, your whole body, resting on the floor (or bed) in this moment. Feel the sensations within and around your body. Feel the air against any uncovered skin, the clothing and coverings against your skin. Feel the floor (or bed) beneath you. Without yet opening your eyes, become aware of your surroundings, your position in the room (as if you were looking at yourself from above). Become aware of any sounds around you.

In a few moments you will be moving out of this Dark Moon Yoga Nidra practice, but before you do, just allow yourself to savour these last few moments of deep relaxation, deep rest, deep healing. Know that when you awaken from this practice you will feel refreshed and renewed, your nervous system nourished, and your mind calm.

Begin to bring movement into your body. Move the fingers and toes, wrists and ankles. Stretch and yawn, gradually awakening the energy in the body. When you feel ready, without any sense of hurry, roll to the right-hand side and rest there for a few breaths in a foetal position.

Always remembering to be gentle with yourself.

Then, use your top left hand to press into the ground and roll yourself up to sitting, head rolling up last. Finish this practice sitting quietly in a comfortable position for you—spine erect, shoulders relaxed back and down, and face and belly soft. Keeping your eyes closed, place your right hand on your lower belly (womb-space) and your left hand at the centre of the chest (heart-centre) in the Heart-Womb Mudra (see Figure 2, p.59).

Feel this gesture as a reminder of how much you cherish this time to yourself for self-care, self-nurturing. Honour yourself as you connect with the softness and feminine energy of your womb-space and heart-centre, for how well you are taking care of yourself during your Dark Moon time, and know how the benefits will flow on outwards to those around you. People will respond positively to you as the highest possible manifestation of your feminine self.

Namaste.

Dark Moon Yoga Sequences

POSTURES AND PRACTICES TO SUPPORT YOUR MENSTRUAL PHASE

CLASSICAL DARK MOON MENSTRUAL SEQUENCE

Best time to practise

This practice is great for any time during the menses, but it's particularly lovely early on, when your flow is heaviest and your energy is generally at its lowest.

Sequence duration

The whole sequence will take you around 60 minutes. If you are short on time, just practise one or two of your favourite postures from this sequence, or try the Express Dark Moon Practice (see p.156).

Sequence benefits

Use this lush practice to create your own yogic red tent. The Classical Dark Moon Sequence rejuvenates and refreshes your energy when you feel tired and heavy and supports optimal menstrual balance and health because it includes a number of therapeutic postures, including the Classical Women's postures (see Appendix 2), to boost circulation and energy flow in the pelvic area and help alleviate menstrual cramping and sore lower back. The overall effect of this sequence is grounding, relaxing and nurturing.

Props for this sequence

A yoga mat, 1-2 blankets or thick towels, 1-2 yoga bolsters and yoga blocks—if practising the Variation B: Double Block Child Pose (see Figure 55)—1 yoga strap (or long scarf if you don't have a strap), 1 chair (a simple kitchen chair will do), an eye-bag (if you like), and additional blankets or shawls to cover you if the weather is cool.

1. Constructive rest position (CRP)

Benefits

- Releases the psoas muscles, which may help with menstrual cramping.
- Relaxes and releases the lower back.
- Restful, rejuvenating and grounding.
- Helps bring breath into the belly; the variation—Constructive Rest Position with Arm Raises, helps bring breath into the chest.
- Good position to practise the Soft Belly Breath (see p.100) and the Apana Breath (see p.102).
- See page 95 for more information on the benefits of this posture.

Props for this posture

A yoga mat, a thin, folded blanket or thick towel to go under your pelvis and torso if the floor is hard, a folded blanket or towel to go under your head (if you like), and an eye-bag (if you like).

Recommended timing

Stay in the static position for anywhere between 2–10 minutes. Then, practise the Arm Raise Variation for up to 10 repetitions.

How to practise

Lie on your back, on your yoga mat, on the floor. If the floor is hard, you may need an extra single or double folded blanket to place under the pelvis and torso. Place a half or triple folded blanket under your head if you feel the need (if your head is thrown back and your shoulders feel tight), otherwise it's quite nice to practise this posture with no support under the head.

Bend up your legs and position your feet flat on the floor, hip distance apart and parallel. The feet need to be a comfortable distance from the buttocks so that pelvis sits in neutral (tipped neither forward nor backward) and you are maintaining the natural curve of the spine at the lower back. When you have the feet positioned correctly (neither too close nor too far away from the buttocks) it should feel completely effortless to hold the legs here; there is a feeling of the thigh bones and shin bones resting upon one another like two playing cards forming a triangle, allowing the muscles of the thighs, hips, buttocks and abdominals to be as relaxed as possible.

Once you feel comfortable and aligned, rest your hands slightly out from your body, palms facing upwards (see Figure 34) or, if you prefer, place your palms on your lower belly (see Figure 35) to deepen your womb-space connection and to support a sense of self-nurturing (particularly nice if you are feeling crampy there). If you choose to rest your hands on your belly, make sure the elbows remain heavy into the floor and you consciously release any holding in the shoulders. Close your eyes, covering them with an eye-bag if you wish.

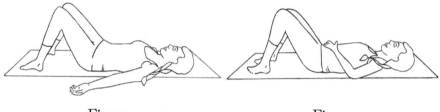

Figure 34   Figure 35

Initially, just allow yourself to completely relax and surrender back into the floor. Feel your head heavy, shoulders releasing back and down, and the back ribs softening and spreading into the floor. See if you can begin to allow the lower, back ribs to release down and connect with the floor. Feel the sacrum broad and light into the floor, and a melting in the front of the hips at the hip creases (where the thighs meet the torso). Finally, check that you are relaxed through the pelvic floor.

Stay for as long as you feel comfortable and supported, progressively allowing your body to let go of tiredness and heaviness. This is a good time to practise the Soft Belly Breath (see p.100), breathing softness and spaciousness down into your womb-space, and you can also practise the Apana Breath here (see p.102).

Variation: Constructive Rest Position with Arm Raises

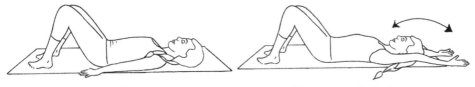

| Figure 36 Exhaling | Figure 37 Inhaling |

When you are ready, remove any support from under your head, and your eye-pillow, to prepare for the Arm-Raise variation.

Start with your hands by the hips, palms down, shoulders drawing down away from the ears—exhale here (see Figure 36). As you inhale, raise the arms all the way up and over to bring the backs of the hands on the floor overhead, if you can—go gently if you have any shoulder tightness or injuries (see Figure 37). Exhaling, lower the hands back down to your side where you started (see Figure 36).

Continue for up to 10 repetitions synchronizing breath and movement. As you inhale, feel the breath opening up into the front and sides of the upper rib cage as the belly gently stretches and the spine begins to lengthen—all combining to bring a sense of energy and spaciousness. As you exhale, feel the lower rib cage gently glide towards the hips, and get a sense of releasing all the air out of the lungs. Keep the pelvis still and stable and in neutral throughout.

2. Apanasana (knees to chest pose)

Benefits

- Promotes the energy of *apana* that is predominant during menstruation.
- Supports the healthy functioning of the digestive, urinary and sexual organs.
- Massages the lower back, helping with menstrual low back pain and sacral tenderness.
- Variation C (knees circling separately) lubricates and opens the hip joints, and stretches the groin area.

Props for this posture

See props for Posture 1 above.

Recommended timing

Variation A (knees in and out)—do up to 10 repetitions.
Variation B (knees circle together)—do up to 10 circles in each direction.
Variation C (knees circle separately)—do up to 10 circles in each direction.

How to practise

Variation A (knees in and out)

From Constructive Rest Position (Figure 34) bend up your knees to draw your thighs in towards your chest, keeping your knees together. Take a knee-cap in each hand, fingers pointing forward. Start with your elbows extended, knees moving away from you (so that your thighs are perpendicular to the floor), but still holding onto your knees (see Figure 38). As you exhale, draw your knees towards your chest, bending the elbows (see Figure 39). Inhale, and return your knees to the starting position (Figure 38).

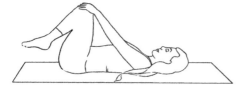

Figure 38 Inhaling   Figure 39 Exhaling

As you exhale, gently squeeze the air out of your abdomen as your knees move in. As you inhale, fill up the belly with breath again. It is a very slow, meditative movement.

Do up to 10 repetitions in your own breath-time, feeling how this simple posture massages the lower back and the abdominal organs.

Variation B (knee circles together)

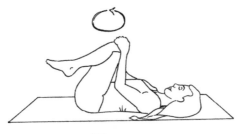

Figure 40

Still holding onto your knees, circle your knees together like you are tracing a circle on the ceiling with your knee caps, gently massaging the sacrum and lower back into the floor (see Figure 40).

Variation C (knee circles separately)

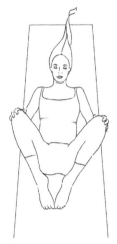

These are sometimes called 'femur circles' because the movement involves rotating the head of the femur (thigh bone) in the ball and socket joint of the hip. Begin by circling the knees away from each other (see Figure 41). Then, reverse the direction of the circles. Do up to 10 slow circles in each direction.

Figure 41

3. Single knee to chest hip flexor stretch

Benefits

- Releases the hip flexors and the psoas, which can create more space in the belly and pelvic area, and can help with cramping and lower back pain that can be caused by tight hip flexors.

Props

A yoga mat and maybe a folded blanket under your head if it's more comfortable for your neck.

Recommended Timing

Hold for 3–5 breaths on each side

How to practise

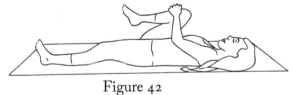

Figure 42

From the previous posture, Apanasana, keep your right leg bent up, hands interlaced on the outside of the shin, just below the knee, and extend your left leg along the floor. Keep the shoulders relaxed on the floor as you gently draw the right knee in towards the right side of the chest, while at the same time extend actively away through your left leg—the foot dorsi-flexed (toes drawing back towards you, heel away), and feel the back of the extended leg working towards the floor (see Figure 42).

As you hold it here, breathe open the hips and groin area, visualise where the psoas runs through the body (extending from the mid back spine, through the core of your body, wrapping over the front of the hips and pelvis and into each inner thigh) and how you are balancing the positioning of your pelvis in relation to your spine when you stretch these deep muscles, plus, you are helping create more openness and space for your uterus and ovaries to function optimally.

Stay her for 3–5 long breaths before changing sides.

4. Supta padangusthasana I & II (reclining big toe pose)

Benefits

- Supta Padangusthasana I stretches the hamstrings and back of the hip and can relieve lower back pain, including sciatica.
- Supta Padangusthasana II opens the hips and groin region, and brings circulation to the pelvic organs, creating space in the pelvic-belly. It's a Classical Women's posture (see Appendix 2)—and can relieve menstrual discomfort.

Props for this posture

A yoga mat, a folded blanket under your head to support your neck alignment if necessary, and a yoga strap or long (strong) scarf.

Recommended timing

Hold Padangusthasana I for 5–10 breaths, and hold the supported version of Padangusthasana II for 1–3 minutes, on each side.

How to practise

Supta Padangusthasana I

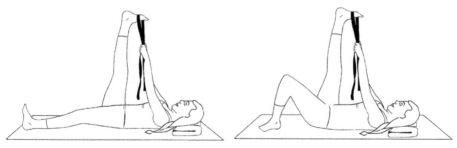

Figure 43   Figure 44

Start from the Single Knee to Chest Hip Flexor Stretch (Figure 42), with the right leg bent up. Catch a strap around the ball of the right foot and then straighten your leg towards the ceiling. Hold each end of the strap in each hand, a comfortable distance from your foot so you are not straining and lifting your shoulders off the mat, and the neck remains long with the chin dropping down towards the throat (see Figure 43).

Keep the opposite left leg that is on the floor active, heel pushing away, toes drawing back, and also work on keeping the outer right hip drawing down so you have space in the right hip socket.

For an easier variation, you can bend up that left leg and place the sole of the foot on the floor (see Figure 44), which is also a more supportive version for the stability of your pelvis—good if you have sacroiliac pain or instability—and also appropriate for beginners, or those with tight hamstrings.

Hold either variation, and breathe deeply, focusing on lengthening the exhalations as you consciously release the muscles at the back of the leg. Stay in the stretch for 5–10 breaths. Then, release and repeat on the other leg.

Supta Padangusthasana II

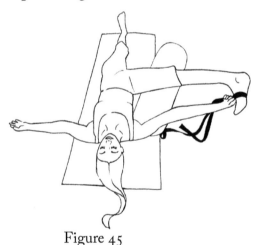

Figure 45

From Supta Padangusthasana I, with the right leg extended, take both ends of the strap in the right hand as you slowly lower the leg out to the right side. Make sure you have placed a bolster next to your outer right hip so that you can rest the thigh on it for this supported version (see Figure 45). By supporting the leg in this way, you're able to stay comfortably for a longer timing because the inner thigh muscles can relax and soften rather than harden and shake in an attempt to keep the leg there. This, in turn, helps relax and soften the lower belly.

As you hold and rest in the pose (stay for 1–3 minutes), breathe into the right hip and groin and right side of the pubic belly as you feel how much space and softness you are encouraging here. Also, become aware of, and breathe into, the right ovary, imagining each breath as the *prana* (life force) that brings healing and balancing energy to your ovary. Release by bending the leg back to the centre. Repeat on the other leg.

After completing both sides, rest onto the floor with the feet falling out to the sides, hands on to the belly in the Corpse Pose. Take a few Soft Belly Breaths here (see p.100), noticing perhaps your increased awareness and sensitivity in your womb-space.

Safety Note

If you suffer pain and instability in the sacroiliac joint (SIJ), do a variation (see Figure 46), bending up your left leg to counterbalance and centre through the pelvis.

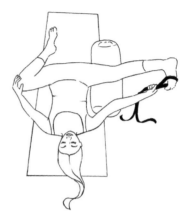

Figure 46

5. Cat-cow pose

Benefits

- Mobilises the spine, opens the chest (heart-centre) and upper back, and gently stretches and creates space in the belly.
- The All-fours Hip Circle Variation releases aching hips and lower back, and brings energy into the lower energy centres (the base and sacral chakras).

Props for this posture

A yoga mat and a thin folded blanket to place under your knees if the floor is hard.

Recommended timing

Do 5-10 repetitions of the Cat-Cow Pose and about 6 All-fours Hip Circles in each direction.

How to practise

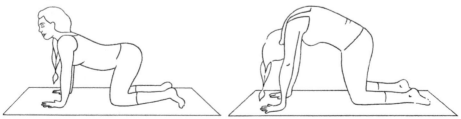

Figure 47 Inhaling   Figure 48 Exhaling

From Supta Padangusthasana II (Figure 45), roll to the side and come up slowly to sitting and then on to all-fours. In the table-top, all-fours position make sure your hands are shoulder distance apart and your knees hip-distance, and start with the spine in neutral—one long line from crown of head to the tail. Spread the fingers wide to evenly distribute the weight across the hands to support the wrist joints.

To begin, inhale and draw the chest through the hands, forward and up, rolling the shoulders back, stretching the throat, and gently arching into the lower back as you roll the sitting-bones up to the ceiling (see Figure 47). Then, as you exhale, start from the tail bone, as you tip the top of the pelvis back, rounding the lower back and then the upper back, pressing the hands into the floor to spread and lift between the shoulder blades, head dropping and chin towards chest (see Figure 48).

Repeat 4–9 times in your natural breath rhythm, as you feel the spine loosening up; enjoying the gentle stretch and spaciousness in the belly as you inhale, and the release of lower back tightness and compression as you exhale.

Variation: All-fours Hip Circles

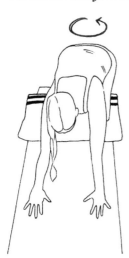

From the all-fours position begin to circle the hips by moving the hips back towards heels, over to the left, forward on the left, across towards to the right and back on the right (see Figure 49). In other words— imagine you have a pencil in the tip of the tailbone and you are trying to trace a big circle with it, behind you. Repeat up to 6 times in each direction.

Figure 49

6. Forward virasana (forward facing 'heroine' pose)

Benefits

- Stretches the spine and back of the body, which can release lower and upper back tightness and pain.
- Opens the hips and groins and gently stretches the perineum.
- Calms the nervous system—because the forehead rests to the floor.

Props for this posture

A yoga mat and a folded or rolled up blanket to place between your buttocks and your heels if necessary (i.e. if your buttocks don't comfortably rest back onto the heels).

Recommended timing

8–10 breaths.

How to practise

From the all-fours position, bring the tops of your feet on the mat, and your big toes to touch whilst your knees stay wide. Then, move your buttocks back to sit onto your heels with your palms resting on the floor, still shoulder distance apart, and your arms extended forward. Rest your forehead into the mat, chin tucked, back of the neck long. In the final position your knees will be about mat-distance apart, big toes touching, heels apart (see Figure 50).

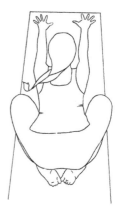

Figure 50

Safety note

If the buttocks don't easily connect down to the heels, place a rolled up or folded blanket between the buttocks and heels. This will also help if you are feeling any discomfort in your knees in the position. Or, for knee pain, you can try placing a thin-fold blanket right up into the knee-fold (between the back of the thigh and the calf) to create more space for the knee joint.

Stay for a up to 10 breaths, breathing into the sacrum, directing the *prana* to sooth any pain or tightness, and create a feeling of ease and spaciousness there. Also feel the pelvic floor soft and open in this stretch.

You can try some Apana Breaths (see p.102) here, drawing the inhalations down the back of the lungs into the adrenals and kidneys and into the sacral centre, then, as you exhale, send the breath flowing down the buttocks into the earth.

Note, that this posture—Forward Virasana—can also be used as a resting posture in between Cat-Cow pose and the All-fours Hip Circles—if you like.

Coming out

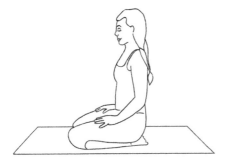

Walk your hands slowly back towards you till you come up to kneeling. Bring your knees to together and sit quietly in Vajrasana (Seated Kneeling thunder bolt Pose—see Figure 51) for a few breaths.

Figure 51

7. Supta baddha konasana (reclining bound angle pose)

Benefits

- Relieves menstrual cramps and spasms and heaviness in the uterus.
- Creates space in and takes pressure off the pelvic area.
- Opens the chest, quiets the mind, calms the nerves.
- See Appendix 2 for additional benefits.

Props for this posture

A bolster and 2 blankets (1 folded blanket to support your head and 1 blanket rolled up (long-ways) to wrap around the legs to support the knees.

Recommended timing

Stay here as long as you are comfortable; this could be anywhere between 3–10 minutes.

How to practise

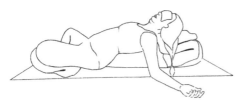

Figure 52

Setting up
Sit in front of the short end of a bolster in Baddha Konasana (legs bent with soles of the feet together and a comfortable distance from the groins). Make sure your bottom is not right up against the bolster; usually at least an inch or two away allows for you to have a comfortable neutral positioning in the spine when you lie back. Wrap a long blanket

roll around the tops of the shins and ankles and tuck it under the knees (see close-up diagram in Figure 21, p.97). Then, lie back along the bolster and rest your head on a folded blanket (see Figure 52).

Once in the position, or even as you lie back, you may need to adjust the positioning of the pelvis by lifting the buttocks a tiny bit off the floor and slightly lengthening the tail-bone under toward the pubic bone, so you feel entirely comfortable through the lower back. Rest your arms to the side, palms facing upwards, fingers lightly curling. Or, if you prefer, place your palms on your belly to connect in to your womb-space.

Being there

Feel the gentle stretch and opening through the pectoral muscles in the chest as your arms hang heavily, shoulder-heads rolling back, shoulder blades melting down the back.

In the lower body, be aware of completely letting go into the support of the blanket beneath your knees, which allows you to soften the muscles of the inner thighs, pelvic floor and the belly.

You can practise the Soft Belly Breath here (see p.100) and/or the Apana Breath (see p.102), or, simply feel the natural breath flowing in and out of your torso, allowing the body to progressively relax in this supported, opening position.

Coming out

To come out of Supta Baddha Konasana, press your hands into the floor next to your hips and use the strength of the arms to support yourself directly up to sitting—avoiding twisting or leaning to either side. Or if you prefer, roll to the side and come up from the side. Either way, there should be minimal, if any, exertion of the abdominal muscles.

Safety note

If you know you get pain in the sacroiliac joint (SIJ) make sure you have a generous distance between your buttocks and the bolster—at least a hand-span away will provide more support for your sacrum and lower back when you lie back. You may also need to provide extra support for the pelvis by placing bricks under the knees (see Figure 20, p.96) in addition to the rolled blanket; play around with finding the right props for you.

8. Supported child pose (forward virasana with a bolster)

Benefits

- Gently massages the abdomen with the pressure of the bolster, particularly as you breathe in.
- Activates the parasympathetic nervous system (the relaxation response), so is deeply calming, nurturing and rejuvenating.
- Stretches out the lower back and releases tension along the spine and into the upper back, neck and shoulders.
- Can help with menstrual cramping—try placing a heat pack or hot water bottle on the sacrum whilst in the pose to soothe strong menstrual cramps.

Props for this posture

Variation A (Simple Variation— Figure 53/Figure 54)

A bolster. You may also need an extra lengthwise folded blanket to put on top of the bolster if it is too low or flat. And you may need another rolled or folded up blanket, or a cushion, to place between the buttocks and heels if you find that you can't easily rest the buttocks on the heels.

Variation B (Double Block Variation—Figure 55)

A bolster and 2 yoga blocks. You may also need an extra rolled or folded up blanket, or a cushion, to place between the buttocks and heels if you find that you can't easily rest the buttocks on the heels.

Recommended timing

Stay for as long as you are comfortable—anywhere between 3–10 minutes.

How to practise

Setting up

Place a bolster lengthwise along your mat, the short end facing you. If you are practising Variation B (Double Block Variation—Figure 55), place the bolster on two blocks, on their flattest edge, one at each end of the bolster.

Sit on your heels in Vajrasana (kneeling Thunderbolt Pose—Figure 51), then move your knees apart, about mat-width distance, whilst keeping your big toes together (heels open and apart). Draw the bolster right up between your legs, into your groins (or shuffle yourself forward into this position for Variation B). As you inhale, walk your hands forward along the mat on either side of the bolster, lengthening your spine and feeling an opening and extension through the sides and the front of the torso. Once you've walked your hands as far forward as you can without lifting the buttocks off the heels, and your spine is fully extended out of the hips, rest your chest and the front of the torso onto the bolster as you exhale. But before you settle in, take another inhalation as you raise the chest slightly off the bolster to get even a little more length if you can through the torso, so that you feel the sternum lengthen away from the navel, and the navel lengthen away from the top of the pubic bone. Then, as you exhale again, rest back down and turn your head to the side, resting onto one cheek.

For the position of the arms, in the Variation A (Simple Classical Variation), your forearms rest on the floor, further forward than your shoulders (see Figure 53), and in Variation B (Double Brick Variation), thread your arms under the bolster so that they are just in front of the top brick, and fold the forearms so you are hugging the bolster (see Figure 55).

If you prefer for your neck, you can interlace your hands and rest your forehead on your hands (see Figure 54), an adaptation which is suitable for both Variations A and B.

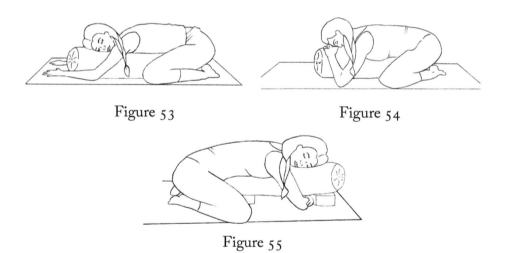

Figure 53   Figure 54

Figure 55

Being there

Now, just let go!

This has to be one of the most nurturing Restorative Yoga postures. It's so comforting—like snuggling into a giant teddy bear!

Initially, the main focus is on relaxing and continuing to let go with each out-breath, feeling the forearms melting into the floor as you consciously release any holding through the arms and shoulders. Then, you can begin to shift the focus to the sensations of the breath in this posture. Notice how the breath is restricted in the front of the body due to the bolster, but how you now have more space and awareness to breathe into the back of the body. Send the breath into the back of the lungs, the back of the heart-space, and even down into the sacrum.

From here, you can practise the Falling-Out Breath (see p.104)—with each releasing breath out through the mouth you can feel your body dropping deeper into the support of the bolster—arms, shoulders, hips releasing. Or you can just continue to breathe naturally and quietly through the nose, and let go; allowing this posture to work its magic on your body and soul.

Important notes

Midway through your timing in the posture, make sure you turn your head to the opposite side to evenly stretch your neck.

Practise whichever variation feels most comfortable to you—Variation A (Simple Classical Version—Figure 53), or Variation B (Double Block Variation—Figure 55). These two variations offer slightly different emphases: Variation B provides a little more traction for the lower back and gentle pressure into the belly, whereas, the Simple Classical Version A, opens the hips a little more. You might want to try a different version each time you practise, to mix things up a little.

Coming out

When you are ready to come out of the posture, slowly walk your hands back towards your knees and come up to sitting. Move the bolster to the side, and sit quietly, with your eyes closed, for a few breaths in Vajrasana (Kneeling Thunderbolt Pose—see Figure 51).

9. Supported bridge pose with 1-2 bolsters

Benefits

- Relieves anxiety, irritability and fatigue.
- Good for depression and tension headaches.
- Relieves upper back and shoulder tightness and facilitates deeper breathing in the chest and frontal and side lungs.
- Creates space in the pelvic belly—relieves tension in the abdomen and heaviness in the uterus.
- The Variation B (T-Shaped Variation) in particular can help alleviate menstrual cramping.
- Regulates your cycle.

Props for this posture

Variation A (Single Bolster Variation—Figure 56)

A bolster and you may also need an extra lengthwise folded blanket if the bolster does not feel high enough, and a thin-fold blanket to cushion your head and shoulders if the floor is hard.

Variation B (T-Bolster Variation—Figure 57)

2 bolsters of the same size and thickness. You may also need a thin-fold blanket to cushion your head and shoulders if the floor is hard.

Recommended timing

Stay in either variation for as long as you are comfortable—anywhere between 4–10 minutes.

How to practise

Setting up: Variation A (Single Bolster Variation

Sit roughly in the middle of the bolster (this will depend on the size of your bolster and your body), legs bent and feet hip-distance apart and flat into the floor. Lie back, positioning yourself so that your head and shoulders are on the floor and the rest of the torso and buttocks

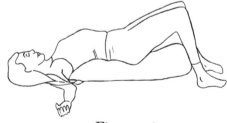

Figure 56

stay on the bolster. You may need to adjust slightly (moving forward or back) so that in the final position just the head and tips of the shoulders rest into the floor with the bolster lifting up into the 'bra-strap' area of your upper back to open the chest, while the lower back and pelvis stay in neutral. Just like in the active Bridge Pose, the back of the neck elongates as the chin tucks into the throat—activating the thyroid and parathyroid glands (see Figure 56).

You can position the arms out to the side, a comfortable distance. Or for a deeper opening into the thoracic, bend them up overhead. Either way, check that you are loose and relaxed through the elbow, wrist and finger joints, palms upper-most.

Setting up: Variation B: (T-Bolster Variation)

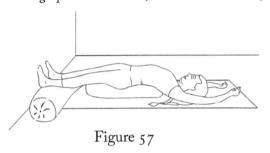

Figure 57

Place a bolster at the wall so that the long edge is parrallel with the wall and place another bolster perpindcular to the wall about 20 centimetres away from the first bolster. The distance between the two bolsters may need to be altered once you try the pose as it depends on both the length of your bolster and your body proportions.

To come into the pose, sit roughly on the middle of the second bolster (the one in the middle of your mat) and lie back to rest your head and shoulders on the floor, keeping your torso on the bolster —in the same way as Variation A.

In the final pose, the head and shoulders should rest down on the floor, and the end of the bolster should lift up and open the area of the upper back around the 'bra-strap' region, and, the soles of your feet should be fully into the wall (and hip width apart) with the legs full extended (see Figure 57).

If your feet don't end up flush agains the wall, you will need to move yourself closer to the wall.

If your head and shoulders are not off the bolster, you may need to roll to the side and come out of the pose and play with moving the perpinducular bolster closer or further to the other one.

There is a bit of fiddling to get it right, but I promise you, once you do, you will be in bliss! The gentle opening through the chest and shoulders feels so lovely for tight, aching neck and shoulders; the gentle stretch through the pelvic belly feels so soothing for your Dark Moon time, and,

The Dark Moon: being with the flow

the pressure of the soles of the feet into the wall is wonderfully grounding and nourishing.

You can position the arms out to the side, a comfortable distance. Or, for a deeper opening into the thoracic, bend them up overhead. Either way, you are loose and relaxed through the elbow, wrist and finger joints, palms upper most.

Being there: Variations A and B

Once you are set up and comfortable in the posture, just enjoy the lovely opening through the heart-centre and sense of gentle stretching and space in your pelvic-belly. You can let the breath flow naturally, or, this is also an ideal position for enhancing the quality of the inhalation. Focus on full deep, in-breaths, drawing the breath right up into the collar-bone chest, at the very top lobes of the lungs, and as you exhale, feel the belly, buttocks, pelvic floor, and walls of the vagina soften.

You could also work with the Soft Belly Breath (see p.100)—focusing on feeling the release of any tension or gripping in the belly area in this lovely, open posture. The Apana Breath (see p.102) is also nice to practise in this posture. As you breathe out your grounding exhalations, visualise the breath (*prana*) moving down the legs into the wall and into the earth in the Variation B (T-Bolster Variation), and in the Variation A (Single Bolster Variation), feel the breath directly grounding through the soles of the feet that rest on the floor.

Coming out: Variations A and B

To come out of the posture or adust your positioning, do not try to sit directly up, as this may strain your back or overuse your belly muscles. Instead, make sure you roll off the bolster to the side. Once you've come out of the pose, rest for a few breaths on your back. If you like, as a counter-pose for your lower back, you can bend your knees up into Apanasana (see Figure 39, p.125).

10. Supported upavista konasana (wide angle seated pose) with a bolster and chair

Benefits

- Eases menstrual cramps.
- Facilities menstrual flow and can also relieve heavy bleeding and heaviness in belly.
- Calming and nurturing.
- See Appendix 2 for additional benefits.

Props for this posture

A yoga mat, a chair, bolster, and possibly a folded blanket to sit on if you find you can't sit up easily without.

Recommended timing

3–5 minutes

How to practise

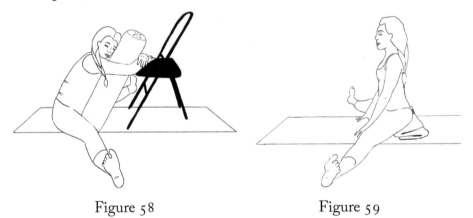

Figure 58   Figure 59

Setting up

Position the seat of the chair facing you on the end of your mat and lean a bolster up against the chair as pictured (see Figure 58). The bolster is tilted forward at an angle that you can adjust depending on how deep you can comfortably go into the Forward Bend—for example, for a deeper Forward Bend, tilt the top of the bolster further away from you as well as moving the chair further away.

Sit in front of the bolster and open the legs wide into Upavista Konasana (Wide Angle Seated Pose). If you find it difficult to sit up tall because your pelvis is rolling back (usually due to tight hips and hamstrings), perch your sitting bones on the edge of a small cushion or a triple-folded blanket (see Figure 59).

To prepare, inhale and raise your arms overhead feeling your waist lifting long out of the hips, and at the same time feel your sitting bones grounding into the floor (or folded blanket) beneath you. As you exhale, tilt forward from the top of your pelvis so that your spine remains long and wrap your arms around the bolster as you lay your torso along its length, resting one cheek onto the bolster (see Figure 58), and…melt! In the final position, the spine needs to still be elongated. Avoid rounding the upper or lower back, or hunching the shoulders.

Being there

Begin the timing here with a few rounds of the Falling-Out Breath (see p.104) to allow yourself to deepen—focusing particularly on releasing tension through the tops of the shoulders—and enjoy the interior journey of this nurturing Forward Bend.

Don't forget to turn your head halfway through your timing in the posture, to evenly stretch the neck in both directions.

Some alternatives

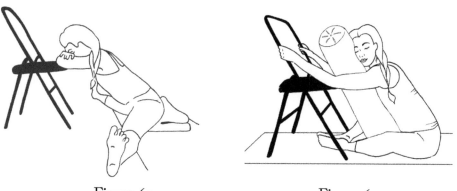

Figure 60   Figure 61

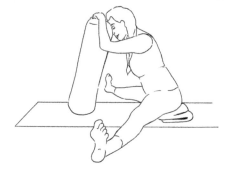

Figure 62

If you are not deliciously comfortable here then you will need to adjust your support so that there is absolutely no strain in the position. If you still can't find a way to be comfortable by adjusting the tilt of the bolster and the position of the chair, then try one of the following modifications or alternatives : -

- Bend the legs (to take the hamstrings out of the equation).
- Remove the bolster and just rest onto the chair (see Figure 60).
- Change to supported Baddha Konasana with a bolster and chair (see Figure 61).
- Remove the chair and tilt the top of the bolster towards you to support the forehead (see Figure 62).

Safety notes:

- If the chair feels like it's not stable and it may slide away (although that's why it's on the sticky yoga mat), position the chair against a wall to ensure the stability of your propping.
- If you have a history of pain and instability in the sacroilliac joint (SIJ), just go very gently, minimising the Forward Bending, listening to your body. If your SIJ is currently flared up, avoid going forward at all, simply sit in upright Upavista Konasana (see Figure 59) for a few breaths, or avoid this posture for today.

Coming out: counter-pose

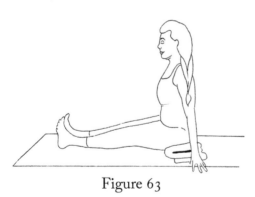

Figure 63

To come out of the pose, sit upright again and move your bolster (and/ or chair) to the side. Sit quietly for a few breaths with the eyes closed, before bringing the legs together in front of you into Dandasana (Staff Pose—see Figure 63). Sit quietly for a few breaths in Staff Pose, allowing time to counter-pose the hips by actively drawing the legs towards each other, and even get a feeling of the legs internally rotating with the thighs rolling in and down.

11. Chair savasana (final relaxation pose)

Benefits

- Rejuvenates and relieves fatigue.
- Alleviates tired, achy legs and eases lower back pain.

Props for this posture

A chair, a folded blanket, and an eye-bag to cover your eyes if you like. You may want to support your head with an extra folded blanket or small cushion.

Recommended timing

5–15 minutes. Or as long as you need!

How to practise

Place a folded blanket on the seat of the chair (half or triple folded) and then lie down and raise your calves onto the chair, making sure the backs of the knees come right up into the edge of the chair. Place an eye-bag on your eyes, and rest your hands to the side or onto your belly (see Figure 64).

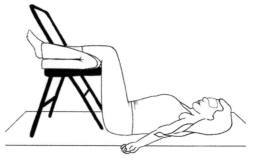

Figure 64

Begin to settle here with a few Soft Belly Breaths (see p.100). Over the timing, feel your body letting go, as you go even deeper than you have in any of the previous Restorative postures so far. Let the weight of your legs be heavy into the chair, and the torso, head and arms heavy into the floor. Feel your eyes soft and descending in their sockets, the throat and jaw relaxed. Breathe evenly and naturally through the nostrils now, as you allow yourself the time and space to rest and integrate at the end of your Dark Moon practice.

Note: You can use this Chair Savasana to practise either the Surrender to the Darkness Relaxation (see p.113) or the Dark Moon Yoga Nidra (see p.116).

Coming Out

When you are ready to come out of the relaxation, start by gently moving the fingers and toes, wrists and ankles. Then, draw your knees into the chest (pushing the chair or yourself away to create enough space), and rest for a few breaths in Apasana (knees to chest —Figure 39, p.125). From here, you can either roll to the side and come to sitting to finish your practice, or if you feel like it, you can practise the gentle Supine Twist Counter Pose below before you come to sitting.

Counter Pose: Gentle 'Windscreen Wiper' Supine Twist

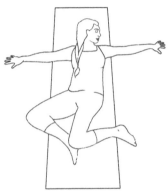

Figure 65

This is a gentle, menstrual-friendly Twist that focuses on releasing the muscles in the upper back and hips rather than twisting into the belly and lower back.

Still lying down, place your feet about mat width apart, knees bent. Bring your arms out to the side in a T-shape. As you exhale, let your kees fall over towards the right, so that your right knee opens out, in external rotation, and your left knee moves onto or towards the floor, in internal rotation (see Figure 65). Lengthen your left knee and hip-bone away from you to deepen the stretch through the front of the left thigh and into the groin and hip flexor area. At the same time, reach through the fingertips of both hands to open the upper back and draw the opposite left shoulder blade into the floor. You can also turn your head in the opposite direction towards the left hand.

You can try an alternate arm variation of stretching the left arm overhead which makes the movement more sensuous—like you are waking up in the morning—as you extend the spine and languidly stretch through the left armpit and the left side of the torso. Then, to come out, inhale and and bring your legs back to the centre and repeat the gentle twist to the other side.

To finish

Sit quietly for a few breaths, in whatever position is comfortable for you, with your hands on your lower belly (womb-space—see Figure 66).

Take these last few moments of your practice to check in with yourself and notice how you feel now after your Dark Moon Menstrual practice compared to how you may have felt before this nurturing practice. Then, place your hands together into prayer position at the heart centre (see

Figure 67), bowing your head, feeling gratitude for the beauty of yoga to nourish your body and soul during this sacred time in your month.

Namaste.

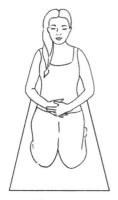

Figure 66

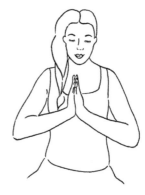

Figure 67

DARK MOON LATE MENSTRUAL SEQUENCE

Best time to practise

This sequence works as a good transition practice to do as you near the end of your menses—for example, around days 4 or 5—before you move into your Waxing Moon phase.

Sequence benefits

The Dark Moon Late Menstrual sequence is designed to begin to get your body moving a little bit more as you near the end of your period and you start to open your awareness outwards again. It can therefore help shift any stagnant energy that may have accumulated, yet is still gentle enough to keep you calm and soothed and follows all the guidelines of a safe, appropriate Dark Moon practice.

Sequence duration

This is a shorter sequence than the Classical Dark Moon Sequence—it takes around 30 minutes, and is more practical for later in your menses when you may be taking on more outside commitments again as your energy returns and your bleeding declines.

Props for this sequence

A yoga mat, 1–2 yoga bolsters, a yoga block, 1 blanket or cushion for your head for Savasana and an eye-bag—if you like.

1. Feminine Nadi Shodhana (alternate nostril breathing)

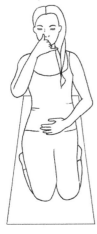

Benefits

This breathing practice cleanses the subtle channels of the body and has a combined calming and uplifting effect on the body-mind. Beginning your yoga practice with Nadi Shodhana is an excellent way to focus the mind, helping you to prepare to go inwards for your Asana (posture) practice.

Props for this practice

Something to sit on—a bolster or a cushion or folded blanket.

Figure 68

Recommended timing

Do between 5–10 rounds of Nadi Shodhana, always taking care not to strain in any way. If at any time you feel dizzy or uncomfortable, cease the practice at once, and return to normal breathing.

How to practise

See page 105 for instructions.

2. Dark moon flowing vinyasa

Benefits

A gently dynamic sequence of postures (Vinyasa) to promote the flow of breath and movement to warm up and energise the body.

Props for this Vinyasa sequence

A yoga mat and something to place between the buttocks and heels (block/ folded blanket/ bolster) if you have trouble sitting in Vajrasana (Figure 69) on your heels.

Recommending timing

Do the Basic Kneeling Vinyasa 2–5 times, then add the variations. Do each variation once.

How to practise

Basic Kneeling Vinyasa

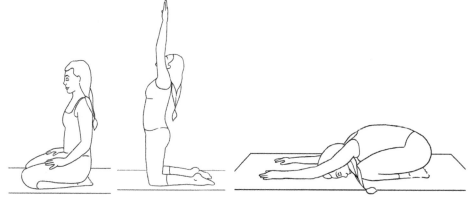

Figure 69
Inhaling
and exhaling

Figure 70
Inhaling

Figure 71
Exhaling

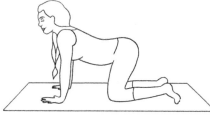

Figure 72 Inhaling

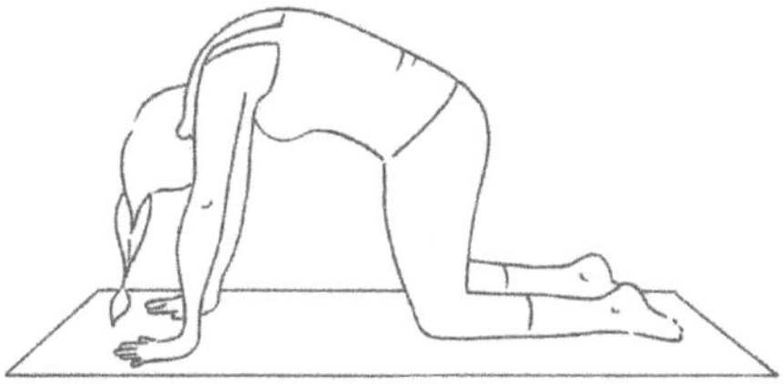

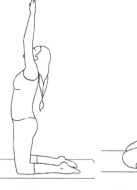

Figure 73 Exhaling

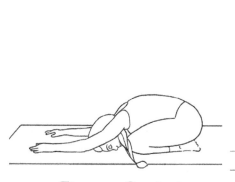

Figure 74 Continuing
to exhale

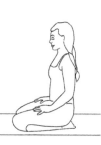

Figure 75
Inhaling

Figure 76
Exhaling

Start in Vajrasana (seated kneeling) with the hands resting on the thighs (see Figure 69). Take a few deep breaths to prepare. Then, as you inhale, raise your arms forward and up overhead as you lift your buttocks up off your heels and come up into High Kneeling Position (see Figure 70), with your gaze up towards your hands, if your neck is OK with this (otherwise look forward).

Then, as you exhale, bend forward from the hips to rest the hands and the forehead onto the mat into Extended Child Pose (see Figure 71). Inhale, and come up onto all-fours, hands shoulder distance and knees hip distance apart, and arch the spine into the Cow Variation of Cat-Cow (see Figure 72). Exhale, and round the spine into Cat Stretch (see Figure 73) as you move the hips to the heels back into Extended Child Pose (see Figure 74).

Inhale, raise the arms forward and up, coming back into High Kneeling Position (see Figure 75). Then exhale, back to the starting position—kneeling, buttocks on the heels in Vajrasana (see Figure 76). Repeat this whole sequence another 1–4 times.

Variations: Postures to build onto the Basic Kneeling Vinyasa

Thread the Needle

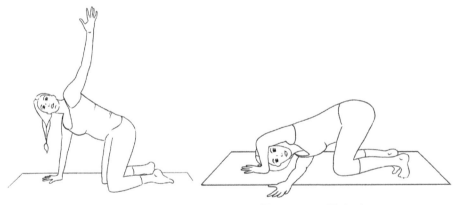

Figure 77 Inhaling   Figure 78 Exhaling

Do Thread the Needle (see Figure 77 & Figure 78) after the Extended Child Pose (Figure 71)—instead of the Cow Pose—from an all-fours/table-top position—then complete the Basic Kneeling Vinyasa back to Vajrasana (Figure 76).

Breathing Pattern: Inhale—stretch the arm up to the ceiling, opening the chest (see Figure 77). Exhale—thread the arm through and rest onto the cheek (see Figure 78). Repeat the Thread the Needle sequence 2–4 times on each side.

Kneeling Lunges

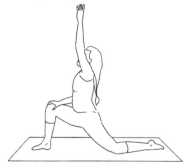 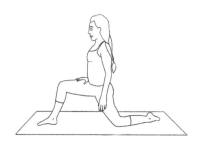

| Figure 79 Inhaling | Figure 80 Exhaling |

Do these Kneeling Lunges after the Extended Child Pose (Figure 71)—instead of the Cow Pose—from the all-fours/table-top position. Then, return to table-top/all-fours and finish the Basic Kneeling Vinyasa back to Vajrasana (Figure 76).

Breathing Pattern: Inhale—lunge the right knee forward and raise the left arm (same arm as back leg) feeling the stretch along the left groin up into the left side of the belly and chest (see Figure 79). Exhale—come back to neutral lunge (see Figure 80). Repeat several more times.

Down Dog to Virabhadrasana I (Warrior I) with 'Goal-Post Arms'.

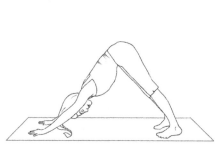 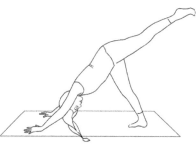

Figure 81 Inhaling and exhaling   Figure 82 Inhaling

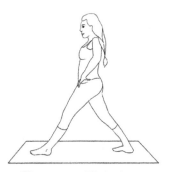 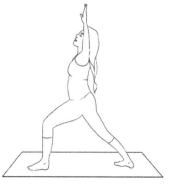

Figure 83 Exhaling   Figure 84 Inhaling

Do this variation-sequence after the Extended Child Pose (Figure 74), and then after completing it, return to the Extended Child Pose (Figure 74) and finish the Basic Kneeling Vinyasa.

Breathing Pattern: Inhale and exhale—into Down Dog (Figure 81). Inhale—raise one leg (Figure 82) and step forward and come up into preparation for Warrior I (both legs straight to start—Figure 83), exhale here. Inhale—lunge into Warrior I, arms in 'goal-post' shape (arms bent up with elbows in line with shoulders, forearms parallel, palms facing forward —Figure 84). Exhale—straighten your front leg back into the preparatory position (Figure 83). Inhale—lunge back to Warrior I (Figure 84) breathing right up into the brim of the lungs as you move the forearms back to create space in your chest and upper back.

Repeat this dynamic movement in and out of the Warrior Pose another 2–3 times. Then, exhale, bending forward to place both hands on either side of the front foot, and then step it back into Down Dog (Figure 81). Inhale here, then exhale return to Extended Child (Figure 74). Repeat this whole variation Vinyasa on the other side, starting by inhaling and exhaling back into Down Dog (Figure 81).

3. Gomukhasana (cow face pose) supported forward bend and open twist

Benefits

Now that you've built up a little heat in the body, it will feel good to stretch out the hips and spine with these two variations of Gomukhasana— especially since you've probably been fairly inactive over the first few days of your menstrual period.

Supported Forward Bending variation of Gomukhasana (Figure 85 & Figure 86)

- Stretches the deep hip and buttock muscles, which provides a good counter-balance to a lot of the Classical Women's postures that we practise during the menses that open the inner thighs and groin.
- Has a quieting effect on the brain and nervous system.

The Open Twisting Variation (Figure 88)

- A gentle twist appropriate for menstruation that releases tension in the muscles along the spine, particularly in the upper back.

Props for these postures

- A block or bolster to sit on (unless your hips are quite flexible, in which case you can just sit on the floor)
- A block and/or bolster to rest your head on for the Supported Forward Bending variation, or even a chair if you need more height.

Recommended timing

Forward Bending Variation

1–3 minutes on each side.

Open Twisting Variation

3–5 breaths on each side

How to practise

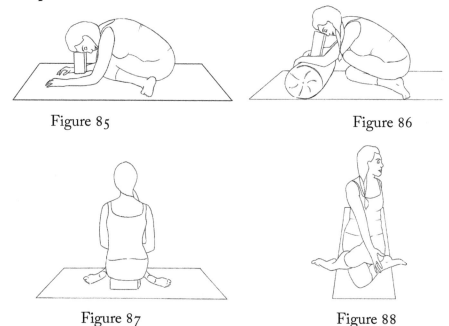

Figure 85

Figure 86

Figure 87

Figure 88

Sit on the long end of a block or the short end of a bolster with your legs bent up in front of you (see Figure 87). Thread your left leg underneath your right leg and bring the left foot around to the outside of the right hip, or as close to it as you can get. Then, with the right leg on top, slide that foot around to sit next to the left hip, or as far as you can get it. In the final pose, your right knee will stack on top of your left knee and your feet will be like the Cow's ears to the side of each hip (see legs in Figure 88).

Then, bend forward from the hips, and lengthen the chest and sides of the torso forward to rest your head on a tall brick in front of you (see Figure 85). If necessary, make the support higher by sitting a block on a bolster (see Figure 86), or even resting the forehead onto the seat of a chair. The forearms can rest towards or onto the floor with the elbows and shoulders soft.

If you are quite flexible in the hips and you're looking for a deeper stretch for the hips you can bring the hands behind you, close to your hips.

Rest here and enjoy how this posture releases tightness in the hips and lower back and brings your focus inward.

When you are ready, come up slowly and take a deep inhalation to prepare for the twist. As you exhale, turn the torso around to the left so that your right wrist or forearm crosses over the top left outer knee (see Figure 88). Hold here for several breaths, feeling for more space through the spine with each inhalation, and just allowing the head to gently follow the direction of the Twist.

When you are ready to come out, turn to face the front and unravel the legs and switch the legs to repeat on the other side—first the Forward Bend, then the Twist.

If you find that this posture is too challenging for you due to tight hips, try the alternative postures below.

Alternative Postures: Supported Cross-Legged Forward Bend and Cross-Legged Twist

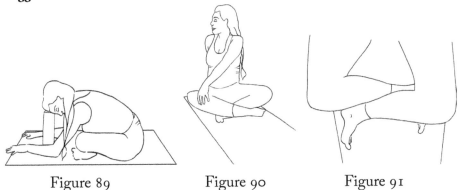

Figure 89   Figure 90   Figure 91

These variations are appropriate if you find it too challenging to get into the pretzel position of Gomukhasana.

How to practise the Variations:

Sit in an open cross-legged position, possibly perching your sitting bones on a folded blanket if you need extra support in helping you sit up tall. Have the legs crossed at the shins, so that when you look down there is a large triangle between the legs (see Figure 91). Inhale and raise the arms overhead as you extend the torso out of the hips, then, as you exhale fold forward, tipping the pelvis forward to rest your head onto a support: block/ block and bolster/ bolster/ chair—whichever supports you without strain or rounding into the spine (see Figure 89). Stay here for as long as you are comfortable—up to 5 minutes. Then, when you are ready, inhale and come up.

To come into the Twist, inhale and again raise your arms overhead, lengthening out of the waist, then, as you exhale place your left hand on your right knee, left hand behind you (see Figure 90). Inhale again to find more length through the spine, and then exhale and either deepen or just maintain the twist.

Go gently in the twisting action—focusing more on the action of creating length and space through the spine and torso rather than twisting strongly from the belly.

After a few breaths, release out of the Twist and change legs to do the Forward Bend on the other side.

4. Supported bridge pose with a block

Benefits

- Relieves anxiety, irritability and fatigue.
- Good for depression and tension headaches.
- Releases tightness in the lower back and stabilises the SIJ (sacroiliac joint).
- This variation with a block tones the kidneys and adrenals.

Props for this posture

A yoga mat and a yoga block.

Recommended timing

Stay here as long as you are comfortable —anywhere between 3–10 minutes

How to practise

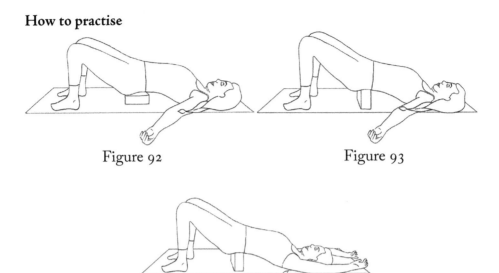

Figure 92   Figure 93

Figure 94

Lie on the floor with a block next to you and your legs bent up, feet into the floor, hip distance apart, and feet parallel. Lift your hips up to slide the block underneath the sacrum (the sacrum is the large, flat, triangular, bony plate at the base of the spine). Begin with the block on its lowest edge (see Figure 92)—you may stay like this for the whole time. Or, if it feels comfortable, turn the block on its side edge after a few breaths (Figure 93). That said, if you have a larger-sized yoga block, the side edge, rather than the lowest, flat edge, may be too high if it tips the uterus, taking the pelvis out of a neutral position (and therefore turning the pose into an Inversion). If this is the case, just stay on the lowest edge of the block for this posture when performing it during your period.

In the final position, have the hands to the side (Figure 93), or bent up overhead, palms facing upwards (Figure 94).

Allow yourself to feel supported by the block so that you are totally relaxed in the buttocks, lower back, legs and pelvic floor muscles. Take some breaths down into your belly. This will help ground your awareness back into the pelvis after the preceding more dynamic postures.

To come out of the pose, lift the hips again and slide the block out and come to rest with the buttocks back on the floor. You can do a counter-pose for the lower back by drawing the knees up into Apanasana (see Figure 39, p.125) and/ or doing the Gentle Windscreen Wiper Supine Twist counter pose (see Figure 65, p.144).

5. Savasana (final relaxation) with bolster and wrapped blanket

Benefits

- Savasana helps relax and balance your nervous system before you re-enter your day. This variation with the legs wrapped in a blanket feels particularly comforting, and having the legs raised on a bolster is very restful for tired, aching legs.
- Can also help relieve pain in the lower back.

Props for this posture

A bolster, a yoga blanket or thick towel. Possibly another folded blanket, towel or small cushion to rest your head on, and an eye-bag to cover your eyes (if you like).

Recommended timing

Stay here as long as you feel you need to in order to feel rejuvenated. This could be anywhere between 5–15 minutes.

How to practise

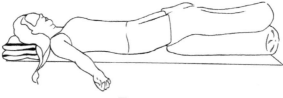

Figure 95

Setting up

Place a bolster lengthwise along your yoga mat and prepare a folded blanket or cushion to put under the head (if you like); have an extra blanket folded in a wide open fold next to your bolster. Come to lie on your back and rest your calves on the bolster and wrap the blanket around your shins and tuck it underneath the bolster to keep it securely in place (see Figure 95). Make sure the end of the bolster comes right behind the knees. Then, lie back and rest your head on the floor (or the support) and cover your eyes. Let the arms rest next to your body—allowing a bit of space between the arms and the body to facilitate a sense of spaciousness for the heart-centre and release for the shoulders, as the shoulder heads roll back and down.

Being there and coming out

Begin to settle here with a few Soft Belly Breaths (see p.100). Over the timing, feel your body letting go. Let the weight of your legs be heavy into the bolster, and the torso, head and arms heavy into the floor. Feel your eyes soft and descending in their sockets, the throat and jaw relaxed. Breathe evenly and naturally through the nostrils, as you allow yourself the time and space to rest and integrate at the end of your Dark Moon practice.

Note: You can use this Savasana to practise either the Surrender to the Darkness Relaxation (see p.113) or the Dark Moon Yoga Nidra (see p.116).

To finish

Roll gently to the side, taking your feet off the bolster. Come up slowly into a comfortable seated position—kneeling or cross-legged. Place your hands on your lower belly connecting down to your womb-space (Womb-space Mudra— Figure 66, p.145) and feel the energy there behind the palms, and notice how you feel as you drop your awareness right down into your belly and your womb-space—feeling the softness and spaciousness of your belly.

Then, place your left palm at the centre of your chest—your heart-centre—whilst keeping your right palm on the belly and feel the connection between these two energy centres (Heart-Womb Mudra—Figure 2, see p.59) and how you have fostered the movement and circulation of energy between the womb and the heart-spaces with this practice.

Lastly, bring your palms together in a gesture of honouring and gratitude (Anjali Mudra—Figure 67, see p.145). Honouring yourself for working so sensitively and compassionately as you near the end of your sacred moon-time for this cycle.

Namaste.

EXPRESS DARK MOON SEQUENCE

Best time to practise

This is a great practice for when you're short on time but need a menstrual-pick-me-up. The Express Dark Moon Practice can be practised at any time during your Dark Moon menstrual phase, although it's particularly nice earlier when your flow is at its heaviest and your energy is usually at its lowest.

Sequence benefits

This practice is designed to help relax you and bring you into your body in the shortest time possible! The postures will help ease menstrual discomfort and rejuvenate your energy.

Sequence duration

Depending on how long you choose to stay in the postures, this sequence will only take around 15 minutes. I've deliberately chosen the simplest versions of the classical menstrual Restorative postures to help save on time fiddling around with your props.

Notes

If even 15 minutes is too long to fit into your busy day, you can do even more of a 'quickie' by reducing the practice to just the first two postures (Postures 1 and 2) and this will take you only about 10 minutes.

Alternatively, for the swiftest menstrual-fix of all, you can just practise the Constructive Rest Position for 5 minutes. See Posture 1 in the Classical Dark Moon Menstrual sequence (see p.122).

Props for this sequence

A yoga mat, a bolster, 2 blankets, and a yoga block.

1. Supta baddha konasana (reclining bound angle pose)

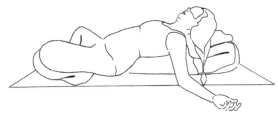

Figure 96

See Supta Baddha Konasana—Posture 7—in the Classical Dark Moon Menstrual Sequence, page 132, for the benefits, props, and instructions on how to practise.

Recommended timing

4-5 minutes

2. Supported child pose (forward virasana) with a bolster

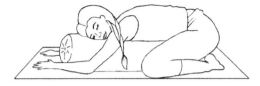

Figure 97

See Posture 8—Supported Child Pose Variation A (Classical Simple Variation)— in the Classical Dark Moon Menstrual Sequence, page 134, for the benefits, props, and instructions on how to practise.

Recommended timing

4-5 minutes

3. Supported bridge pose (setu bandha sarvangasana) with a single bolster

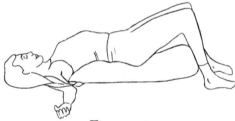

Figure 98

See Posture 9—Supported Bridge Pose Variation A (Single Bolster Variation)—in the Classical Dark Moon Menstrual Sequence, page 137, for the benefits, props, and instructions on how to practise.

Recommended timing

4–5 minutes

To finish the sequence

After coming out of the Supported Bridge Pose come to sit in a comfortable position. Bring both palms onto your lower belly—womb-space (Womb-Space Mudra—Figure 55, p.145) and take some deep breaths into your belly.

Then, keep one hand on your womb-space and place the other onto the centre of your chest, your heart-space (Heart-Womb Mudra—Figure 2. p.59).

Take a few moments to feel the connection between your womb and heart spaces and embody how nurturing this gesture is for your body and soul.

Finish by bringing both palms together at your heart-centre into the prayer gesture (Anjali Mudra—Figure 67, p.145), giving thanks for the transformative powers of yoga—that, even in a short, simple practice like this, you can feel the positive shift in how you feel physically, mentally and emotionally.

Namaste.

CHAPTER FIVE
THE WAXING MOON: RE-EMERGING

The waxing moon begins to gather strength and brings with it the energy of potency, regeneration, and rejuvenation.

—MAYA TIWARI[195]

The Waxing Moon phase is the spring of your cycle. It's when a woman emerges from the hibernation of the Dark Moon menstrual phase and moves more actively towards ovulation.

During this phase, your ovaries are busy growing a number of potential follicles (that house the eggs) and the uterine lining begins to build and thicken. Your immune system is also strengthening as circular collections of immune system cells, called 'lymphoid aggregates', begin to develop within the wall of the uterus.[196] Correspondingly, your physical-emotional-mental energy tends to shift to an upward spiral during your Waxing or 'dynamic' phase.[197] Maya Tiwari suggests that, during this phase, a woman may experience an 'abundant surge of creative and sensual energies, vibrantly growing in tandem with the moon as she becomes brighter and brighter.'[198]

From an Ayurvedic perspective, a woman's *ojas* naturally increases during this Waxing Moon phase.[199] *Ojas* is vital energy that nourishes your tissues

---

195   Maya Tiwari, *Women's Power to Heal through Inner Medicine*, p.65

196   According to the Christiane Northrup, M.D., article, 'The Wisdom of the Menstrual Cycle' (at http://www.drnorthrup.com/wisdom-of-menstrual-cycle/#sthash.dZiZanzw.dpuf), 'Recent research has found that the immune system of the reproductive tract is cyclic as well, reaching its peak at ovulation, and then beginning to wane'.

197   As mentioned, this is a term coined by Miranda Gray in her book, *The Optimized Woman*

198   Maya Tiwari, *Women's Power to Heal Through Inner Medicine*, p.70

199   Ibid. p.238

and organs, and is represented by a healthy glow, overall vitality, sexual virility and fertility.

According to Miranda Gray, you can be sure you have moved from your reflective (internal, Dark Moon phase) to your dynamic (outward, Waxing Moon phase) phase when you 'wake up feeling more confident and mentally sharp, and more motivated and enthusiastic'.[200] After the heaviness of menstruation, this post-menstruation to pre-ovulation phase feels light, as your energy begins to increase again.

The Waxing Moon phase is all about action and 'doing' which is in strong contrast to your Dark Moon phase which was all about letting go, 'un-doing', and just 'being'. If you gifted yourself rest and retreat time during your Dark Moon menstrual phase, you will find you have extra energy to burn during your Waxing Moon phase.

OUR MASCULINE PHASE

Taoist master and a specialist in Chi Kung for women's health, Mantak Chia, says that the energy of your ovaries is at its most *yang,* or hottest, during this phase of the cycle.[201] Since *yang*-energy is associated with solar, masculine energy, this ties in with the idea that this is a woman's most masculine cyclical phase. You are now very outcome-focused and this can make you feel that, during your post-menstruation-ovulation, Waxing Moon phase—more than any other phase—that you are in tune with the 'man's world'. 'The dynamic phase gives us the opportunity to experience a more masculine energy and perception which, in the modern achievement and success-oriented business world, can be a huge advantage,' writes Miranda Gray.

However, Gray also cautions that you should remember that this is just *one* phase of your cycle and not to try to override your other phases. This is because you risk losing out 'not only on some amazing abilities and opportunities for growth, but more importantly on the feelings of completeness, fulfilment and well-being generated by living in tune with each of our phases'.[202]

---

200 Gray, *The Optimized Woman*, p.81

201 Mantak Chia, *Healing Love through the Tao: Cultivating Female Sexual Energy,* Kindle edition: location 760

202 Gray, *The Optimized Woman*, p.82

PACE YOURSELF

With the renewed vigour that accompanies your Waxing Moon phase, it can be tempting to power through your to-do list with little consideration for slowing down. However, it's important to remind yourself to keep the balance, even during this more dynamic phase of your cycle. You need to ensure you stay grounded and nourished; it is easy to get carried away and do too much, especially if you have not taken the vital time to rest and rebuild your energy in the previous Dark Moon phase.

I have personally experienced the pitfalls of getting over-excited about my newly regained energy, and have suffered crash-and-burn when I end up overdoing it during my Waxing Moon phase. This ultimately means I have had to take a step back to administer self-care. It is so much more preferable (and productive!) if I can anticipate this and proactively take care of myself, as I go, before I inadvertently exhaust myself.

Like all the other menstrual phases, it's vital to listen to your body and follow your *true* energy needs. This may change from day to day in your Waxing Moon phase, and it's important to pace yourself. In this way, you can gear-up or gear-down your expectations of productivity depending on how you're feeling on any given day, or throughout the day, and therefore maintain the balance for your nervous system, which will ultimately bolster your overall health and vitality.

YOGA FOR YOUR WAXING MOON PHASE

Principles and guidelines for a Waxing Moon yoga practice

The Waxing Moon phase is the time in your cycle about which I have the least to say. This is because it epitomises the masculine way of 'doing' that is already inherently built into our societal—and therefore the dominant yogic—paradigm: i.e., yoga by men for men. In this most masculine of your menstrual phases, the recommendation is to generally just do the yoga that is normally practised.

Therefore, this is the time to work on a more dynamic practice, particularly in the latter part of this phase, when your body and mind are usually at their most robust. You can enjoy building your strength and stamina with Standing poses, dynamic Vinyasa (flowing, linked sequences), arm balances, and the stronger, more Active Inversions.

163

This is also the best time in your menstrual month to attend the standard, more dynamic, one-size-fits-all yoga classes; the group energy can be invigorating.

Contraindications and cautions for a Waxing Moon yoga practice

There are just two precautionary guidelines to help support you in a safe and appropriate Waxing Moon practice.

1. Make a graduated return: early Waxing Moon practice

It's important that you ease yourself gradually and mindfully back into a stronger practice after bleeding. The first day or two after your menstruation has finished is a little similar to the postnatal period after a woman has given birth. After all, as I explained in chapter four, you have just undergone your monthly 'mini birth'. This means that you will need to allow time for your uterus and the pelvic floor to return to their premenstrual tone. You can support this process by practising a gently strengthening and stabilising practice that may look and feel like a blended yoga-pilates practice (see the Waxing Moon Post-Menstrual sequence at the end of this chapter).

You will also want to include gentle Inversions to help tone and support the uterus and pelvic floor and to flush fresh blood into key glands of the hormonal system as your body gears up again in preparation for the next phase—ovulation (the Full Moon phase).

2. Keep the balance

Even though this is your most dynamic phase, I recommend you maintain a balanced yoga practice that still includes postures and practices to nourish and calm your nervous system. Include one or two Restorative and restful postures to centre you at the beginning of your practice, or to calm and integrate at the end—or both! Balance also means that if you notice that on some days you don't feel so energetic, or you have just worked a long, tiring day, reward yourself with a gentler, more feminine practice to ensure you don't risk burnout.

To help you keep the balance, you can practise the Busy Days Nurturing Waxing Moon sequence (at the end of this chapter). Alternatively, you can insert one or several Restorative Yoga postures into your standard, dynamic Waxing Moon practice (see Appendix 3), and you may also want to consider occasionally practising a restful and rejuvenating Yoga Nidra practice (deep guided relaxation)—try the Dark Moon Yoga Nidra (see p.116), or the Waning Moon Yoga Nidra (see p.268).

If you are focusing on your fertility and hoping to conceive, I recommend you practise the Classical Women's postures (see Appendix 2), as well as the Waxing Moon Post-Menstrual Sequence in order to support your body in producing healthy eggs during this follicular phase.

Waxing Moon Pranayama

Ujjayi Breath

Ujjayi means 'victorious', and this breathing technique works well with the more *yang*, Waxing Moon practice. It involves constricting the throat slightly to lengthen and deepen the breath, and is simultaneously relaxing and energising.

This Pranayama generates internal heat while keeping you calm and focused, and makes it an excellent practice to accompany Asanas (postures).

How to do it

When you're first learning this Ujjayi Breath, adopt a simple cross-legged or kneeling seated position, or even a supported supine Restorative posture (see Appendix 3). Once you are familiar with this breathing practice, you can also incorporate it within your dynamic, flowing posture practice.

Begin by taking a few Soft Belly Breaths (see p.100) to deepen and slow down the breath. When you are ready, bring your awareness upwards, to become aware of the breath as it passes through your throat, as you breathe in and out gently through the nose. Then, slightly constrict the throat as you inhale—so it's like you're breathing in through a straw (but with your mouth closed).

Now, as you exhale, just for the first few rounds, breathe out through the mouth making a gentle, whispering 'haaa' sound, from your throat, like you're trying to fog up a mirror that is just in front of your mouth. Then, close your mouth again and continue to cultivate this sound as you now breathe in and out through the nostrils; it's as if you are breathing through the throat. The classic sound of the Ujjayi Breath will be an ocean sound— like the sound of the sea when you hold a seashell up to your ear.

Continue Ujjayi Breath as long as you like, and as with all Pranayama practices, if you feel dizzy or uncomfortable in any way, cease the practice.

Breast self-massage: a balancing Waxing Moon self-care ritual

This is essentially a nurturing, self-massage technique and not a breathing technique, but it can be done in conjunction with mindful breathing to encourage relaxation and release of tension.

Breast self-massage is a good practice to do during your Waxing Moon phase as it not only reminds you to give yourself plenty of self-love and self-care, balancing the outward, active energy of this phase, but it also subtly encourages you to soften into your heart-space. With the outcome-focused nature of this phase, you may find you lose touch with your own feeling centre—the heart-centre—as well of that of others. Mantak Chia says it's important for women to cultivate this connection, and writes:

> Energy can be stored in the heart centre, which is a powerhouse for a woman. It is the seat of love, joy and happiness, and is the centre of rejuvenation, because it is the site of the thymus gland, which plays an essential role in the immune system. With this centre open you will experience all of these positive emotions and will be provided with abundant healing energy to heal yourself and others.[203]

Breast self-massage is also said to help alleviate PMS symptoms and to benefit your overall health as a woman.[204] By practising it earlier in your cycle, during your Waxing Moon phase, you set yourself up for a smoother remainder of your menstrual month, which can help you be more prepared for your turbulent Waning Moon (premenstrual) phase.

How to do it
You can do a dry massage through your clothes, or do it before or after your shower, using oil.[205] I often incorporate a dry massage as I sit quietly in meditation or contemplation at the end of my yoga practice.

Here are two suggested ways of doing breast self-massage.

---

203 Mantak Chia and William U. Wei, *Chi Kung for Women's Health and Sexual Vitality: A Handbook of Simple Exercises and Techniques*, location 703 (Kindle edition)

204 Claims have been made that breast massage increases your prolactin levels (which can increase the size of your breasts) and oxytocin levels (which makes us feel relaxed and loving). It's definitely been proved that it raises your oxytocin levels—see this study: https://www.ncbi.nlm.nih.gov/pubmed/8187915 . Also see this informative article about the benefits of breast massage that may include breast cancer prevention/ awareness: https://www.honeycolony.com/article/6-reasons-to-massage-your-breasts-today/

205 Any type of natural oil is fine—black sesame oil is very nourishing, particularly if you are trying to balance your *vata dosha* (see Appendix 1) but this oil is very dark and can stain clothes and sheets. Coconut oil is lighter and is especially good in summer, or if you are trying to balance your *pitta dosha*. Personally, I like to also use a Weleda oil: 'Pomegranate Regenerating Body Oil'.

Option one: Taoist technique

I have adapted a breast self-massage technique that I learnt from Taoist Sexology teacher Willow Brown,[206] which involves crossing the arms (see Figure 99) and massaging the breasts in a circular action in one direction for 36 times and then in the opposite direction for a further 36 times.[207]

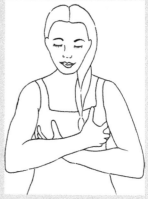

Figure 99

As you circle the hands, move as much of the breast as you can in order to encourage circulation into the breast tissue and lymph glands. During your self-massage, you can simply breathe deeply, perhaps with some Soft Belly Breaths (see p.100), or Falling-Out Breaths (see p.104).

Alternatively, a more complex breast self-massage practice is to focus on breathing through the 'microcosmic orbit', which is a Taoist energy-circuit. The microcosmic orbit practice involves drawing the energy up the back of the body, from the back of the perineum—anal area—all the way up the back, to the crown of the head, during your inhalation. As you exhale (touching the tip of the tongue to the roof of the mouth to seal the energy), feel the energy cascading down the front of the body, through the throat, heart centre, solar plexus, womb-space, back down into the perineum. This technique will take some practice—it's a bit like the right-left brain challenge of patting your head with one hand and circling your other hand on your belly.

Option two: affirmation integration

In this breast massage practice, place each hand onto each breast and begin by circling your hands away from each other (see Figure 100). In other words, you're moving your right hand in an anti-clockwise direction and your left hand in a clockwise direction, with your hands both moving down on the outsides of the breasts at the same time. This outward motion of the

---

206   Willow Brown L.Ac is an acupuncturist and Taoist Sexology practitioner and teacher. You can find out more about her work here: http://thetaoistway.com/

207   The number 36 is a sacred (and oft-used) number in Taoism. I have not been able to ascertain for sure why this is so. What I have discovered is that there are 36 'Heavens' in Taoism (see: http://taoist-sorcery.blogspot.com.au/2014/03/36-heavens-of-taoism.html) and also 36 x 3 = 108, a universally sacred number in Hinduism and Buddhism.

hands represents a detoxing; an opportunity to relinquish negative energy, thoughts or habits that are not serving you. As I do this outward massage, I imagine words or qualities that I'd like to let go of, such as anxiety, fear, stress, anger, ill-health, pushing, striving, and so on. At the same time, I focus on releasing exhalations, Falling-Out Breaths (see p.104). If you like, you could even work with full sentence-mantras, such as, 'I am letting go of tension and holding in my life'.

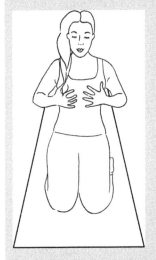

When you're ready, you can reverse the direction of your hands, so they are now circling inwards, towards each other, both moving up the outside of your breasts at the same time, with the right hand now moving in a clockwise direction and left hand in an anti-clockwise direction. This now represents a nourishing, drawing-in energy; it's an opportunity to contemplate those positive habits and qualities you'd like to manifest in your life. I like to imagine qualities like love, flow, ease, good health, and so on. Or, you could repeat a full sentence affirmation or mantra like, *I am attracting all the abundance I need in my life*.

Figure 100

This self-massage practice can be done at the end of your yoga practice or, I like to do it after a shower, with some nourishing oil. If you're in a hurry, you need only do 10–15 repetitions in each direction to help engender the loving (including love of self and others) heart connection that is so potent in this practice.

Waxing Moon Yoga Sequences

POSTURES AND PRACTICES TO SUPPORT YOUR POST-MENSTRUAL PHASE

WAXING MOON POST-MENSTRUAL SEQUENCE

Best time to practise

This is a graduated sequence that works to gently support you in the transition from your menstrual cocoon and back out into the world. Therefore the best time to practise this Waxing Moon post-menstrual sequence is straight after your period has finished and all bleeding has ceased.

Sequence duration

This sequence will take approximately 35 minutes.

Sequence benefits

- Includes gentle Inversions to lift and tone the uterus after menstruation.
- Gradually re-awakens the body with gentle stabilising, strengthening and stretching following your monthly hibernation.

Props for this sequence

A yoga mat, a yoga bolster, a yoga strap, a yoga block, and an eye-bag to cover your eyes (if you like).

1. Constructive rest position (CRP)

Benefits

- Grounds, centres and relaxes you in preparation for your Waxing Moon sequence of postures.
- See page 95 for further benefits of CRP.

Props for this posture

A yoga mat and a thin-fold (single or double) blanket to place under the sacrum if the floor is hard.

Recommended timing

Let your awareness drop out of the head and into the belly as you breathe and soften here for 3–5 minutes

How to practise

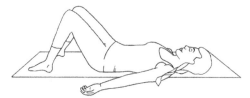

Figure 101 CRP

See Posture 1 in the Classical Dark Moon Menstrual Sequence on page 122 for instructions on practising CRP.

Note

As you work with the Soft Belly Breath here (see p.100) emphasise the hollowing action of the belly back towards the spine as you exhale to begin to bring a sense of toning in the deep abdominal muscles.

Then, do the following variations:

Variation: Constructive Rest Position with arms crossed

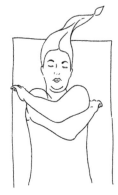

Fold the arms across the upper chest to feel the upper back—the space between the shoulder blades—softening and releasing (see Figure 102).

Figure 102

Variation: Constructive Rest Position with Arm Raises

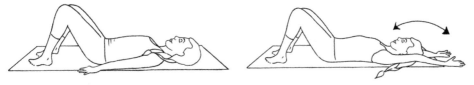

Figure 103 Exhaling   Figure 104 Inhaling

Follow the instructions for this variation on page 124.

2. Pelvic tilts and pelvic clock

Benefits

- These simple pelvic movements gently tone the deep abdominal muscles (transverse abdominis).
- Warms up the body and loosens the lower back and pelvic area.

Props for this posture

A yoga mat and a thin-fold (single or double) blanket to place under the sacrum if the floor is hard.

Recommended timing

Do about 10 repetitions of the Pelvic Tilts and about 6 in each direction for the Pelvic Clocks

How to practise

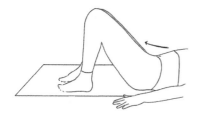   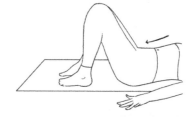

Figure 105 Exhaling   Figure 106 Inhaling

Still with your body in the Constructive Rest Position, place your palms on the floor by your hips, drawing the shoulder blades down, away from the ears, to bring a sense of stability through the shoulder-girdle, and to prepare for the Pelvic Tilts and Pelvic Clock.

As you exhale, feel the navel draw back towards the spine, hollowing the belly, and tilt the pelvis so the top of the pelvis moves back, tailbone moves up towards the knees and the ceiling, and the lower black presses into the floor ('posterior pelvic tilt'—see Figure 105)—you may also get the subtle sense of engaging the pelvic floor muscles. Then, as you inhale, release the lower back gently away from the floor, tailbone and sitting bones moving towards to the floor ('anterior pelvic tilt'—see Figure 106). Repeat up to 9 more times.

The Pelvic Clock movement involves the same tilting back (posterior tilt) and forward (anterior tilt) of the pelvis but also includes adding a circling action through the pelvis (going to each side of the pelvis as well). Imagine your pelvis is like a bowl and there is marble in the bottom of the bowl and you're trying to circle the marble right around the circumference of the bowl.[208] Or, another way to think about it is that you're pressing around the outside of sacrum, like you're moving around the numbers on a clock.

The breath can be free with these Pelvic Clock movements, although you can focus more on exhaling when the top of your pelvis is tilting back and tail is tilting up and belly is hollowing (posterior pelvic tilt), and inhaling when the pelvis is tilting forward and the tailbone is tilting back towards the floor (anterior pelvic tilt). Circle the pelvis about 6 times in each direction.

3. Abdominal apanasana

Benefits

- Tones the deep abdominal muscles providing stability and support for the core and lower back.
- Heats and warms up the body.

Props for this posture

A yoga mat and a thin-fold (single or double) blanket to place under the sacrum if the floor is hard.

Recommended timing

Do 10-12 repetitions

How to practise

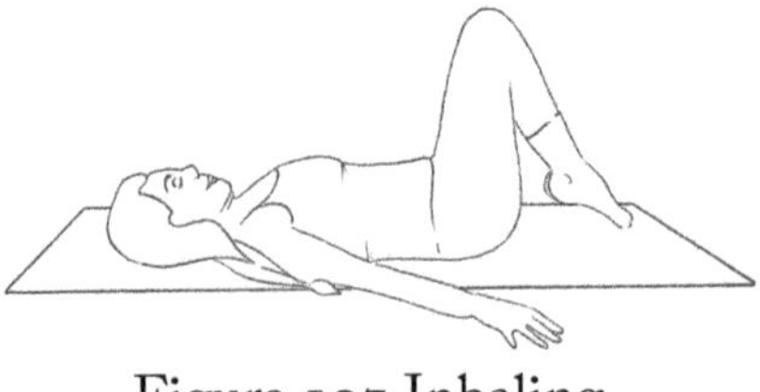

Figure 107 Inhaling

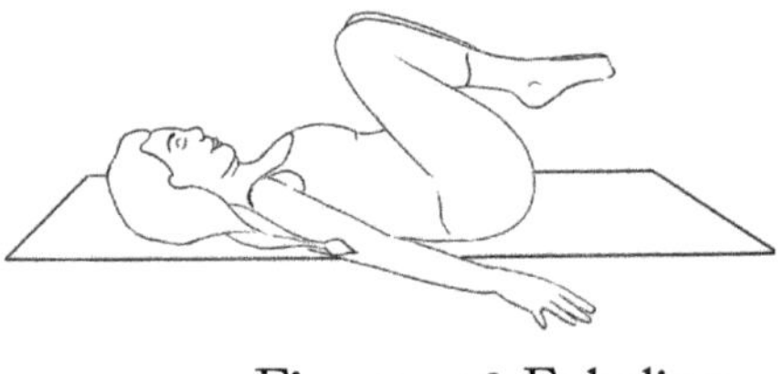

Figure 108 Exhaling

---

208 I have borrowed this analogy from yoga therapist and yogalates teacher, Maria Kirsten. You can find out about her work here: https://www.yogaforgrownups.com/

Draw the thighs into the chest, feet relaxed towards the buttocks, hands still resting on the floor beside the hips, palms down. As you inhale move the knees away from you so they point up towards the ceiling and the thighs are perpendicular to the floor (see Figure 107). As you exhale, using the scooping action through the belly, move the knees back towards your chest (see Figure 108). Repeat another 8-11 times, slowly and mindfully.

As you inhale and move the knees away from you, try not to lose neutral spine and pelvis; see if you can maintain a sense of gently pressing the lower back ribs towards the floor.

4. Crescent psoas release

Benefits

- Stretches the deep psoas muscle, providing relief for the lower back, and also nourishing the nervous system and reproductive organs.
- Stretches the lateral-body, warming up the body.

Props for this posture

A yoga mat and a thin-fold (single or double) blanket to place under the sacrum if the floor is hard.

Recommended timing

Stay on each side for 5–10 slow breaths.

How to practise

Bring the legs back into Constructive Rest Position. Then move both feet over a few inches to the left side of your mat. Extend your right leg along the foot and move it about a foot or so over to the left side of your mat. Scoot your head and shoulders about a foot over to the left as well. You are aiming to end up with your body in a crescent/c-shape (see Figure 109). Roll the right leg in so it internally rotates at the hip, moving towards the big-toe side of the foot. Holding this inward-spiral through the leg, relax it as much as you can from the hip through to the foot. Fold the arms over head and hold (see Figure 109), breathing some long, slow exhalations into the area that should be feeling the stretch and opening—the front of the right hip

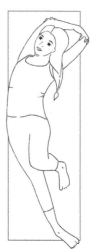

Figure 109

and groin, and ultimately into the psoas muscle.[209] You should also feel a beautiful stretch radiating up the whole right side of your torso, into the waist, ribs and even the armpit.

When you are ready, straighten up the torso and centre the legs, and repeat on the other side.

5. Forward virasana (forward facing 'heroine' pose)

Benefits

- Stretches the spinal muscles and creates space between the vertebrae; creates neutrality through the back after the previous asymmetrical lateral stretch.
- Opens up the upper back/thoracic region.

Recommended timing

5 slow breaths.

Props and how to practise

See Posture 6—Forward Virasana—in the Classical Dark Moon Menstrual Sequence, page 130, for information on props and how to practise.

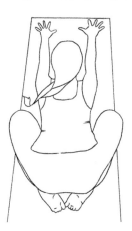

Note

There is no need to come out of the pose; simply transition into Down Dog (see below) from here.

Figure 110

---

209   I was first introduced to this wonderful passive psoas stretch by psoas-savvy expert, Kylian Martin, who has trained with Liz Koch. Find out more about Kylian's work here: https://www.kylian.com.au/

6. Down dog pose

Benefits

- Stretches the entire back and spine; opening the upper and lower back.
- Releases tightness and stiffness through the shoulders.
- Stretches the calves and hamstrings.
- Lifts and tones the uterus and pelvic floor.
- Quiets the mind and stimulates the circulation.
- Balances the hormonal system.

Props for this posture

Just your yoga mat.

Recommended timing

5-10 slow, deep breaths

How to practise

From Forward Virasana turn the toes under and lift the hips up and back into the upside-down 'v' shape of Down Dog (see Figure 111). The feet should be hip-width apart, with the toes turned in slightly, heels out; the hands should be shoulder width, fingers spreading, with even weight into the thumb and little finger sides of the hands.

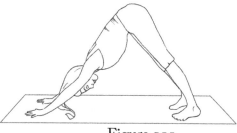

Figure 111

To warm-up in the pose, try 'Walking Dog'—bending one knee and stretching the opposite heel into the mat, alternating. And then when you're ready hold the pose statically, releasing the head and neck, pressing the floor away from you, firming the outer edge of the shoulder-blades into the back, side ribs, and reaching the hips up and back, heels descending onto or towards the mat. You can bend the legs a little (or a lot!) if the hamstrings and/or calves are very tight; the main focus should be on extending the spine, the extension of the backs of the legs can come in time.

7. High lunge pose

Benefits

- Stretches the groins and frontal thigh muscles.
- Strengthens and tones the legs and buttocks.

Props for this posture

Just your yoga mat.

Recommended timing

Hold for 5 breaths on each side.

How to practise

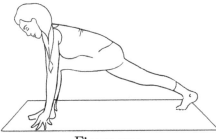

Figure 112

From Down Dog (see above) step your left foot between your hands. If that is difficult to do smoothly, try doing it in several steps or lower your knees down into table-top first and step through from there. Make sure you've stepped your left foot far enough forward so that the knee aligns over the ankle (see Figure 112). Have your fingertips on the floor on either side of the foot and lift the chest away from the front thigh as you extend strongly through the back leg, all the way out through the back heel; at the same time, descend your hips towards the floor as much as you can. After 5 breaths or so, step the left foot back into Down Dog and change sides.

After holding the pose on the second side for another 5 breaths, rather than stepping your right foot back into Down Dog step your left foot forward to join it so you are coming into the next pose, Uttanasana.

Variation: Low Lunge Pose

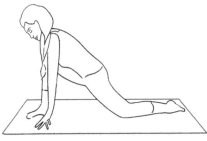

Figure 113

If the High Lunge Pose is too strong for you—you find it impossible to drop your hips and straighten the back leg—or if you prefer a gentler practice, try the Low Lunge variation. This involves keeping your back knee on the ground as you lunge forward with your front knee (see Figure 113).

8. Uttanasana (standing forward fold)

Benefits

- Stretches the back and hamstring muscles; and releases the neck muscles.
- Relaxing and cooling.
- Good transition pose.

Props for this posture

Just your yoga mat.

Recommended timing

2-3 breaths in Uttanasana and 1 breath (inhalation) in the variation: Urdhva Uttanasana.

How to practise

From the Lunge Pose, step the back foot forward to join the front foot and position the feet parallel and hip-width apart. Hang the torso forward, folding from the hips, resting the fingertips on the floor in front of you, or even on either side of each foot (see Figure 114). If it's difficult to reach the floor or you have low back pain or sensitivity bend your knees as much as

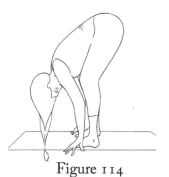

Figure 114

you need to. Let the head hang, gently shaking it out, or turning it from side to side to completely release any tension in the neck.

Variation: Urdhva Uttanasana (Lifted Standing Forward Fold)

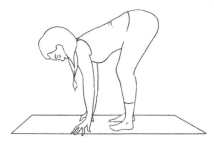

Figure 115

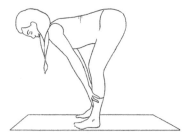

Figure 116

On your next inhalation, bring the fingertips in front of you and lift your chest and head, so that you are looking a foot or so out in front of you on the floor. Lift your chest forward and away, but keep the back of the neck long (see Figure 115).

If it's difficult to have your fingers on the floor, a modification is to have your hands on your shins (see Figure 116).

Then, as you exhale, fold back into Uttanasana (Figure 114).

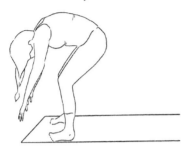

On your next exhalation, roll up through the spine to standing. As you roll up, draw the navel up and back to the spine, head rolling up last, arms dangling (see Figure 117).

Figure 117

9. Tadasana (mountain pose) with a block

Benefits

- Helps with postural alignment.
- Using the block helps to tone the inner thigh muscles (adductors) and the pelvic floor muscles.
- The arm movement mobilises the shoulders and stretches the spine; it also helps link your breathing with your movement, serving to deepen the breathing and calm the mind.

Props for this posture

A yoga mat and a yoga block.

Recommended timing

Raise and lower the arms 2–4 times

How to practise

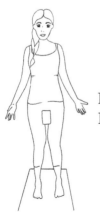

Figure 118
Exhaling

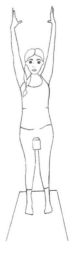

Figure 119
Inhaling

When you come to standing, grab a yoga block and bring it between the thighs right up against the pubic bone and come to stand into Tadasana (Mountain Pose)—feet parallel (with the outer edges of the mat) and as close to together as the block will allow, hands to the side, shoulders drawing down the back, chest lifted and broad, navel lifting up and back gently into the spine (see Figure 118).

As you inhale, bring the arms up and overhead, palms facing each other, shoulder blades continuing to move down the back ribs (see Figure 119).

Repeat several more times—arms sweeping up the side and overhead on the inhalation, then back down to the floor as you exhale.

10. Utkatasana (standing squat pose) with a block

Benefits

* Strengthens and tones the legs, buttock muscles and the core.
* Using the block helps to tone the inner thigh muscles (adductors) and pelvic floor muscles.
* Builds stamina.

Props for this posture

A yoga mat and a yoga block.

Recommended timing

Hold Utkatasana for 5-8 slow breaths. Repeat if you have the energy.

How to practise

From Tadasana turn the block around so the long edge of the block runs parallel to the thigh bones and also move it a little lower down the leg so it is positioned on the lower thigh region (see Figure 120). Initially with the hands on the hips, bend the knees, moving the buttocks back and down to come to sit into/towards an imaginary chair behind you. As you bend your knees, you will need to begin to hinge from the hips and tilt your torso forward, ensuring your chest stays lifted and your lower back in neutral—avoid sticking out your butt. Keep the direction of the buttocks moving backwards as much as you can so that the knees stay as much over the heels as you can. Keep squeezing the block, and

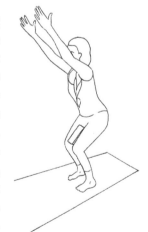

Figure 120

pressing down through the heels into the floor. If you have the stamina, raise the arms to complete the pose—upper arms beside the ears, energy running out through the arm-lines, through the fingertips (see Figure 120).

After 5-8 breaths here, straighten the legs, lower the arms, and come up. Repeat if you are feeling like some extra challenge today.

11. Down dog pose with a block

Benefits
The same benefits as for Posture 6 (Down Dog) in this sequence, but with the additional benefit of toning the inner thigh and pelvic floor muscles.

Props for this posture
A yoga mat and a yoga block.

Recommended timing
5-10 breaths, depending on your stamina and energy.

How to practise

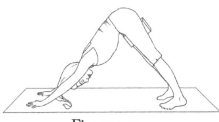

Figure 121

In Tadasana (after straightening the legs and coming out of Utkatasana), change the position of the block again so the short end faces forward and it's right up against the pubic bone, as in Posture 9—Tadasana with a block (see Figure 118). Then, inhale and raise the arms overhead, and exhale and fold forward into Uttanasana (the Standing Forward Fold—see Posture 8 in this sequence).

From Uttanasana walk your hands forward and your feet back to come into Down Dog, still with the block between your thighs.

Work in Down Dog for a further 5-10 breaths before taking the block out and resting into the next pose—Child Pose with a block.

12. Child pose with a block

Benefits
- A resting pose.
- Calms the mind and nervous system—resting the forehead on a block increases the calming, cooling effects.
- Rests and balances the muscles of the lower back and shoulders.

Props for this posture

A yoga mat and a yoga block. You may also need a folded blanket to place between your buttocks and heels (if your buttocks don't rest easily onto your heels).

Recommended timing

As long as you like! Anywhere between 1-4 minutes.

How to practise

Lower your knees onto the floor coming out of Down Dog Pose into table-top (all-fours) position and take the block out from between your thighs and put it in front of you. Then, move

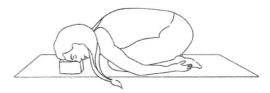

Figure 122

your buttocks back to your heels and fold forward into Child Pose with the forehead resting on the lowest edge of the block, and your hands resting by the feet palms facing upwards (see Figure 122). If your buttocks don't easily reach the heels you can place a folded blanket between the buttocks and the heels.

Rest here for as long as you need, just letting the breath settle and quieten.

When you are ready, roll up through the spine, drawing the navel back towards the spine, head rolling up last, to come up to a kneeling position.

13. Trianga mukhaikapada pascimottanasana (three-limbed forward bend)

Benefits

- Stretches the hamstrings and calf muscles of the extended leg; stretches the quadriceps and hip muscles of the bent leg.
- Gently stretches out the deep lower back of the side that the leg is extended (quadratus lumborum muscles).
- A safe, stabilising Forward Bend—best option if you have SIJ (sacroiliac joint) pain or instability.
- Cooling and calming for the body and mind.
- Nourishes the digestive organs.

Props for this posture

A folded blanket to go under one hip, and a yoga strap.

Recommended timing

Stay in this Forward Bend for 5–10 slow breaths

How to practise

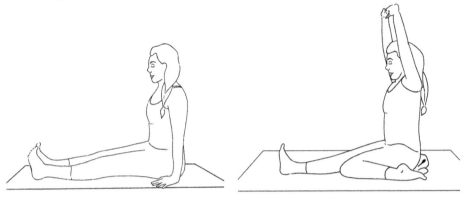

Figure 123

Figure 124

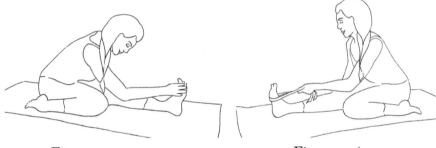

Figure 125

Figure 126

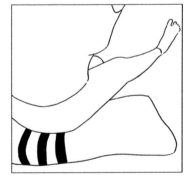

Figure 127

Setting up

Extend your legs out in front of you in Dandasana (Staff Pose—Figure 123). Then bend up your left leg, rolling the calf muscle away from the back of the knee and out to the side as you do, into half-Virasana (Hero pose)— toes pointing backwards, heel on the outside of the hip, weight towards the little-toe side of the top of the foot (see Figure 124). Once you've bent up the leg, you will find that the hips become uneven and most of the weight drops into the hip of the leg that's extended (right side). So, to balance out the hips, place a folded blanket underneath your right sitting bone (see Figure 127). If you know that you're tight through the hamstrings and hips, you may want to have a strap looped around that right foot so you can hold it for the modified version of the pose (see below).

Going into the pose and being there

To prepare for the pose, inhale as you interlace the hands overhead (see Figure 124), pushing the palms up towards the ceiling and feeling for length through the spine and the sides of the torso; at the same time feeling both hips grounding back evenly into the floor. As you exhale, bend forward from the hips and take the edge of the foot with your right hand, and keep your left hand on the floor beside you to ground you and stop you tipping into that side (see Figure 125). If you are unable to reach the foot and keep the spine long and chest lifted, take both ends of a strap that is looped around your right foot, and hold it a comfortable distance away from the foot (see Figure 126).

Stay for 5-10 breaths, feeling for length through the spine, lifting the sternum up and away from the navel, as you inhale, and softening and yielding into the Forward Bend as you exhale. Also, keep the extended leg active, toes drawing back (particularly the little-toe edge of the foot), and focus on pressing both sitting bones and hips back evenly, grounding the pose from your hips.

When you're ready, raise your torso upright and release your foot or the strap and prepare to transition straight into the next pose, Bharavadjasana (Sage Pose Twist—see Posture 14 below) on the first side, before then coming back to complete Trianga Mukaikapada Pascimottanasana on the second side.

14. Bharavadjasana (sage twist)

Benefits

- Releases the spinal muscles, relieving upper and lower back tension.
- Mobilises the hips.
- Tones the internal organs—reproductive and digestive—and also nourishes the adrenal glands.

Props for this posture

A folded blanket or small cushion to put under one buttock. You may also choose the option of a block to rest your back hand on, which will give you more lift out of the lower back.

Recommended timing

Hold the twist for 5-10 slow breaths, before coming out and doing Trianga Mukhaikapada Pascimottanasana (see Posture 13 above) on the second side, and then complete the second side of Bharavadjasana.

How to practise

Variation A: Simple Version

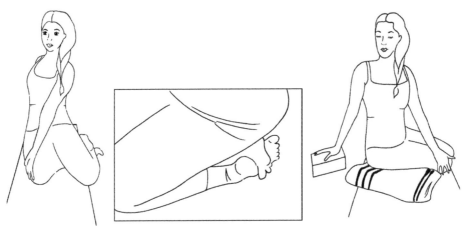

Figure 128   Figure 129   Figure 130

From Trianga Mukaikapada Pascimottanasana with the right leg extended, bend up right leg to the left side to join the other leg. Rest the top of your right foot on the in-step of the left foot (see Figure 129).

Inhale as you raise both arms overhead to aim for as much extension through the spine and torso as possible. Then, as you exhale, place your left hand on the outside of the right knee, right hand behind you on the floor (see Figure 128), or on a block, if that's more comfortable (see Figure 130). With each inhale, create space throughout the spine, lifting and broadening across the chest; with each exhale, gently deepen the twist, or just maintain, and soften. When you're ready come out of the twist, straighten both legs out to the front into Dandasana (see Figure 123) and get ready to do Trianga Mukaikapada Pascimottanasana (Posture 13) on the second side before repeating Bharavadjasana on the second side.

Variation B: Advanced (Half Lotus) Version

Note

This advanced variation is only suitable if you can comfortably perform the Half-Lotus position, if not, do variation A: the simple version of Bharavadjasana, shown above.

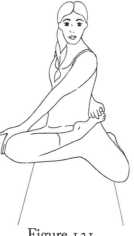

From Trianga Mukhaikapada Pascimottanasana with the right leg extended, bend up the right leg drawing the foot into Half Lotus—heel up to the top of the left thigh, spiralling the hip and thigh open (never force the knee). Inhale, and raise the right arm. Then, wrap the arm behind the back reaching for the right heel (see Figure 131). If you can't reach the heel, just have the right hand on the floor or a block behind you. Bring the left hand to

Figure 131

hold onto the right knee, or even bring the back of the hand against the outside of the knee if you can. Inhale again, finding length through the torso, then as you exhale, twist gradually around to the right to look over the right shoulder.

After staying here for a few slow breaths, turn just the head back to gaze over the left shoulder (see Figure 131), stretching the neck briefly. Then slowly release from the pose and stretch the legs out into Dandasana (see Figure 123) and do the second side of Trianga Mukhaikapada Pascimottanasana (Posture 13).

15. Half shoulderstand

Benefits

- Shoulderstand, the 'queen' of all yoga postures, nourishes the thyroid glands as well as the other hormonal organs to bring about balance and health to the hormonal system.
- Cooling and calming—nourishes the nervous system; good for adrenal fatigue.
- Tones the abdominal organs and lifts and tones the uterus, and takes the weight off the pelvic floor; good for the digestion.
- Boosts the circulation and lymphatic flow—beneficial for health, vitality and immunity.

Props for this posture

Just your yoga mat.

Recommended timing

Up to 5 minutes if you can stay comfortably

How to practise

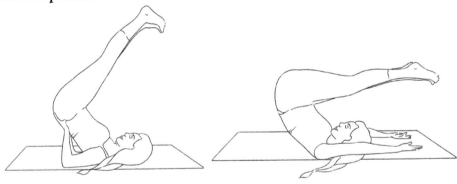

Figure 132   Figure 133

Come to lie on your back along your mat and then swing the legs overhead, bending up the elbows to rest the sacrum into the palms of the hands, fingers pointing upwards. To make the posture relatively effortless, draw the elbows in as close as possible (just a little wider than shoulder width), so that most of the weight rests into the elbows and not so much into the head and neck. Let the feet drop slightly overhead so you are forming a side-'v'-shape (see Figure 132). This is a gentle variation of the traditional, full Shoulderstand that is easy on the neck (and nervous system) yet still offers all the benefits of Shoulderstand.

While in the pose, make sure your breathing remains even and steady, focusing in particular on lengthening the exhalations.

To come out of the pose, lower your feet further overhead behind you into a full or modified Plough Pose—either with the feet touching the floor behind your head, if you can, or just have the feet hovering overhead and bring your arms overhead (see Figure 133). Stay here for several breaths, if you can comfortably, then roll down through the spine (using your abdominal muscles to brace you) with control until you are lying flat on your back, legs extended.

Safety and Comfort Notes

If you have trouble getting into the pose, bring yourself about a shin-distance away from the wall and walk your feet up the wall before bringing the feet overhead into the full pose. This makes the transition into the posture more easeful, decreasing any chances of straining the neck or the back getting into it. Likewise, when you're ready to come out of the posture, you can walk your feet down the wall and come to rest onto your back, pushing yourself away from the wall to lie out straight.

If this posture feels too strong for you, especially on your neck, you can do a Restorative version of the Shoulderstand. Try the Supported Bolster Shoulderstand (see p.292) or the Chair Shoulderstand (see p.300). And if you have any kind of neck injury or discomfort, avoid any variation of the Shoulderstand and just do Supported Bridge Pose (see p.137).

16. Matsyasana (fish pose)

Benefits

- A counter-pose for the neck from the previous posture, Shoulderstand.
- Opens the chest and facilitates deeper breathing—energises and uplifts.
- Strengthens the neck.
- Stimulates the thyroid.
- Can release tightness in the jaw and tone the facial muscles around the chin and jaw.

Props for this posture

Just your yoga mat.

Recommended timing

Open and close the mouth up to 8 times and take several breaths before/after.

How to practise

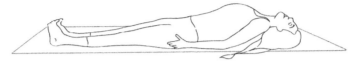

Figure 134

Lying on your back with your legs stretched out, come up on to your forearms, hands beside the buttocks and arch your head back so you are resting lightly on the crown of the head, throat stretching, chest expanding (see Figure 134). Make sure you keep the forearms in close to the body. Once in the pose, open and close the mouth, up to 8 times, like a fish. Then, take several breaths, filling up the space in the chest. Draw the chin in, slide the head back, and lower down off the elbows to mindfully come out of the pose.

Safety Note and an Alternative Neck Release

Avoid this posture if you have any neck pain or injury. Instead, simply lay on your back and gently tip your chin up towards the ceiling as you inhale, as if you were trying to look at the wall behind your head, and then as you exhale, drop the chin towards the throat, lengthening through the back of the neck. Repeat several times.

17. Simple supine twist

Benefits

- Releases the lower and upper back.
- Detoxes the digestive and reproductive organs.
- Another good counter-pose to Shoulderstand—balances and neutralises the body.
- Can subtly tone the abdominal muscles if you keep a slight tail-tuck when in the twist and also focus on engaging your deep abdominals when bringing the knees to centre.
- Stretches the outer thigh muscles and fascia (iliotibial band).

Props for this posture

Just your yoga mat.

Recommended timing

Stay for around 5 deep breaths on each side

How to practise

Place the feet into the floor as if you were going to do Constructive Rest Position—legs bent, soles of the feet into the floor. Bring the arms up shoulder height, palms facing upwards. Bring the feet together and lift the feet and the buttocks about a foot or so towards the right side of your mat. From there, lower the knees gently over to the left side of your mat so that your right knee ends up on top of your left. Reach actively through your oppo- site, right arm, pressing the back of the shoulder into/towards the floor, and turn your head to look at your right hand (see Figure 135).

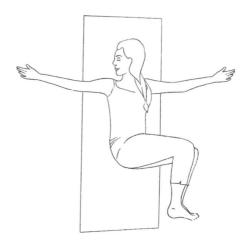

Figure 135

With each exhalation, twist gently from the belly with a sense of wrapping the side abdominal muscles in towards the centre-line of the body. Also, have a slight tuck under of the tailbone to keep the abdominal muscles switched on and to protect the lower back. The twisting action should be focused in the upper back (thoracic) area and, as you lengthen your top right knee and hip-bone away from you, you should feel a gentle opening through the outer (lateral) right thigh and hip.

After about 5 breaths, use your exhalation to draw your knees back to centre, to face the ceiling, and realign your buttocks and feet to the centre of the mat, to repeat on the other side.

18. Savasana (final relaxation)—simple variation

Benefits

- Helps relax and balance your nervous system before you reintegrate into the outside world.
- Rejuvenates your energy.

Props for this posture

A folded blanket or small cushion for the head, a bolster (or rolled blanket) for under the knees, and an eye-bag for the eyes (if you like).

Recommended timing

5–10 minutes

How to practise

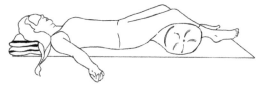

Figure 136

Setting up

Place a folded blanket under your head, making sure it's not so high that your head is pushed forward out of alignment with the natural curve at the back of the neck. Also, make sure the support is not too low that you find you are thrusting your chin up to the ceiling, shortening the back of the neck. Place a bolster under the knees to support the lower back. Cover your eyes with an eye-bag if you wish, or lightly close the eyes, and let the arms fall a little out from the sides of the body with the palms facing up (see Figure 136).

Being there

Take a few deep, conscious breaths to allow your body to settle into the floor. Feel all the parts of the body that make contact with the floor and props merging more deeply into these supports. Continue to scan your awareness through the body looking for areas of tension and holding and using your conscious exhalations to release this tension out and away.

Coming out

When you are ready to come out of Savasana, begin by gradually moving and awakening the body—moving the fingers and toes, wrists and ankles, gently rolling the head from side to side. Then draw the knees up to the chest and roll over to your right hand side. Rest on your right hand side in a foetal position for several breaths and then roll up to sitting throught the spine, from side-lying (pressing your top left hand into the floor in front of your chest).

To finish

Come to a comfortable sitting position—kneeling or cross-legged—and sit quietly for a little while before you transition back into your day or evening.

Place your hands on your lower belly connecting down to your womb-space (see Figure 66, p.145). Feel the energy there behind the palms, and notice how you feel as you drop your awareness right down into your womb-space—feeling the softness and spaciousness of your belly.

Then, place your left palm at the centre of your chest—your heart-centre—whilst keeping your right palm on the belly (Heart-Womb Mudra, see Figure 2, p.59) and sense the connection between these two energy centres and how you have fostered the movement and circulation of energy between the womb and the heart-space with this practice.

Lastly, bring your palms together at the heart-centre in prayer position, in a gesture of honouring and gratitude (Figure 67, p.145); feeling a deep sense of gratitude overflowing from your heart-centre down into your womb-space, nourishing you deeply.

Namaste.

BUSY DAYS NURTURING WAXING MOON SEQUENCE

Best time to practise

This sequence is good for unwinding at the end of a busy day (or even to punctuate a busy day) when you may have been powering through your to-do list and need a little balance so that you don't burn out during this more dynamic phase of your cycle—or so that you don't pay the price later in your cycle.

Sequence duration

The Busy Days Nurturing Waxing Moon sequence is designed to be short enough to fit into a busy schedule. It should take about 15-20 minutes, depending on how long you choose to spend in the Restorative Postures.

Sequence benefits

- Rejuvenating and balancing
- Releases tension in the upper and lower back

Props for this sequence

A yoga mat; ideally 2 yoga bolsters, but if you only have 1 bolster you can choose to do the Prone Savasana with Transverse Bolster variation. You may also need to slip a folded blanket or small cushion between your buttocks and heels if you're not able to sit comfortably in the kneeling Vajrasana position.

1. Vajrasana (thunderbolt pose) with shoulder stretch vinyasa

Benefits

- The kneeling posture (Vajrasana) limbers the hips, knees and ankles and is said to be beneficial for your digestion.
- The Shoulder Stretch Vinyasa (sequence) warms up the shoulders and upper back and deepens the breathing, calming and energising the body-mind.

Props for this posture

Possibly a folded blanket to place between the buttocks and heels for the first pose, Vajrasana—to help with the comfort of your knees and/or ankles.

Recommended timing

Repeat the whole sequence 2-3 times.

How to practise

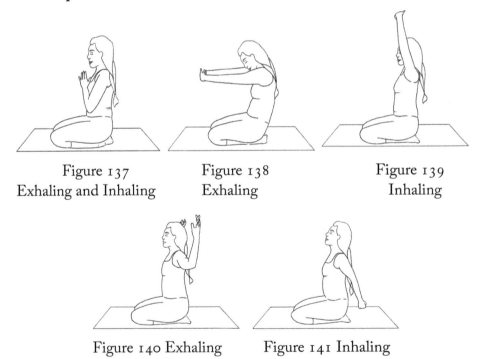

Figure 137
Exhaling and Inhaling

Figure 138
Exhaling

Figure 139
Inhaling

Figure 140 Exhaling   Figure 141 Inhaling

Sit into a kneeling position onto your heels. If you're uncomfortable sitting on your ankles or there is discomfort in the knees try placing a folded blanket or even a bolster between the buttocks and heels.

Start by placing the hands into Prayer (Anjali) Mudra at the centre of the chest, and inhale deeply here, feeling the chest expanding behind the thumbs (see Figure 137). As you exhale, interlace the hands, push the palms away from you and round the upper back, concaving the chest (see Figure 138). On your inhalation, raise the arms overhead and press your palms towards the ceiling, lengthening your spine at the same time as you ground your sitting bones down to the earth (see Figure 139). On your exhalation, release the hands and float the arms down to the sides, slightly behind the line of the body, as feel the inner edges of the shoulder blades move into the back ribs (see Figure 140). As you inhale, interlace the hands behind your back, backs of the knuckles face away from you, shoulder blades draw towards each other, chest expands (see Figure 141). Finally, on your exhalation, bring your palms back to the centre of your chest into Anjali Mudra (see Figure 137). Repeat this whole sequence another 1-2 times.

2. Down dog pose

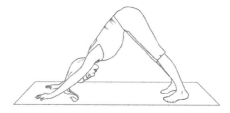

Figure 142

See Posture 6 in the Waxing Moon Post-Menstrual Sequence, page 175, for instructions.

3. Double-bolster child pose-savasana

Benefits

- Nurturing, calming and deeply relaxing.
- Therapeutic for lower back and sacral pain—gently lengthens, creates space and releases the lumbar and sacral areas.
- Releases tension in the neck, shoulders and upper back.
- Encourages the breath into the back of the lungs.

Props for this posture

2 yoga bolsters and a thin-fold blanket to support knees.

Recommended timing

5-10 minutes

How to practise

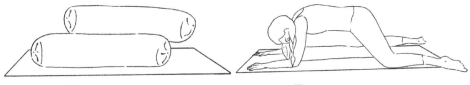

Figure 143   Figure 144

Stagger two bolsters as in Figure 143. The top bolster is set back about 10cm from the bottom bolster. You can place the two bolsters onto a thin-fold blanket as well if you'd like to cushion the legs (and the arms) if the floor is hard.

Come to straddle and lie prone upon the top bolster. The whole front of your torso needs to be supported and the legs are softly bent, hips opening enough for your big-toe side of the shins to rest on the floor. Your head hangs forward, chin tucked slightly so that your forehead rests on the bottom bolster. Move the top bolster forward or back if you're not entirely comfortable and to facilitate the correct position to rest your forehead on the bottom bolster and so that your neck is lengthening.

Begin by taking a few Falling-Out Breaths (see p.104) here as you allow yourself to relax and surrender your weight into the bolsters beneath you. Let the arms hang heavily and the legs heavy and loose from the hip socket

With each Falling-Out Breath, feel that you're letting go of any tension and holding across the shoulders, breathing it out and away down through the arms, out of the hands into the earth beneath you.

As you spend time here you may feel a sense of unravelling within the sacrum and/or the lower back.

When you are ready, sit up slowly to kneeling.

Alternative: Prone Savasana with transverse bolster under pelvis
This is a good alternative option if you only have one yoga bolster.

Benefits of this posture

- Relaxing and nurturing—lying face-forward engenders a feeling of safety.
- Releasing and therapeutic for the lower back pain—gently tractions/ lengthens out the lower back.

Props for this posture

A bolster and a thin-folded blanket. You can also place a sandbag on the sacrum (weighting in the direction towards the tailbone)—if you like.

Recommended timing

5–10 mins

How to practise

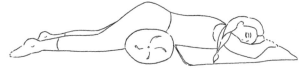

Figure 145

Place a bolster in the middle of your mat, the long end parallel with the short end of your mat. Also, spread out a thin-folded blanket in front of the bolster, or even over the whole mat area to cushion your body, especially if the floor is hard. Then lie over the bolster so that is directly underneath your pubic bone. When you have the position right it should feel like your lower back is gently lengthened, reducing the lordosis of the lower back. Have your arms bent up in front and your head turned to the side, resting on one cheek (see Figure 145).

Rest here with your eyes closed as long as you like. Just make sure you turn your head the other direction half way through the timing to evenly stretch your neck.

To finish

Once you come out of either variation of Savasana, come to a comfortable sitting position and place your right palm then your left on top into Womb-Space Mudra (see Figure 66, p.145). Take some deep Soft Belly Breaths here (see p.100) allowing your awareness to stay grounded deep in your belly and womb-space, so that when you re-enter your day you can stay connected and centred.

CHAPTER SIX
THE FULL MOON: SOFTENING INTO THE FEMININE

The Full Moon phase occurs around the time of ovulation and spans the two or three days before and after a fertile egg bursts from the ovary. When the moon is full and the world is bathed in its silver light, you may feel more inclined to go outdoors and enjoy its beauty and energy. In the same way, you tend to feel more energetic and more outward focused during this phase of your menstrual month.

The ripe and juicy qualities of the Full Moon phase symbolize the summer of your cycle. If your body is in tune with the moon, and literally aligning with the full moon (a 'white moon cycle'[210]), you are considered to be at your most fertile.

Of course, not everyone ovulates in tandem with the full moon, which is totally legitimate too. No matter which phase of the moon your ovulation coincides with, you can view your mid-cycle, ovulatory phase as your *metaphorical* Full Moon time. By engaging with this metaphor of the full moon, you are able to more deeply appreciate the very fullness of this phase; with the ripening of the follicles and the peak in hormones, ovulation represents the zenith in your cycle.

THE BIOLOGICAL IMPERATIVE TO PROCREATE

Ovulation occurs when there is a surge of oestrogen (stimulated by the pituitary gland's production of FSH—Follicle Stimulating Hormone), which causes the rupturing of a follicle from an ovary. Your cervix lifts up high and opens.[211] You may feel that your whole vaginal passage becomes more open and spacious, and the vagina produces the slippery, fertile

---

210   See chapter two, page 37 in this book for more information on a 'white moon' and 'red moon' cycle.

211   'As you approach ovulation, your cervix becomes soft, high, open and wet', says Amin Gafar, Fertility Treatment Expert . see: https://www.babycentre.co.uk/x561007/how-do-i-check-my-cervix-for-signs-of-ovulation

mucous that facilitates the passage of sperm up into the uterus. This all leaves no doubt that, during this menstrual phase, your biology is doing everything it can to get you pregnant—whether you intend to, or not!

During your Full Moon, ovulatory phase, your 'mojo' is at its peak, and women report feeling sexier than usual. Along with oestrogen, there is a surge in testosterone around mid-cycle, which may contribute towards the heightened libido that is common during this phase.[212] It is not surprising to discover that studies have shown that women's bodies emit pheromones[213] that make us more attractive to the opposite sex during the ovulation phase. A famous study was conducted by researchers from the Department of Psychology in the University of Mexico that concluded that strippers—professional lap-dancers—earned higher tips when ovulating![214]

THE 'BIG INHALE': THE SOCIALLY ACCEPTABLE PHASE

In flowing, we learn to inhale, how to take things in:
compliments, put-downs, gifts, intuitive hunches, moods, music,
space—whoever or whatever else is going on around us.

—GABRIELLE ROTH[215]

The Full Moon ovulation phase is the polar opposite of the Dark Moon menstrual phase. The Dark Moon phase represents the darker side of femininity: it's all about releasing, letting go (the 'big exhale'), turning inwards, and being unavailable to others. The Full Moon phase, on the other hand, is all about receptivity—taking things in, both physiologically (in terms of our uterus sucking up sperm) as well as emotionally. During the Full

---

212 'Some believe this may be an in built stimulus to increased sexual activity in women close to ovulation and therefore nature's way of enhancing sexual activity close to ovulation and therefore increasing the likelihood of conception,'—this is according to Monash University's Womens Health Program (see: http://med. monash.edu.au/sphpm/womenshealth/docs/androgens-in-women.pdf)

213 Northrup, *Women's Bodies, Women's Wisdom*, p.105

214 As cited by Jean Kittson in *You're Still Hot to Me*, location 840 (Kindle edition) and also as summarised in Scientific American at https://www.scientificamerican.com/ article/news-bytes-week-ovulating-strippers-bigger-tips/ : '…participants scored $335 per five-hour shift while ovulating compared with $260 per shift during the luteal phase after ovulation and $185 while menstruating'.

215 Gabrielle Roth, *Sweat your Prayers: Movement as a Spiritual Practice*, p.54

Moon phase, a woman's body is in a physical as well as an emotional place of 'holding', as the lining of her womb has now thickened in preparation to potentially receive a fertilised egg.

It follows that from a patriarchal point of view, the ovulation phase is the most acceptable phase of a woman's cycle because the qualities of availability, passivity and receptivity are traditionally more socially valued feminine behaviours. A 1930s study, cited by Christiane Northrup, M.D.,[216] concluded that during ovulation women were more 'relaxed and content and quite receptive to being cared for and loved by others.' This is in stark contrast to qualities recognized in the luteal (premenstrual Waning Moon) phase, when progesterone peaks, and when women were found to be more 'focused on themselves and more inward-directed activity.'[217]

A woman's predisposition towards spending time with others during her Full Moon phase has also led to it being called the 'mother phase'.[218] We tend to be more tuned into others during this phase of our cycle: we are more receptive to receiving care and also more active in nurturing others. Gray writes, 'nature is preparing us to become mothers; to care about a child and to create the social connections through which our child and ourselves are supported by others.'[219]

Miranda Gray also suggests that this is your peak time for expressing your innate '"female" creative abilities' that may include the more traditional, feminine tasks like cooking, sewing, gardening and crafts. Gray labels this as the 'expressive' phase, and writes, 'The reduced drive of the ego and the heightened ability to empathize makes this the Optimum Time to talk to people'.[220] I have observed, when tracking my own cycle, that after my Waning Moon and Dark Moon phases in which I have prioritised my personal space and creative time, and my Waxing Moon phase, in which I have been more outcome-focused and have thrown myself into my work, my Full Moon time is when I finally feel the urge to redress the social balance, and I naturally want to socialize with friends and reconnect with my husband, re-fostering our intimacy.

---

216 The study cited by Northrup, *Women's Bodies, Women's Wisdom* (p.109) was by Dr Therese Benedek and Dr Boris Rubenstein—'Correlations Between Ovarian Activity and Psychodynamic Processes: The Ovulatory Phase', 1939

217 Northrup, p.109

218 Miranda Gray in *Red Moon*, p.38, suggests the archetype of the good mother or Queen for the ovulation phase.

219 Gray, *The Optimized Woman*, p.96

220 Ibid., p.98

Science concurs that this phase of higher oestrogen seems to cause more sociable behaviour in women. Neuropsychiatrist and author of *The Female Brain*, Louann Brizendine, M.D., explains how in teenage girls there is a correlation between higher oestrogen in the first phase of their cycle (that includes the Full Moon phase) and a heightened interest in socializing. She also explains that the teenage girls that were studied exhibited more relaxed, stress-resilient behaviour during this phase. This is in contrast to the second phase of the cycle (the premenstrual, Waning Moon phase) when oestrogen levels drop and progesterone levels are high instead, and girls were 'more likely to react with increased irritability and will want to be left alone.'[221]

Another interesting finding is that this rise in oestrogen at ovulation may have an effect on our brain functioning, causing an increase in left-hemisphere activity (associated with verbal fluency) and a decline in right-hemisphere activity (connected with visuo-spacial competencies like being able to mentally re-position 3D shapes).[222] This increase in verbal fluency might explain why this is truly our most expressive phase and why Gray advocates this as the best time in your cycle to have heart-to-heart dialogue with those close to you, as your ability to express yourself with compassion and tact is at its highest at this phase.[223]

---

221   Louann Brizendine, M.D., *The Female Brain*, p.35

222   I came across this assertion in Northrup's, *Women's Bodies, Women's Wisdom*, when she cites a research study by E. Hampson and D. Kimura, 'Reciprocal Effects of Hormonal Fluctuations on Human Motor and Perceptual Skills', which then led me to another study: 'Altered Functional Brain Asymmetry for Mental Rotation: Effect of Estradiol Change across the Menstrual Cycle' (see: https://www. ncbi.nlm.nih.gov/pmc/articles/PMC4549195/) This study seemed even more conclusive stating, 'Better performance in the LF (late follicular) than the EF (early follicular) phase was associated with a pattern of reduced recruitment of the right hemisphere and increased recruitment of the left hemisphere. The increased recruitment of the left hemisphere was directly associated with greater changes in estradiol. Given that the right hemisphere is the dominant hemisphere in visuo-spatial processing, our results suggest that estradiol is associated with reduced functional asymmetry, consistent with recent accounts of hormonal modulation of neurocognitive function.'

223   Gray in, *The Optimized Woman* writes, 'The *Expressive* phase provides us with the ability to strengthen the relationships that strengthen us, and it also gives us the ability to communicate in such a way as to get the best from these relationships,' p.99

ON TOP OF THE WORLD

The peak in oestrogen during this ovulation-phase also seems to positively affect a woman's mood. This could be related to the complex connection between oestrogen and the production of neurochemicals in the brain like serotonin and endorphins, both of which make you feel happy and counteract depression. The presence of oestrogen in a woman's body also promotes the production of allopregnanolone, a hormone that has strong anti-anxiety effects.[224] As well, during this phase, women tend to feel on top of their game physically because their immune system is at its most robust during ovulation.[225]

Maya Tiwari writes that the ovulation phase denotes the most feminine aspect of your cycle and says, 'The full moon cycle is the natural time for you to enjoy and celebrate your womanhood'. Tiwari recommends incorporating practices that nurture and beautify, such as, 'oil massages, aromatherapy, warm baths, moonlight dips in the water'.[226] Personally, I've noticed that when I ovulate, I have a natural inclination to go clothes shopping, which invariably delivers even more pleasure for me during this phase than any other. If I'm going to do a spontaneous splurge on clothes, this is the point in my cycle when I am most likely to do it! Obviously the Full Moon phase urge to beautify oneself (and appear attractive to the opposite sex)—by enhancing my wardrobe—is unconsciously being enacted here! [227]

224 These facts come from an article, 'Estrogen in Psychiatry', from the website, PsycheEducation.org—http://psycheducation.org/hormones-and-mood-introduction/basic-information-about-estrogen-in-psychiatry/ —which also refers to two studies that have shown that oestrogen can treat depression in peri-menopausal women.

225 'Recent research has found that the immune system of the reproductive tract is cyclic as well, reaching its peak at ovulation, and then beginning to wane'—this is according to Christiane Northrup, *Women's Bodies, Women's Wisdom*, p.106

226 Maya Tiwari, *Women's Power to Heal Through Inner Medicine*, p.238

227 In a fascinating article in the *Daily Mail*, 'Forget PMT—here's the real time of the month that that sends us women crazy: From sex to shopping binges, new research reveals how your moods are dictated by your ovulation day'. The author, Clair Goldwin, refers to studies that have shown women are more competitive during their ovulation phase that results in this kind of shopping-behavior, particularly for the high-status, 'impulse buy'. Goldwin says that, according to Professor Karen Pine, a development psychologist at the University of Hertfordshire, this is called the 'Ornamentation Effect', and is intended to send out a clear signal to men that you are an alpha female. See: http://www.dailymail.co.uk/femail/article-2648907/Forget-PMT-heres-real-time-month-sends-women-crazy-From-sex-shopping-binges-new-research-reveals-moods-dictated-ovulation-day.html#ixzz4u1OvayHb

It should be noted that not all women experience their ovulation as a high. Some women suffer ovulation pain, or 'mittelschmerz', which can feel like a sharp stabbing pain or twinging in the pelvic area. According to Dr Andrew Orr, a specialist in reproductive medicine and women's health, ovulation pain is a sign that there may be an underlying cause—like endometriosis, PCOS (polycystic ovarian syndrome), or adhesions from previous surgery—and needs to be investigated by your gynaecologist.[228]

YOGA FOR THE FULL MOON PHASE

Principles and guidelines for your Full Moon yoga practice

The One Who Is at Play Everywhere says,
There is a space in the heart where everything meets.
Come here if you want to find me.
Mind, senses, soul, eternity—all are here.
Are you here?
Enter the bowl of vastness that is the heart.
Listen to the song that is always resonating.
Give yourself to it with total abandon.
Quiet ecstasy is here,
And a steady, regal sense
Of resting in a perfect spot.
You who are the embodiment of blessing,
Once you know the way,
The nature of attention will call you to return.
Again and again, answer the call,
And be saturated with knowing,
"I belong here, I am at home"

—RADIANCE SUTRA:26[229]

---

228   See: https://www.bellybelly.com.au/conception/ovulation-pain/

229   Lorin Roche Ph.D, *The Radiance Sutras*, p.61

Open the heart and the womb

You are better able to enhance your experience of this archetypically feminine phase of your cycle if you indulge in postures and practices (breathing, relaxation and meditation) that nourish and activate the two most feminine of your energy-centres: the heart-centre and the womb-space.

Choose Active and Supported Backbends, or what I call the 'Heart-Opening' poses, to work with the innately loving and uplifting energy of this more outwardly nurturing and expressive phase. And, to maximise your fertility and 'juiciness' and strengthen your *shakti prana*[230] at this time when you are potentially producing a fertile egg, play with Womb-Salutes (feminine Lunar Salutes—see the Classical Feminine Flow Full Moon Sequence at the end of this chapter) that include circling, flowing movements through the hips and pelvis, as well as connecting with your sacrum (the back of the pelvic bowl).

At any time in your yoga practice, most particularly when you are resting in a Restorative posture, or at the beginning or end of your practice, you can also incorporate the simple practice of the Soft Belly Breath (see p.100) with your hands resting on your lower belly—your womb-space—to more deeply ground your awareness there.

Connect the womb and the heart

> We all have moments of living below the waist
> or above the waist, but true empowerment—and
> your magnetic presence—come alive when both
> "power centres" communicate with each other.
>
> —RACHAEL JAYNE GROOVER[231]

As well as individually nurturing the energy within the two feminine Chakras—the heart and womb-spaces—it's also beneficial to foster the connection *between* them, particularly if you're hoping to get pregnant.

According to Chinese medicine there is an important meridian (energy channel) that flows between the heart and the uterus called the 'Chong Mai' meridian that must be open for conception to occur. In an interesting article by acupuncturist and chiropractor Dr John Veltheim, he explains

---

230   *Shakti prana* means 'feminine energy'. See p.55 in chapter three for more of an explanation of this term.

231   Rachael Jayne Groover, *Powerful and Feminine*, p.82

the importance of the Chong Mai Meridian for our health and vitality as women and that if the energy in this meridian is disrupted by hysterectomy or depleted by stress this can have negative repercussions:

> In modern times, where there is continuing stress exhaustion, it is often the Chong Mai meridian that suffers the most. The Chong Mai works at its best when the body has abundant energy and is stress-free. In a sense it is considered the energy system indicative of good health because when the Chong Mai is "full" the whole abdominal cavity is filled with nurturing energy, the organs are vital, the breasts are full, the lungs are strong, and the face is wrinkle free.[232]

One of the simplest ways to engender the womb-heart connection is by practising the Heart-Womb Mudra (right hand on the womb-space, left hand at the centre of your chest—see Figure 2, p.59). This Mudra can be performed at the beginning or end of your Full Moon yoga practice, in a sitting, standing or lying position, to help centre and ground you, bringing an immediate connection between these two sacred feminine centres. You may also want to practise the Womb-Heart Meditation on page 59.

Be creative and playful

> *Flowing is more than a rhythm; it's a specific energy field in which the feminine aspect of the soul is revealed in all its awesome beauty, fierce power, and animal magnetism. Deep within each one of us is a mother longing to nurture, a mistress impatient to flirt, and a madonna serene in her wisdom. And they all bop out when the beat kicks in.*

> —GABRIELLE ROTH[233]

---

232 Dr John Veltheim from an article called, 'The Penetrating Meridian (Chong Mai)'— https://www.bodytalksystem.com/learn/news/article.cfm?id=761

233 Gabrielle Roth, *Sweat Your Prayers*, p.54

One of the qualities of femininity is playfulness,[234] and this can be embodied in your Full Moon Feminine Yoga practice. In a spirit of feminine frivolity, you may want to broaden your movement practice beyond the confines of what is considered 'traditional' yoga and include some free-flowing movements and even some dance.

During my Full Moon phase, I find myself intuitively working with lots of flowing hip-circling movements—what I call 'Womb-Circles'—in various sitting and standing positions (see Figure 159, p.223 and Figure 187, p.230). These movements free up the energy in the pelvis and stimulate the root and sacral (womb-space) areas, facilitating optimal fertility, and naturally aligning with your heightened sensuality at this time of the month.

A free-dance technique known as 'Five Rhythms', created by Gabrielle Roth, offers an exploratory framework for what Roth has identified as the qualities or energies that form the undercurrent of our lives. It's one of these rhythms, the 'Flowing Rhythm', which serves as a key inspiration for my Feminine Yoga approach to the Full Moon phase. I believe that the movements we naturally adopt during our Full Moon phase—flowing, juicy, playful, sexy—are the same as those that are explored in the Flowing Rhythm dance practice. The grace and natural femininity of the Full Moon phase informs the Vinyasa (linked posture) sequences I find myself creating during this phase.

It can be liberating and balm-like to your feminine soul to sometimes break out of the confines of your yoga mat completely, put on some of your favourite Full Moon inspiring tunes[235] and dance with abandon—playing with feminine, flowing moves that may instinctively include lots of hip circling, swaying and undulations. Let your free-flowing dance-yoga movements reflect your innate joy and natural creativity at this time of the month.

---

234   Dr Azra Bertrand and Seren Bertrhand, authors of *Sacred Womb Rituals: Nourishing the Feminine Soul*, list the gifts of the feminine essence, and point #7 is described as, 'Joyfulness, **playfulness**—the ability to infuse any situation with these qualities, and lift any person into this state of being. **Laughter**, heartfelt smiles, having **fun** and daring to dream your happiness into being and imagine **magical** possibilities unfolding in every moment. To play with life and have an adventure'. See: https://www.thefountainoflife.org/womb-awakening/what-is-womb-awakening/gifts-of-the-feminine-essence/

235   See Appendix 4 for some Moving with the Moon playlist suggestions.

Come back to earth

> *The aspect of the soul that is mother lives in your*
> *hips and grounds you in an earthy, instinctive way. Not*
> *to be grounded is to be like an uprooted tree.*
>
> – GABRIELLE ROTH[236]

Alongside Heart-Opening postures and practices, and flowing, sensual movements, a Full Moon yoga practice also embodies an earthy energy that inspires deep, hip opening postures like the Pigeon Pose (see Figure 149, p.208) and what I consider to be the quintessential Full Moon posture, Malasana (The Earth Squat Pose—see Figure 147).

Classical Full Moon Pose: The Earth Squat

The Earth Squat circulates and strengthens *shakti prana* within the pelvic bowl as well as connecting you to the grounding and nourishing energy of 'mother earth'.

The optimum time to do this posture is during your Full Moon phase. It can be practised on its own or incorporated within a Full Moon Womb-Salute (see the Classical Feminine Flow Full Moon Sequence). I also like to do this pose on the beach—it seems to heighten the earthy, grounding effects. And, a little tip—if you have trouble squatting, you'll find that squatting in the sand is so much easier and more supportive for tight ankles and hips.

How to do it

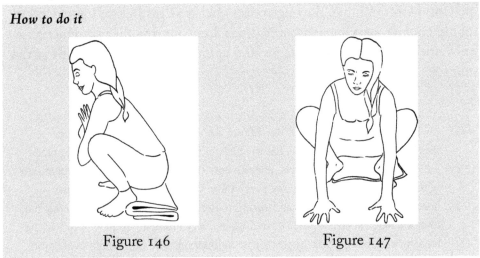

Figure 146   Figure 147

---

236   Gabrielle Roth, *Sweat Your Prayers*, p.60

Place your feet hip width apart, turn the toes out slightly and lower down into a squat. If your heels don't easily reach the ground, place a support (folded blanket or rolled mat) under your heels (see Figure 146).

To begin, place your palms on the ground in front of you, between your legs (see Figure 147). Take a few breaths here sensing the energy of the earth beneath your palms. Then, place your palms into a prayer position (see Figure 146).

Take a deep inhalation and a strong, releasing exhalation (out of the mouth if you like). Then, breathe deeply and smoothly focusing your awareness into your pelvic, womb-space area. Visualise the energy from 'mother earth' filling your womb-space with energising *prana*, boosting your natural *shakti* essence and overall feminine wellbeing. Stay here for as long as you are comfortable.

Contraindications and cautions for a Full Moon Yoga practice

As already touched on, there is a surge in oestrogen that triggers ovulation, but as soon as you have ovulated, your oestrogen levels begin to drop quite dramatically. Not only can this affect your mood as you begin to transition into the post-ovulation (Waning Moon) phase of our cycle, but it may also lead to a potential vulnerability to injury for the back and pelvis. Oestrogen is associated with providing strength to the muscles and ligaments so that when it departs, we may experience a weakness in the soft-tissue structures that support the lower back and pelvis. According to a BBC news article, 'Menstrual Cycle Injury Risk Link', a study conducted by Portland Hospital surveying 1000 osteopaths and 17 women, found that the risk of injury for women occurs not only towards the end of the cycle around early menstruation (as already mentioned in chapter four), but can also occur mid-cycle. The survey found that 21% of the osteopaths' female patients reported pain mainly in the lumbar and pelvic area during days 12–14 of their cycles—i.e. around ovulation time.[237]

This means that in your Full Moon yoga practice you need to take care in any of the stronger Heart-Opening or Backbending postures, and also in any deep hip-opening postures.

In concrete terms: when practising the more active, Dynamic Backbends during this phase of your cycle, such as Urdvha Dhanurasana (Wheel Pose—Figure 14, p.91) or Ustrasana (the Camel pose—see Figure 148) make sure you have warmed up sufficiently. Engage your abdominals

---

237   See: http://news.bbc.co.uk/2/hi/health/6354303.stm

and core, keep the knees parallel, avoid torqueing the pelvis, and focus on achieving opening and space in the thoracic spine, rather than facilitating all of the movement from the more mobile and vulnerable lumbar spine. In the hip-opening postures, take care, especially if you have a history of sacroiliac instability (SIJ). Don't go into the poses too deeply and always keep an awareness of symmetry and integrity in your pelvis. Note that in the Pigeon Pose (see Figure 149) I always recommend having a prop such as a folded blanket, block or bolster underneath the buttock of the front leg to avoid any potential injury (or exacerbation) to the sacroiliac joints.

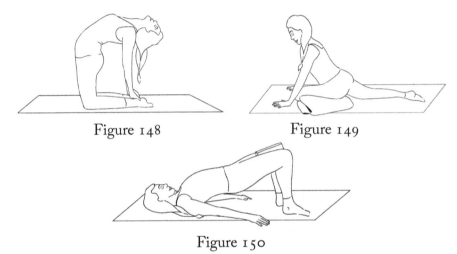

Figure 148   Figure 149

Figure 150

Additionally, to help balance and maintain the integrity of your sacrum and pelvis during this phase, it's a good idea to continue to do your stabilising movements—for example: Baby Bridge Pose squeezing a block (see Figure 150) or Utkatasana (Chair Pose) squeezing a block between the thighs (see Figure 120, p.179).

Of course, this all points back to the governing Feminine Yoga principle of *ahimsa*—practising 'non-violence' in how you approach your yoga practice. It's always about listening to your intuition on any given day that you practise, no matter which phase of your cycle you are in. If you feel like you have the energy and strength, by all means challenge yourself while still remaining mindful. If you happen to feel less energetic and vibrant, which can occur, even during this peak phase—particularly if your hormones are out of balance[238]—then don't push it or go against

---

238   One reason for having lower energy during your ovulatory phase may be connected to low oestrogen levels, as fatigue is one of the symptoms we can suffer if there is a deficiency in this hormone. See this clarifying article on what can happen if our oestrogen levels are too high or too low: http://www.cycleharmony.com/remedies/hormone-imbalance/signs-of-estrogen-dominance-or-deficiency

your natural lower ebb in energy. In this instance, you could choose to do some of the more gentle, passive Backbends instead (see the Heart-Opening postures in Appendix 3).

Full Moon Pranayama

Focus on the Inhalation

A key intention for Full Moon phase breathing practices is to focus on the inhalation, particularly when you are in the Heart-Opening positions. Breathe right down into your womb-space then allow the breath to fill all the way to the centre and then to the brim of the chest, the top lobes of the lungs. As you breathe this way, consciously foster spaciousness, energy and joy.

Feminine Ovarian Breathing

Ovarian Breathing could be classified as both a breathing technique and a meditation practice and it comes from the ancient Chinese Taoist and Chi Kung traditions. I enjoy it because it really helps me settle and soften my awareness into my womb-space, quiets my busy mind, and it leaves me with a feeling of dreamy femininity that particularly seems to suit the energy of my Full Moon phase. It can however be practised at any other phase in your cycle—except your Dark Moon menstrual phase. In fact, if boosting fertility is your focus, Mantak Chia suggests you do this practice during your post-menstruation–pre-ovulation (Waxing Moon) phase.[239]

Ovarian Breathing is said to regulate imbalances in the menstrual cycle and aid fertility.[240] Chia says it 'tones the pelvic diaphragm' and also writes, 'The whole lower abdomen is deeply massaged each time the pelvic diaphragm flexes. Life force flows into the region on periodic waves of breath which stimulates the glands and vital organs'.[241]

---

239 Mantak Chia, *Healing love through the Tao*, location 760 (Kindle edition)

240 'When practiced four to seven times a week, women have noticed changes in their menstrual cycles, such as less bleeding, decreased cramping, and a reduction in breast pain,' writes Mantak Chia in *Healing Love through the Tao*, location 730 (Kindle edition)

241 Mantak Chia, *Chi Kung for Women's Health and Sexual Vitality: A Handbook of Simple Exercises and Techniques*, location 741 (Kindle edition)

How to do it

The technique that I describe here has been largely inspired by how I was taught by American Taoist Sexology Teacher Willow Brown.[242] Brown simplifies this traditionally quite complex breathing and energy practice to make it more accessible, and she focuses on returning the energy to the womb-space (rather than the navel-centre) at the completion of the energy-circuit. I find this to be a more feminine approach that honours the womb-space as the centre of power for women.

To get ready for Ovarian Breathing come into a comfortable upright position—Mantak Chia suggests that this practice is best done with the sitting bones perched on the edge of a chair, or standing in the 'Chi Kung' stance (see Figure 27, p.103). The advantage of these positions is that they allow the feet to connect to the earth and for the free movement of the pelvis to rock forward, which can be helpful when you are pumping the energy from the front of the perineum to the anus and sacrum. However, if you feel that you have easy pelvic-rocking movement in a sitting position on the floor, this is fine too.

Begin by placing the hands in an adapted version of Yoni Mudra with your thumbs at your navel and your index fingers extending and touching at the tips to form a diamond-like shape (see Figure 1, p.54). Where your index fingers meet indicates the position of your uterus (deep within your body), or what the Taoists call your 'ovarian palace', and if you spread the little fingers slightly they will be resting over the position of the ovaries. Rub in small circles with your little fingers to warm and activate your ovaries.

Close your eyes and take a few Soft Belly Breaths (see p.100), breathing into your soft, lower belly, and specifically into your ovaries. Become aware of your ovaries as storehouses of latent energy. These are where all your potential for creating new life lies, and has always been. When a baby girl is still curled up in her mother's womb, her tiny ovaries already contain all the eggs she is ever going to use in her lifetime—about 300-500 potential mature eggs with a reserve of 450,000 others! [243]

Gently engage your pelvic floor several times—on your inhalations—as softly and subtly as a flower opening and closing; feeling that you are drawing energy up from the earth into your pelvic floor and into your ovaries, charging them still further with *chi* or life-force.

---

242   Find out more about Willow Brown's work here: http://yinwellness.com

243   Chia, *Chi Kung for Women's Sexual Health and Vitality*, location 159 (Kindle edition)

When you are ready, you will begin the process of pumping the latent energy from your ovaries into your 'ovarian palace' (womb). Do this by taking three short sips of breath in through your nose, then exhale deeply and fully. Then repeat. On each short, sipping inhalation imagine and even try to subtly sense your ovaries pulsing and squeezing as you draw the essential energy or 'ovarian *chi*' into your fallopian tubes and down and across into your womb.

Do these sipping breaths for a number of rounds—say, 6–9 times—until you start to feel that your 'ovarian palace' is filling up with this juicy nectar from your ovaries.

Once your 'ovarian palace' feels really full with this 'ovarian *chi*', take a gentle exhalation and simply allow the energy that you've gathered in your womb to drain down through your cervix (imagine it opening slightly), down through your vagina, through the lips of the labia, to the front of the pelvic floor around the urethra and the clitoris. Take a few moments just to let the energy settle there (without letting it leak further out of the body). Then on your inhalation, in a wave-like action of your pelvic floor, pulse the energy from the front to the back of the pelvic floor—from your urethral area to the anus and up into the sacrum. Do this three times. You can try rocking the pelvis forward as you do—inhaling and gently engaging the pelvic floor in a wave from front to back. From here, just breathe for a round or two feeling the energy at the base of the spine or even up into the sacrum.

Over the next three inhalations, accompanied by a gentle pelvic floor contraction, pump the energy using the back of your pelvic floor (anal muscles) up the spine from the sacrum to the base of the skull (occiput), or what the Taoists call the 'jade pillow'.

From here, you will circulate the energy around inside the head. First, circle 36 times in an anti-clockwise direction and then, 36 times in a clockwise direction. As you circle the energy around inside your head, you can imagine it's like fairy floss (cotton candy) that is gathering up all of the '*citta vritti*' (mind-chatter) so that your mind is becoming increasingly clear and empty. Willow Brown says that this circling, clearing action is very good for your pineal gland that lies deep inside the brain and is an important gland for your hormonal system. The pineal gland corresponds to the Third-Eye Chakra, an energy centre that is responsible for intuition and even psychic ability—qualities that will be enhanced with regular practice of this technique.

Now, bring the tip of the tongue to the roof of your mouth and simply allow the energy to drain down from the centre of the brain, through the throat, the chest and solar plexus, and back into the 'ovarian palace'.

As the energy flows down through the front of the body you can imagine it nourishing all the organs and glands along the way—the thyroid glands, thymus gland, the heart and lungs, the stomach, spleen, liver, and small and large intestines.

Once you have brought the energy down the front of the body back to the womb, you can then get ready to do another round—starting with little pulses of the ovaries, with three short, sipping inhalations, as you draw more ovarian energy into the 'ovarian palace'. Continue as for the first round, but when you get to circling the energy in the brain, first in an anti-clockwise direction, imagine an outward, every-increasing spiral that moves out and above the head, connecting with all-potentiality above you ('heaven energy') and stimulating the Crown Chakra. I like to pause here for a little while as I imagine the most perfect, ideal version of myself—soft, feminine, flowing, peaceful, loving. Then, as you reverse the circling (in a clockwise direction) feel an inward spiral, funnelling the energy back down, inside your head. Once you've finished your second round you can continue for one more round, or finish here.

After you've completed your last round, sit quietly for several breaths before coming out of the meditation, with your hands resting on your lower belly, noticing how you are now feeling as you sense into the soft, fullness—a kind of potent juiciness—there in your 'ovarian palace', your sacred, feminine womb-space.

Full Moon Mudras

Mudras are specific hand gestures that work to direct energy within the body and heal ailments of the body-mind. They are very calming and centring.

Anjali and Hands-to-Heart Mudras

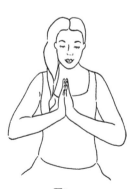

Figure 151

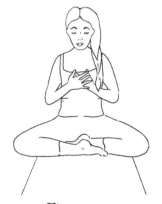

Figure 152

Benefits

These two simple Mudras connect us to our heart.

Anjali Mudra (see Figure 151) is a well-known Hindu gesture of prayer, gratitude and honouring; it signifies that you are honouring the other as well as yourself.

With your heart so open during your Full Moon phase, it's a fertile time to work with gratitude practices. By simply placing the palms together at the heart (centre of chest) and bowing the head we acknowledge all of the gifts in our lives, and this perpetuates an upward spiral of positivity for us and for those around us.

The Hands-to-Heart Mudra, (see Figure 152) or what well known American yoga teacher, Shiva Rea calls 'Svastika Mudra',[244] has a similar effect as Anjali Mudra, but is a little more personal and intimate in focus—it draws us inwards to connect with ourselves and our true heart's intention.

Lotus Mudra

Benefits

This beautiful Mudra relates to the Heart Chakra and symbolizes purity.[245] It therefore purifies and energises the heart-centre, and helps to cultivate feelings of compassion and gratitude. It is an effective Mudra to shift you out of your head into your 'heart'.

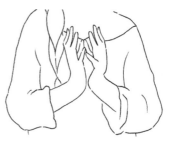

Figure 153

How to do it

Bring the palms together at the centre of the chest (heart-centre) into Anjali Mudra (see Figure 151). Keeping the tips of the little fingers and thumbs connected, fan open the other fingers into a beautiful, lotus-flower shape (see Figure 153).

Inhale into the heart area, behind the thumbs, feeling a beautiful sense of expansion and joyousness there.

---

244   Shiva Rea, *Tending the Heart Fire: Living in the Flow with the Pulse of Life*, p.136

245   Reference: Gertrud Hirschi, *Mudras: Yoga in your Hands*, p.150

Full Moon Relaxation & Visualisation Practices

Heart Cleansing Meditation

This visualization practice is inspired by Dinah Rodrigues, a Brazilian yoga teacher and author of *Hormone Yoga Therapy*.[246] It is best practised lying down. If you like, you can integrate it into your Savasana (relaxation pose) at the end of your practice. I like to also practise this visualization when I'm in a Supported Heart-Opening Restorative posture like the Supported Bridge Pose (see p.450)

How to do it

Once you are totally relaxed and settled into your chosen posture and your breath is gentle and even, you can begin this visualisation practice.

As you inhale, imagine white, healing, cleansing light flowing up from the fingertips of your left hand, up through your left arm, and into your heart. As you exhale, imagine dirty, muddy, sullied, dark light moving out of the right arm, out of the right fingertips, and out of the body. Repeat several times.

Then, reverse the direction: as you inhale, imagine white, healing, cleansing light flowing up from the right fingertips. And, so on.

After a few repetitions, now moving from right to left, you can let go of the visualisation and take some conscious breaths into your now, clean, clear, pure heart-space, before rolling to the side and coming up slowly to sitting.

Light of the Full Moon Yoga Nidra

Yoga Nidra is a deep, psychic relaxation that can be practised at any phase in the cycle in order to restore your energy. This Full Moon Yoga Nidra is designed to complement this joyful feminine phase, and includes a moon-light visualisation to nourish some of the key glands of our hormonal system in order to promote optimum menstrual cycle, and peri-meno-pausal, balance and vitality.

---

246   Dinah Rodrigues, *Hormone Yoga Therapy: To reactivate your hormone production and eliminate symptoms of menopause, TPM, Polycystic Ovaries, infertility*, p.145–146. Rodrigue's version that inspired my more simplified meditation is called 'Energy for Ovaries and Thyroid Yoga-Nidra to clean the nadis' and it involves moving the energy up the arms to the throat (rather than the heart-centre) to nourish the thyroid. She also emphasizes that you include in your awareness the area around the wrists as she claims these are points to activate the ovaries.

How to do it

Lie down on to the floor or your bed, with a small cushion or folded blanket underneath the head and a bolster or pillow underneath the knees. Place an eyebag on your eyes and cover yourself with a blanket or shawl if necessary so you can be warm and comfortable for the duration of the practice. Make sure you have created a space for yourself where you will not be disturbed for the next 15 minutes or so.

Position the arms so that they are a little way out from the sides of the body and not touching the body. The palms are uppermost, fingers lightly curling. The feet are at least hip distance apart and allow them to fall out to the sides so that your hips are loose and relaxed. Make any final adjustments to your posture to ensure that you are as comfortable and supported as possible and so that you will not need to move for the remainder of the relaxation practice.

Now, feel your body settling in. Know that this is your time, just for you. Nowhere to go, nothing to do, nobody you have to be. Just *be*. Time to rest and nourish yourself, soaking up your beautiful Full Moon time.

You can just let go here, softening more deeply into your body, into the embrace of the earth beneath you as you exhale deeply—through your mouth—if that feels good.

Now bring your awareness to your *sankalpa*. This is your positive resolution for change, your deepest, heartfelt desire. You may already have a *sankalpa* that you are working with—if so, bring this to mind now. Or, you can create a new one—a short, positive affirmation in the present tense. If you like, you can cultivate one directly related to your Full Moon time. Here's an example:

I am joyful, grateful and deeply connected to my feminine self.

Mentally repeat your *sankalpa* three times, with conviction. Planted deep into the fertile soil of your unconscious your *sankalpa* is a potent agent for positive change in your life.

Now, let go of your *sankalpa* and become aware again of your breath— the natural rise and fall of your breath through the nostrils. Feel the breath subtle and easeful, without any force or strain. Simply allow the breath to rise and fall of its own accord. Feel the slight coolness of the breath on the inhalation as it draws in through the nostrils, and feel the warmth of the breath, gently heated by the airways as you exhale.

We now begin the rotation of awareness around the body that is a key element of Yoga Nidra. As I name each part of the body, sense into that part of the body—picturing it, feeling it, letting go. If you find that your mind wanders or becomes sleepy, bring yourself back to the practice, even if you must do this many times.

Begin by becoming aware of your left hand thumb, first finger, second finger, third finger, fourth finger. Palm of the hand, back of the hand, left wrist, forearm, elbow, upper arm, armpit, shoulder. Left waist, left hip, upper left leg, knee, lower leg, left ankle, top of the foot, sole of the foot, big toe, second toe, third toe, fourth toe, fifth toe.

Move your awareness to your right hand thumb, first finger, second finger, third finger, fourth finger. Palm of the hand, back of the hand, right wrist, forearm, elbow, upper arm, armpit, shoulder. Right waist, right hip, upper right leg, knee, lower leg, right ankle, top of the foot, sole of the foot, big toe, second toe, third toe, fourth toe, fifth toe.

Moving up through the back of the body. Become aware of the left heel, right heel, back of the left knee, back of the right knee. Left buttock, right buttock. Sacrum, the bones of your sacrum. The lower back—left kidney and adrenal, right kidney and adrenal. The upper back—left shoulder blade, right shoulder blade. Back of the neck. Back of the head. Crown of the head.

Move your attention now to the front of the body. Left side of the forehead, right side of the forehead. Left temple, right temple. Left eyebrow, right eyebrow, eyebrow-centre. Left eye, right eye. Left cheek, right cheek. The nose—left nostril, right nostril, bridge of the nose. The mouth—upper lip, lower lip. Inside of the mouth. Left side of the jaw, right side of the jaw. The tongue. The chin. The throat—swallow and relax the inner walls of the throat.

Become aware of the chest—left side of the chest—left breast, right side of the chest—right breast. Centre of the chest, heart-centre. Now become aware of your abdomen—upper-abdomen (solar plexus), mid-abdomen (navel-centre), lower abdomen (womb-space). Stay here for a few breaths—feeling each inhalation creating a sense of space and ease in your belly and womb-space—each exhalation releasing any tension in the belly.

Finally, become aware of your left hip, right hip, the pelvis—the bones of the pelvis. And now the vagina—walls of the vagina. Feel the softness and openness of the walls of the vagina. And journey up through your vagina to the opening of the womb, the cervix. Sense your cervix—high and open. Feel your body ripe, juicy and fertile.

Now, bring your consciousness into your whole body. Your *whole body,* resting on the floor in this moment. *Whole body awareness.*

Become aware now of the point between your eyebrows—your third-eye-centre. Feel as if you are breathing in and out from this point.

After a few third-eye breaths, picture the full moon in your mind's eye. See the full moon in all its gorgeous, silver-white, radiant splendour. Visualise the shining, silver light of the full moon flowing down into your third-eye, flowing deep into the centre of your brain, bathing your pineal gland with its healing, balancing light.

Continue to feel this beautiful silver light circulating around your brain, nourishing the other important governing glands of your hormonal system—the hypothalamus and pituitary.

Now, watch as this silver, lunar light flows from your brain down through your throat, nourishing your thyroid glands, into your heart-centre, nourishing your thymus gland, and filling your heart-centre with its luminous, healing light and energy.

Take a few breaths at your heart-centre, the centre of your chest, watching the chest fill more and more with the beautiful moonlight, each time you inhale.

Then, allow this gorgeous, silvery light to flow from your heart down into your womb and to wash around your ovaries—nourishing and healing these organs as it moves and flows.

Watch as the glittering, silver moonlight flows throughout your *whole body*—your torso, your arms and legs. Feel how the effulgent moonlight is cleansing and balancing your whole body.

Bring to mind again your *sankalpa*—your heartfelt prayer for positive transformation. And mentally repeat your *sankalpa* three times, with conviction, knowing that, in time, this will come to pass.

Bring your awareness now to your whole body, your whole body, resting on this floor (or bed) in this moment. Feel the sensations within and around your body. Feel the air against any uncovered skin, the clothing and coverings against your skin. Feel the floor (or bed) beneath you. Without yet opening your eyes, become aware of your surroundings, your position in the room (as if you were looking at yourself from above). Become aware of any sounds around you.

In a few moments, you will be moving out of this rejuvenating Full Moon Yoga Nidra Practice, but before you do, just allow yourself to savour these last few moments of deep relaxation, deep rest, deep healing. And know that when you awaken from this practice you will feel refreshed and renewed, your mind calm and your heart open.

Begin now to bring movement into the body. Move the fingers and toes, wrists and ankles. Stretch and yawn, gradually awakening the energy in the body. And when you feel ready, without any sense of hurry, roll to the right hand side and rest there for a few breaths in a foetal position.

Always remembering to be gentle with yourself.

When you are ready, use your top left hand to press into the ground and roll yourself up to sitting. Come to sit quietly in a comfortable position for you—spine erect, shoulders relaxed back and down, and face and belly soft. Keeping your eyes closed, place your right hand on your lower belly (womb-space) and your left hand at the centre of the chest (heart-centre). Feel this gesture (Heart-Womb Mudra—Figure 2, p.59) as a reminder to yourself of how much you cherish this time to yourself—for self-love.

You are deepening your love and connection with your inner self, your inner sanctuary, connecting with the softness and feminine energy of your womb-space and heart-centre. Filling yourself up so you can then share this soft, loving energy with others.

Finish by placing both hands together at your heart-centre in Prayer Mudra (Anjali Mudra—see Figure 151, p.212), bowing down to your own heart and setting the intention to let your boundless love flow from your heart to everyone you come in contact with.

Namaste.

Full Moon Meditations

Smile to your Heart—Chocolate Meditation

This is a delicious, heart-opening meditation inspired by my dear friend and meditation teacher, Supiani Ucui.[247] It evokes feelings of deep contentment and happiness and helps you connect with others from a more loving, heart-felt space.

The magic of this meditation lies in the simple, physical practice of smiling and then feeling the energy of your smile within your heart-centre. To receive the full benefits of this practice you need to keep smiling and smiling—if someone were to walk into the room and see you meditating, they would see you smiling goofily to yourself! It's a discipline! Your natural instinct is most likely to feel silly, smiling to yourself, but I encourage you to persevere.

---

247 Connect with Supiani, Dayahati Healing, here: https://www.facebook.com/dayahati.healing

How to do it

Come into your favourite sitting position for meditation—kneeling, cross-legged, Siddhasana (see Figure 31, p.109), either on the floor or on a chair. Take some time to feel comfortable and relaxed in your body and mind. Relax the muscles around and behind the eyes, the upper and lower jaw; swallow to relax the throat, and feel the shoulders softening and melting, like ice melting into water.

Turn up the corners of your mouth, gently smiling to yourself.

Place your left palm onto the centre of your chest as you bring your attention to your heart-centre. If you like you can place your right palm on top of the left palm as in Hands-to-Heart Mudra (see Figure 152, p.212), or just have the left hand resting there. Take a few deep breaths into your heart-centre.

Then, begin smiling into your heart. While your mouth continues to smile, imagine your heart-centre smiling too. Think about your favourite chocolate—for example, dark chocolate. Think about 70% dark chocolate, smiling into your heart-centre. Now, think about 85% dark chocolate, smile more into your heart-centre. Finally, think about 90% dark chocolate, smile even more into your heart-centre.

Continue to think about the best quality dark chocolate (or milk chocolate, if you prefer!) feeling how it naturally helps you smile into your heart-centre. When thoughts enter your head, simply let them go and come back to focusing on smiling into your heart-centre.

Continue to smile into your heart for at least 5 minutes.

When you are ready to complete the practice, bring both palms together into the Prayer Mudra (Anjali Mudra—see Figure 151, p.212) at the heart-centre, and say a silent prayer of gratitude for all the gifts you have in your life. You might like to finish with Supiani's gratitude-prayer, repeating out loud or mentally:

Thank you Divine Source. Thank YOU!

Full Moon Lotus Meditation

Here is a beautiful, healing meditation to boost your heart-energy, which is lovely to practise at the full moon.

How to do it

Come into a comfortable sitting position and allow yourself to settle and soften for a few breaths. Then, bring your hands up to the heart into Lotus Mudra (see Figure 153, p.213). Bring your awareness into your heart-centre, feeling the space there behind the thumbs.

Visualise a flame deep within your heart-space. Focus on this flame and watch how as you exhale it becomes brighter. Continue fanning the light of the flame brighter for at least another five exhalations.

Then, as you inhale, imagine that you are breathing in positive qualities—such as: love, harmony, bliss and contentment—into your heart-space. Hold the energy of these positive feelings within your heart. As you exhale and the flame brightens, feel that you are offering up any negative qualities—deep-held tensions, fears, worries—to be cleansed and transformed by the fire of your heart.

Continue for as long as you like.

When you are ready to finish, place the palms back to together into the Prayer Mudra (Anjali Mudra—see Figure 151, p. 212), bowing your head in humility, and honouring the purity of your own heart.

Om shanti, shanti, shanti. (*Om Peace, Peace, Peace*)

Full Moon Yoga Sequences

POSTURES AND PRACTICES TO SUPPORT YOUR OVULATION PHASE

CLASSICAL FEMININE FLOW FULL MOON SEQUENCE

Best time to practise

This is a perfect practice for your ovulation phase—the few days when you ovulate, or at any time when you feel like doing a flowing, juicy, heart-centred practice. This is a fairly dynamic practice so it is best done when you feel strong and energetic.

Sequence duration

40-50 minutes, depending on how many rounds of the Full Moon Salutes you do.

Sequence benefits

The Classical Feminine Flow Full Moon Sequence helps you connect with your two sacred feminine energy centres—the heart-centre and the womb-space—and is an utterly delicious, inspiring practice! This sequence can help bring you into an embodied state of total presence that is refreshing and reveals your innate creativity and softness.

Props for this sequence

A yoga mat, a folded blanket, and 2 bolsters.

1. Centering: heart-womb mudra

How to practise

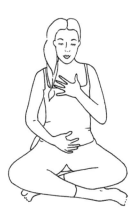

Sit in a cross-legged position and place your right palm on your lower belly (womb-space) and left palm at the centre of your chest (Heart-Womb Mudra—see Figure 154). Take some deeper breaths here, taking time be present in this moment and present to the sensations in your body and mind as you begin your Full Moon yoga practice. Feel how this Mudra helps you connect with the energy in both your heart and your womb and set the intention to nourish these two sacred feminine centres as you move through the practice.

Figure 154

2. Cross-legged warm up postures— Chest Opening Variation, Side-bends, Twists, Womb Circles, Forward Bend

Benefits

- These postures warm up the hips, spine, lower and upper back.
- Deepen the breathing—grounding and centering, and prepare the body-mind for the postures to come.
- The Cross-Legged Forward Bend stretches the hips and buttocks region, freeing up energy in the lower Chakras (energy centres).

Props for this posture

A folded blanket to sit on if you find that you have trouble sitting up straight through the spine (due to tight hips).

Recommended timing

See Posture 7 'Seated Cross-Legged Pose with Variations' on page 416 (from the Women's Pawanmuktasana Sequence) for recommended number of repetitions of each cross-legged warm up pose.

Cross-legged warm-ups: Chest Opening Variation, Side-bends, Twists, Womb Circling Variation

How to practise

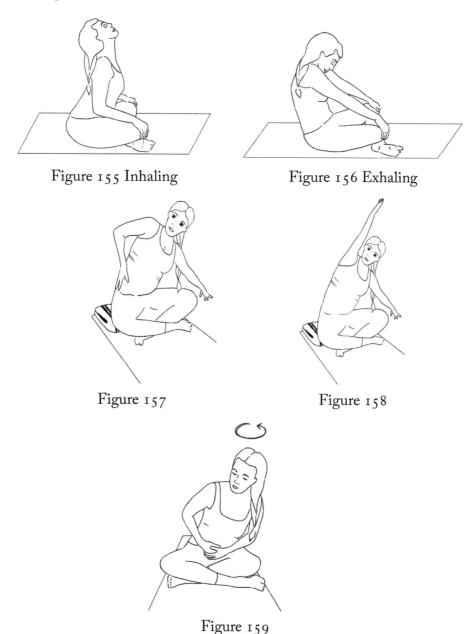

Figure 155 Inhaling   Figure 156 Exhaling

Figure 157   Figure 158

Figure 159

For these Cross-Legged Warm ups—see Posture 7 from the Women's Pawanmuktasana Sequence on page 416, for instructions.

Cross-Legged Forward Bend

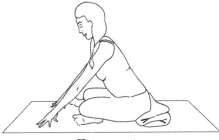

Figure 160

Come into a seated, cross-legged position, sitting on a folded blanket for extra support if you find that your lower back slumps and you can't sit up tall. Make sure you are in an open, cross-legged position, so that when you look down there is a large triangle between the legs; the ankles are not crossed too close towards the groins but more towards the knees (see Figure 91, p.152). Inhale and raise your arms overhead, feeling for length through the entire torso and, at the same time, ground the hips down into the floor beneath you. As you exhale, bend forward, tilting the top of the pelvis forward and place the hands on the floor a few feet in front of you. Inhale again, extending the chest forward, lengthening out the spine as you press the sitting bones back into the floor (or the folded blanket beneath you). Then as you exhale, fold forward more deeply or maintain your current position (see Figure 160).

Stay here in this gentle Forward Bend for another 5 or so breaths, allowing the belly to soften and relax, and sending the breath into any tight areas that you feel in the hips/buttocks or the lower back. Then, come up and change the cross-legs (bringing the other leg in front) and repeat on this side so you that you are evenly stretching into both hips.

3. Full moon salutes

Benefits

- This beautiful, feminine flowing sequence warms up the body and the progressive poses focus on stretching and strengthening target areas. It also aims to be flowing in a way that feels exquisitely sensuous helping you connect with your body and emotions.
- The overall focus of this Full Moon Salute Sequence is heart-opening—it opens the chest area to promote deeper breathing, release tension through the upper back, shoulders and neck, and create an uplifting emotional effect.

Props for this posture

Just your yoga mat.

Recommended timing

Do as many rounds of this Full Moon Salute as feels good for you—anywhere between 4-10 rounds would feel full and satisfying.

How to practise

I recommend you practise this sequence accompanied by some uplifting and inspiring music to really help you flow and 'groove' along. See Appendix 4 for my suggested playlist for this kind of Full Moon Feminine Flow practice.

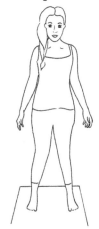

Start with the feet about hip width apart and parallel (outer edges of the feet parallel with the outer edges of your mat) hands by your side, knees slightly soft (see Figure 161). Take a few breaths to settle into the standing Mountain Pose (Tadasana), feeling your connection with the earth as you connect through the soles of the feet (in particular the heels) and lengthen the tailbone to the earth. At the same time feel a rebounding action coming from this connection with the earth in which the spine lengthens and the heart-centre (sternum/chest) lifts and opens.

Figure 161

Part 1: Wave Body Breath

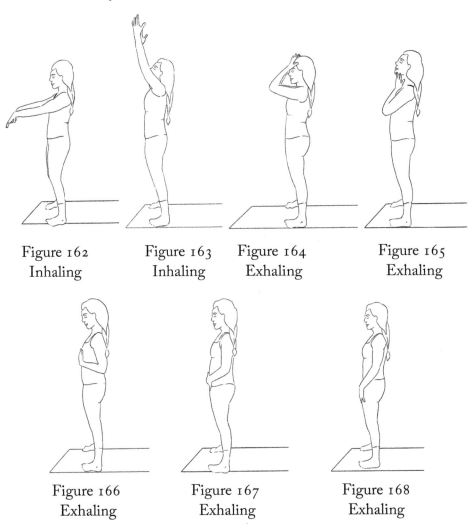

| Figure 162 | Figure 163 | Figure 164 | Figure 165 |
| Inhaling | Inhaling | Exhaling | Exhaling |

| Figure 166 | Figure 167 | Figure 168 |
| Exhaling | Exhaling | Exhaling |

Inhale and raise the arms up (in a wave-like action) in front of you and overhead (see Figure 162 & Figure 163). As you exhale brush the hands back down your body—over the forehead and face (Figure 164), throat (Figure 165), breasts (Figure 166), solar plexus, down to the belly (Figure 167), and all the way to the *yoni* (sacred vagina/pelvic area—Figure 168). Feel how this brushing action is both a nurturing gesture of self-care, as well as a way to connect deeply with your inner, feminine sensuality. Repeat this Wave Body Breath 2-3 times.

Part 2: Basic Lotus Breath Salute—Round One

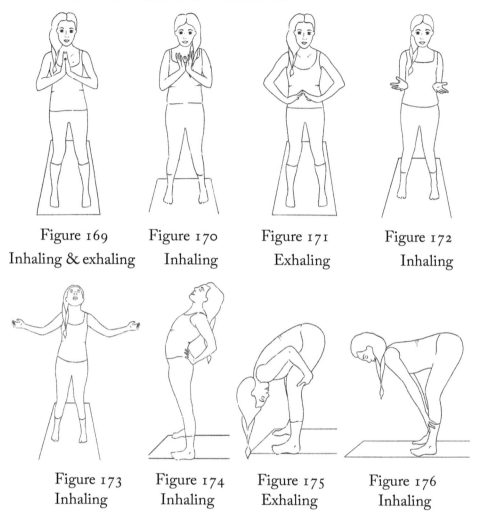

| Figure 169 | Figure 170 | Figure 171 | Figure 172 |
| Inhaling & exhaling | Inhaling | Exhaling | Inhaling |

| Figure 173 | Figure 174 | Figure 175 | Figure 176 |
| Inhaling | Inhaling | Exhaling | Inhaling |

Start this Part 2 of the Full Moon Salutes with your hands in Anjali (prayer) Mudra at the centre of the chest (see Figure 169). Open your hands out into Lotus Mudra—heels of the hands together, little fingers and thumb tips connecting, other fingers fanning out—and inhale here at the heart-centre (see Figure 170). As you exhale, release from Lotus Mudra and touch the tip of the middle fingers together as you push your palms down towards the earth, moving your hands to about navel-height (see Figure 171). Then, as you inhale, bring the hands up a little to just below your breast-height (see Figure 172) and open the arms out to the side (see Figure 173), and bring the hands all the way behind so that the palms are on the sacrum, fingers pointing up, elbows drawing in—continue to breathe in from the heart-centre as you expand the chest and lift the gaze (see Figure 174). On your next exhalation fold forward into Uttanasana (Standing Forward Fold) as you slide the hands down the buttocks and backs of the legs (see Figure 175). You can keep your knees a little bent if you need to so that the spine can hang freely.

As you inhale, lift yourself up into Urdvha Uttanasana with your hands on the floor if you can comfortably, or have your hands on your shins—extending forward from the heart (see Figure 176).

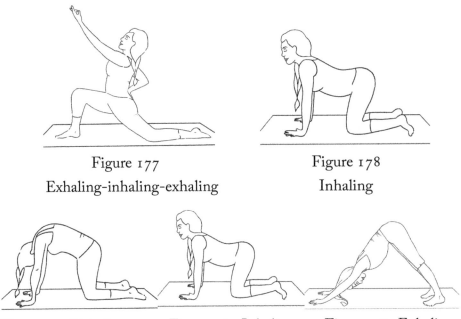

Figure 177
Exhaling-inhaling-exhaling

Figure 178
Inhaling

Figure 179 Exhaling   Figure 180 Inhaling   Figure 181 Exhaling

Then on your out-breath step your left foot back into Kneeling Crescent Lunge with your right hand on your sacrum and your left arm up in front, a little higher than eye-height, finger and thumb together into Jnana Mudra (see Figure 177). Inhale here. As you exhale, windmill the left arm over-head and behind you (tracing the shape of the full moon), and step the right leg back to come into table-top/all-fours, and inhale into Cow Pose (see Figure 178). Then, exhale into Cat Pose (see Figure 179). Inhale again into Cow Pose (see Figure 180) and as you exhale, turn the toes under, press your hands into the floor, lift your knees and extend your legs into Down Dog (see Figure 181). Take a few breaths to unfurl into Down Dog Pose: try 'Walking Dog'—bending one knee and extending the other—and also shifting from hip to hip as you organically, fluidly begin to open into your fullest version of the pose.

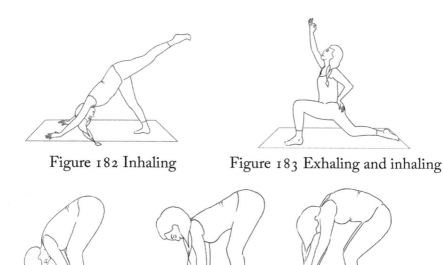

Figure 182 Inhaling   Figure 183 Exhaling and inhaling

Figure 184 Exhaling   Figure 185 Inhaling   Figure 186 Exhaling

From Down Dog Pose, inhale as you raise your left leg up to the sky behind you (see Figure 182) and exhale as you step the foot through to Crescent Kneeling Lunge again (see Figure 183), right arm up. Inhale here in Kneeling Crescent Lunge. Exhale as you step your right foot forward so that you are in Uttanasana (Standing Forward Fold—Figure 184). Inhale as you lift your chest up into Urdvha Uttanasana (hands on the shins or the floor—see Figure 185), and then exhale as you roll up through the spine, drawing the navel in and up, head rolling up last (see Figure 186).

Once you come to standing, inhale and raise your arms overhead, then exhale as you sweep your hands down the front of the body (face, throat, breasts, solar plexus, belly, *yoni* (see the Wave Body Breath—Part 1, Figure 163-Figure 168).

Finish this round by placing your hands or your lower belly (womb-space) taking a few Soft Belly Breaths (see p.100) here. And before you commence another round, do some Womb Circles—with your hands on your womb-space circle your hips, and even work with some figure-8 shapes, in both directions (see Figure 187).

Round 2

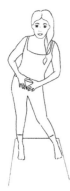

For the second round of your Full Moon Salutes, you can repeat the above basic Lotus Breath Salute (from Part 2, Figure 169) but step back on the right leg and then step forward on the right leg for the lunges.

Figure 187

Part 3: Building on the Lotus Breath Salute (Rounds 3-10)

Add the following additional 'build-postures' as you feel ready, over several rounds.

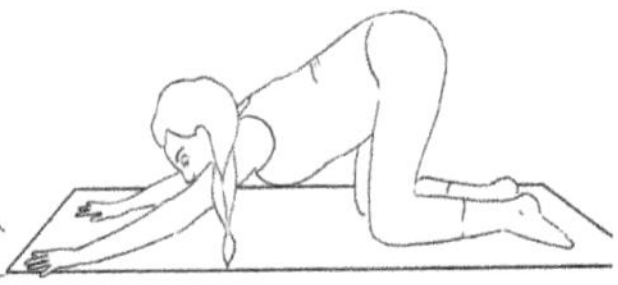

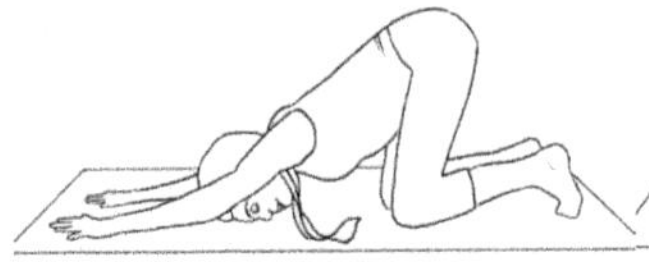

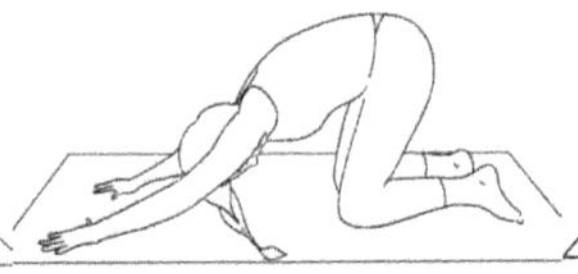

Figure 188   Figure 189 Exhaling   Figure 190 Inhaling

How to practise

Repeat as above until you get to Figure 178 and Figure 179 (Cat-Cow Pose). Instead of Cat-Cow Pose, from the Kneeling Crescent Lunge (Figure 177) step back into an all-fours/table-top position and extend your arms forward as you project the hips up and back to come into Anahatasana (Melting Heart Pose—see Figure 188). Rest here with the forehead onto the mat for a few breaths as you open the armpits towards the floor, feeling the space between the shoulder blades opening and softening.

Then, move into Wave-Anahatasana—exhale as you round the spine (as in the Cat Stretch—see Figure 189), dropping the head; inhale as you open the chest and heart back towards the floor, lifting your gaze slightly and mobilising the spine the other way (see Figure 190). Do this for several breaths feeling the spine fluid and articulating, in coordination with the breath.

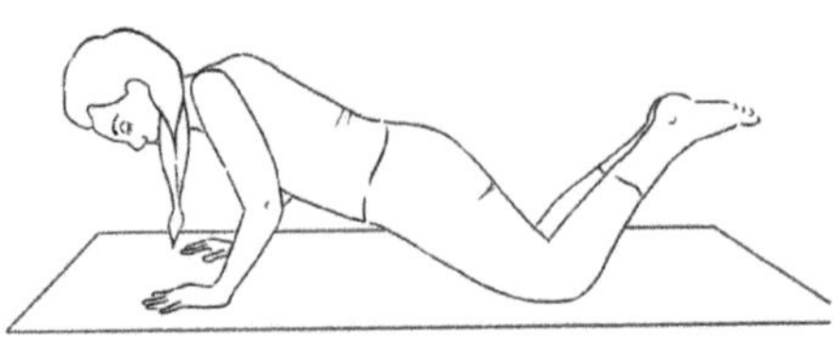

Figure 191 Exhaling 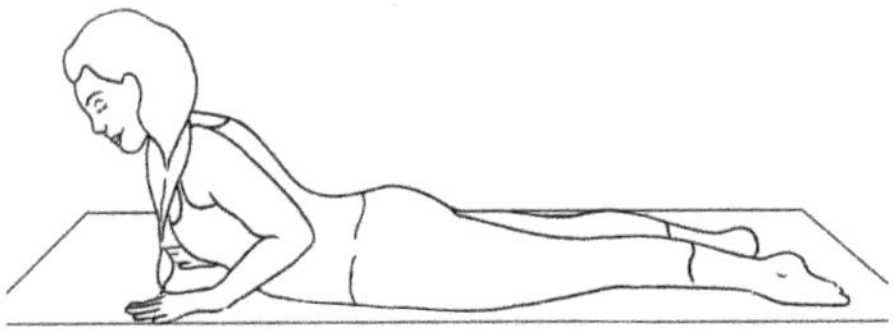   Figure 192 Inhaling

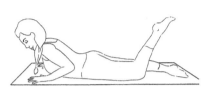

Figure 193 Inhaling and Exhaling

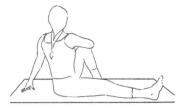

Figure 194 Inhaling and Exhaling

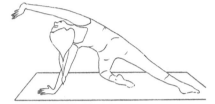

Figure 195 Inhaling and Exhaling

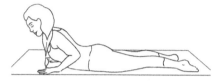

Figure 196 Inhaling and Exhaling

When you are ready bring the shoulders forward in alignment with the wrists and lower yourself down into a Baby Push Up (see Figure 191) as you exhale, keeping the shoulder blades stabilised back towards the hips. With the hands by the shoulders, roll the head and chest off the floor into Baby Cobra Pose (see Figure 192) as you inhale. Make sure you keep your belly on the floor and feel for the Backbend coming more from the upper back rather than the lower spine.

To build on this Cobra Pose you can roll each shoulder alternately, moving a little from side to side like a snake slithering. Then, begin to bend up each leg alternately as you roll each shoulder (see Figure 193). Eventually you'll build up enough momentum that, as you bend up the left leg, you will roll all the way up to sitting, rotating around towards your right.

From here, bend up the left leg and come into the Marichyasana Twist wrapping the right arm around the bent left leg (see Figure 194). Hold for here for a breath or two. Then evolve this pose into Rock Star—lowering the bent left knee onto the floor, bringing the weight into that knee and extending the right leg to bring the right foot onto the floor, and sweeping the right arm in a diagonal line, as you lift the hips forward and up (see Figure 195). Hold here for several breaths. Then, roll back the way you came—back onto your stomach into Baby Cobra (see Figure 196). From here, you can repeat the whole sequence (Cobra-Marichyasana III-Rock Star) on the other side[248]. Or you can come back to the second side after you've done another round of Salutes.

---

248 This little section of the sequence—From Figures 193-196— was inspired by international yoga teacher, Delamay Devi. See more about here work here: https://www.delamaydevi.com/ '

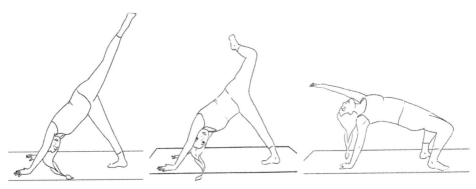

Figure 197   Figure 198   Figure 199

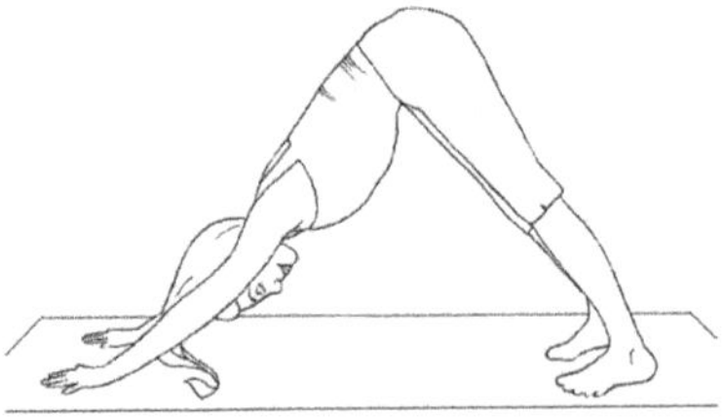

Figure 200

After you've come back into Baby Cobra, you can press your hands into the floor to push back into Down Dog Pose (see Figure 200). From Down Dog, raise up your left leg and then roll the hip up to the ceiling (see Figure 197). From here, bend the left leg, the foot dropping towards the buttock and continue to peel open the left hip up towards the ceiling. Look underneath the left arm as you spiral the belly and chest up towards the ceiling (see Figure 198). Just breathe naturally as you do this.

Then, pivoting on the right foot, keep dropping the left foot further towards the floor, rolling the left hip up, lifting the left hand off the floor so that you end up with your weight into your right hand and both hips facing towards the ceiling. Let the left arm extend up and overhead to get a full opening through the left hip into the left shoulder. This pose is called Wild Thing (see Figure 199). Hold for a breath or three and then pivot around to face back into Down Dog Pose (Figure 200).

From Down Dog Pose step your left foot forward (or if you're on Round 2 or 4, step your right foot forward) into the Kneeling Crescent Lunge (Figure 183) and continue all the way back to Tadasana (Figure 184-Figure 186, then, Figure 163-Figure 168), completing another round.

Continue another full round up, starting from Figure 169—Part 2 Basic Lotus Breath Salute, up until Figure 178 and Figure 179 (Cat-Cow Pose), substituting Anahatasana (Figure 188) for Cat-Cow Pose, and then doing Baby Push Up Pose (Figure 191) and Cobra (Figure 192) into Down Dog Pose .

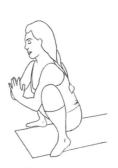

Figure 201

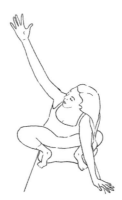

Figure 202

After stepping your right foot forward into Kneeling Crescent Lunge (if it's the second, fourth or sixth round, otherwise stepping the left foot forward), step the other foot forward and come into Malasana (Squat Pose—see Figure 201). If you find your heels don't rest easily on the floor, put a folded blanket under the heels (see Figure 146, p.206), and begin by pressing the palms together into prayer position, the arms between the legs. From here place your left hand onto the floor and extend your right arm up in a diagonal direction, looking up towards the right hand (see Figure 202). As you descend the hips and ground the heels lift up and out of the hips with the chest and torso so there is a lightness through your upper body. Hold this extended arm version of the Squat Pose for several breaths before changing sides and extending the opposite left arm up. Then straighten the legs and lift the hips to come into Uttanasana (see Figure 184) and roll up to standing to complete this round of the Salutes.

Additional postures to add to this sequence are Utkatasana (Standing Squat Pose—see Figure 120, p.179) and Twisting Utkatasana (Figure 203). Do these postures at the start of a new round after Tadasana (Figure 169) and before coming into Uttanasana (Figure 175).

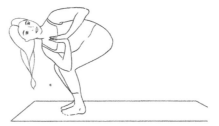

Figure 203

Safety Notes for the Full Moon Salutes

If you have any lower back pain always bend your knees in Uttanasana (Figure 175 and Figure 184) Don't force any position and make sure you feel adequately warmed up before building up to any of the progressive postures (eg: Wild Thing—Figure 199—and Dancing Pigeon—see below).

4. Pigeon pose

Benefits

- Opens the hips—specifically the buttock/piriformis muscles; stretches the psoas muscle (particularly this upright version); Dancing Pigeon Pose also stretches the quadriceps (frontal thigh muscles).
- The upright version opens the heart and deep-belly areas, and the flowing, dynamic sequence (raising and lowering the torso) loosens the spine and frees up the breath.
- Brings circulation to the pelvic area (blood circulation and *shakti prana*) boosting your reproductive health and feminine vitality.

Props for this posture

I recommend you place a folded blanket under the hip (sitting bone) of the leg that is bent up in front (see Figure 149, p.208). Propping the front hip helps prevent knee injury and torqueing in the sacrum, protecting the SIJ (sacroiliac joint).

Recommended timing

Do the dynamic version—raising and lowering the torso with the breath— for 3-5 repetitions. Then, hold the pose for up to 5 slow breaths. For the Dancing Pigeon Variation, hold for a further 5 slow breaths.

How to practise

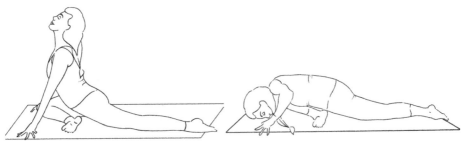

Figure 204 Inhaling   Figure 205 Exhaling

Enter this pose from Down Dog Pose (see Figure 181). In order for your practice to best flow, you may want to do a round of the Full Moon Salute to bring you to Down Dog. From Down Dog raise your right leg and step the knee and shin through so that that the knee is toward towards the right side of your mat and the foot is just in front of your groin, the left leg is extended behind you in line with the hip (see Figure 204). Place a folded blanket underneath the front right sitting bone/buttock to ensure the hips are level (see Figure 149, p.208). Have the hands just in front of your front leg, resting on your fingertips (cupping your hands).

Begin by working dynamically—inhale as you raise your chest, lifting your torso up tall out of the hips and lifting your gaze (Figure 204); exhale as you lower your chest and forehead towards the floor, bowing forward (Figure 205). Repeat this dynamic movement another 2-4 times. Then hold the pose either with the torso raised or the forehead resting on the floor (whichever feels like it gives you the most-needed stretch) for another 5 breaths or so.

From here, you can evolve into the more advanced variation, Dancing Pigeon Pose (see below), or simply press the palms into the floor and step the front leg back into Down Dog Pose.

Variation: Dancing Pigeon Pose

This is a more advanced version of Pigeon Pose. It's a good idea to make sure your muscles are really warm before embarking on this pose.

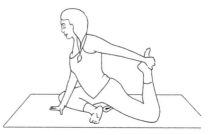

Figure 206

From Pigeon Pose, bend up the leg that is extended. So, if you right leg is in front, bend up your left leg, moving the foot towards the centre of the buttock. Use the left hand to draw the foot into the stretch and support yourself with your right hand into the floor (see Figure 206). Square your hips so you sink into the frontal hip of that left leg and, at the same time, have a sense of lengthening the left kneecap away from the hip, to deepen the stretch through the quadriceps.

Hold for about 5 breaths, during which time you may find that you are able to soften a little more deeply into the stretch and can move the foot a little closer to the buttock. When you are ready to come out of the pose, straighten the left leg and press the palms into the floor by the front leg to push back into Down Dog Pose preparing to do Pigeon and then Dancing Pigeon on the other leg.

5. Ardha matsyendrasana—hand to heart variation

Benefits

- Stimulates the liver and kidneys.
- Boosts digestion.
- Releases tightness in the hips, spinal muscles, shoulders and upper back.
- This 'Hand to Heart' variation helps you connect with the heart— it's grounding and nurturing.

Props for this posture

If you have difficulty sitting up tall in this position you may need to raise yourself so you are sitting on the short end of a folded blanket or even along the wide edge of a yoga block.

Recommended timing

Stay in this Twisting pose for 5 breaths or so on each side.

How to practise

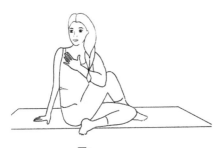

Figure 207

From Down Dog Pose (Figure 181, p.228), jump or step the legs through the hands, via cross-legs, into Dandasana (Staff Pose—Figure 123, p.182). Bend up the left leg to bring the foot around to the outside of the right buttock, the knee pointing forward. Then, pick up your right foot to bring it on the outside of the left knee, sole of the foot into the floor. Bring your right hand onto the floor behind you, close to your spine. Inhale, and raise your left arm up to extend through the spine and both sides of the torso. As you exhale, bring the left arm around the right knee and hug the knee towards the left side of the chest, as you place the left palm onto the centre of your chest (heart-centre) and twist to the right (see Figure 207).

Hold for about 5 breaths; with each exhalation squeezing from the belly, and creating more space through the spinal column. When you are ready to come out, slowly release the twist and straighten the legs. Repeat on the other side.

6. Supported bridge pose with a bolster

For benefits, props and instructions for the Supported Bridge Pose see Posture 9, Variation A from the Classical Dark Moon Menstrual Sequence, page 137.

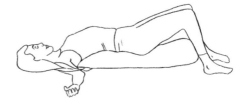

Figure 208

7. Simple savasana (Final Relaxation)

For instructions see Posture 18 from the Waxing Moon Post-Menstrual Sequence, page p.189

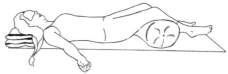

Figure 209

8. Ovarian breathing or smile to your heart—chocolate meditation

See page 209 for instructions on Ovarian Breathing. See page 218 for instructions on the Smile to your Heart—Chocolate Meditation.

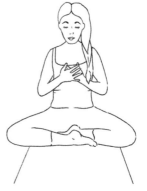

Figure 210

BUSY DAYS NURTURING FULL MOON SEQUENCE

Best time to practise

This sequence is great for any time during your Full Moon (ovulation) phase when you are seeking a nurturing practice that is short enough to fit into your busy day.

Sequence duration

This sequence will take you around 25 minutes, depending on how long you choose to stay in the Restorative postures.

Sequence benefits

A nurturing and rejuvenating heart and belly opening practice that connects you with your innate softness and femininity.

Props for this sequence

A yoga mat, a yoga bolster, a yoga block, and a folded blanket.

1. Supta baddha konasana (reclining bound angle pose)

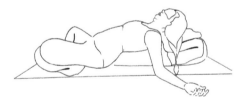

See Posture 7 in the Classical Dark Moon Menstrual Sequence, page 132, for benefits and instructions.

Figure 211

2. Cat-cow pose with variations

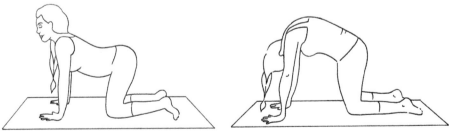

Figure 212 Inhaling   Figure 213 Exhaling

See Posture 5 in the Classical Dark Moon Menstrual sequence, page 129, for props, benefits and instructions.

Variation A: Side stretch Cat and 'Snaky Cat'

After doing Cat-Cow Pose, bring your spine back into neutral (table-top) and as you exhale move your head to the left, looking towards the left hip as you curve the right side of the torso and compress the left ribs towards the hips, squeezing the left

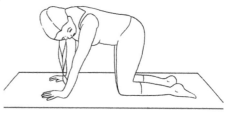

Figure 214

waist muscles (see Figure 214). Inhale and straighten up your spine bringing your head back to centre. Exhale and curve the spine over towards the right as you look towards the right hip. Inhale back to centre. Repeat another 3-5 times on both sides. Then, when you're ready, move into Snaky Cat, moving your tail from side to side as you undulate through the whole spine up unto the head.

Variation B: All-Fours Hip Circles

See page 130 from the Classical Dark Moon Menstrual Sequence for instructions on practising this variation.

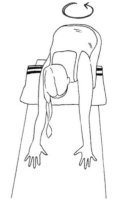

Figure 215

3. Anahatasana (melting heart pose)

Benefits

- Releases tightness in the upper back and shoulders.
- Stretches the spine.

Props

Just your yoga mat.

Recommended Timing

Stay here for 5-10 deep breaths

How to practise

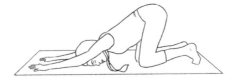

Figure 216

Still in the all-fours position, extend your arms forward, placing your palms about shoulder-width apart, as you project the hips up and back. Rest your forehead onto the mat, toes turned under (see Figure 216). Keep extending through your arms actively as you feel your armpit-chest area softening, 'draping' towards the floor, and the space between the shoulder blades opening.

When you are ready to come out return to the all-fours position.

4. Supported bridge pose with a block

See Posture 4 in the Dark Moon Late Menstrual Sequence, page 153 for benefits and instructions.

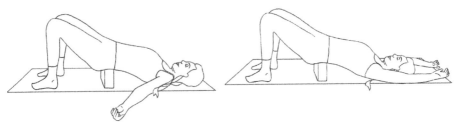

Figure 217   Figure 218

Variation: Block on Tallest End

If it feels comfortable for you, turn the block to its tallest height and lift your hips to rest your sacrum onto it. You can either keep your arms to the side (see Figure 217), have your arms bent up overhead (see Figure

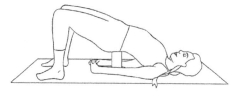

Figure 219

218), or, for a stronger shoulder opening, interlace your hands around the block, little finger-edge of the hands pressing into the floor, shoulder blades drawing in, shoulder-heads rolling under (see Figure 219).

Stay here for as long as you're comfortable—up to 2 minutes. But make sure you change the interlace of the hands (to evenly stretch through the wrists and the shoulders) halfway through your timing.

5. Supported child pose with a bolster

See Posture 8, Variation A, in the Classical Dark Moon Menstrual Sequence page 134 for benefits and instructions.

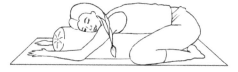

Figure 220

CHAPTER SEVEN
THE WANING MOON: CREATING SPACE

Every month the wildness courses through the female,
enriching her blood and compelling her to follow down
the overgrown pathway into the depths of the psyche. The
wolf stalks, the hawk circles, the mad dog bares the teeth.
Many women try to tame these beasts and control their
fury because they don't understand their meaning or their
message. But one might as well tell the moon not to rise
or the high tide to control its surge and swell. Understand
them or not, make time for them or not, like them or not, the
hormones will rage, for they are part of the blood's power.

Open the door and invite them in. Howl with them. Use
their presence to speak of the disappointments and fears
that have accumulated since they last spent time with
you. Confess your fears, let go of your anger, surrender your
control. Then when the raging is dying down, release your
emotions on the tailwinds of their departing energy.

—JASON ELIAS AND KATHERINE KETCHAM[249]

In the waning phase of the lunar cycle, the moon moves towards darkness. In the same way, within our own bodies, we find that our physical and mental energy wanes as we prepare to menstruate. For some women, this diminishing energy might extend for a week to 10 days before they bleed; for others, it might be that they feel suddenly and exceptionally tired the day before they bleed.

---

249 Jason Elias and Katherine Ketcham, *In the House of the Moon: Reclaiming the Feminine Spirit Healing*, p.178

In medical terms, this is called the luteal phase, which spans from post ovulation to the first day of the menses, and on average is 14 days long. For many women, the latter part of this phase—about the week leading up to menstruation[250]—is the most challenging time in their whole monthly cycle. This is when you may experience the dreaded PMS (Premenstrual Syndrome) symptoms that include moodiness, bloating, tiredness, headaches, food cravings—and that's just a few of the more than 150 potential premenstrual symptoms women can experience![251]

An estimated 80% of women in Australia regularly suffer one or more of these 150 monthly symptoms.[252] In the USA, the American College of Obstetricians and Gynecologists estimates that at least 85% of menstruating women suffer PMS. And about 5% of women suffer an extreme form of PMS called Premenstrual Dysphoric Disorder (PMDD).[253] PMDD can manifest as extreme aggression or rage, anxiety, and blood sugar disturbances. It has been known to lead to psychosis, suicide, and even murder!

WHAT CAUSES PMS?

The jury is out as to what definitively causes these premenstrual symptoms, and in fact if PMS even exists—more on that later! One view is that PMS is potentially related to the fluctuating levels of hormones during your cycle: just before you bleed, the key female hormones of oestrogen and progesterone plunge to their lowest monthly levels. Louann Brizendine, M.D. suggests that for some women, PMS is caused by 'estrogen and progesterone withdrawal in the brain'. Brizendine makes the point that

---

250   'Duration of symptoms each month averages six days, with severity usually peaking anywhere from two days before to the first day of the menstrual flow,'—see this research study: https://www.aafp.org/afp/2011/1015/p918.htmln Although health journalist and author of *28 Days: What Your Cycle Reveals about Your Love Life, Moods and Potential*, Gabrielle Lichtermann suggests that many of us may experience a kind of "pre-PMS" much earlier in our Waning Moon phase. She says in the 1-2 days after we ovulate, due to the drop in oestrogen 'you'll likely feel slightly fatigued to downright lethargic, have intermittent irritability, be mentally foggy or forgetful and have a significantly lower sex drive.' See: https://www.myhormonology.com/hormonology-road-map/

251   See: http://www.webmd.com/women/pms/premenstrual-syndrome-pms-symptoms

252   See: http://www.abc.net.au/health/features/stories/2005/12/08/1836110.htm

253   Ibid.

women who naturally produce more oestrogen and progesterone are more resistant to stress because the brain produces higher levels of serotonin (the 'feel-good' chemical). She goes on to explain that of the 80% of women who experience PMS symptoms, about 10% say they get extremely 'edgy and easily upset … Those women with the least estrogen and progesterone are more sensitive to stress and have fewer serotonin brain cells.' She adds, 'For those stress-sensitive individuals, the final days before their period starts can be hell on earth.'[254]

Dr Brizendine suggests that the hormonal changes, and related plunge in serotonin, can affect the proper functioning of your prefrontal cortex in the brain (the brain's seat of judgment) causing 'dramatic, uncontrolled emotions' to 'push through more easily from the primitive parts of our brains.'[255] I'm sure many women can relate to the feeling that they have temporarily lost their usual rational capabilities and are almost completely beholden to their emotions leading up to 'that time of the month'!

Sara Gottfried, M.D. suggests that PMS symptoms like rage, headaches, insomnia and anxiety may be present in those women who have low levels of progesterone during this second (luteal) phase of their cycle, causing an oestrogen dominance. Interestingly, progesterone has a calming and sedating effect on your body and emotions. Gottfried writes, 'Progesterone literally soothes you when you get enraged. It helps you sleep. When you produce the right amount you feel more level headed and relaxed.'[256]

Other factors that may contribute to the occurrence of PMS in your cycle are: depletion of vitamins and minerals; and poor diet, including too much salty food (causing fluid retention) and too much alcohol and caffeine, which can alter your moods and energy levels.[257]

Stress and pre-existing emotional problems do not seem to necessarily cause PMS, but doctors and health professionals concur that they can make it worse.[258] John Eden, associate professor in reproductive endocrinology at the University of New South Wales says, 'If you've got a high-powered job and lot of stress in your life, that aggravates everything.'[259]

---

254 Louann Brizendine, M.D., *The Female Brain*, p.47

255 Ibid

256 Sara Gottfried M.D., *The Hormone Cure*, location 2191 (Kindle edition)

257 See: https://www.womenshealth.gov/a-z-topics/premenstrual-syndrome

258 Ibid.

259 Cited at: http://www.abc.net.au/health/features/stories/2005/12/08/1836110.htm

Dr Christiane Northrup says that premenstrual symptoms are related to 'cellular inflammation, resulting from a complex interaction of emotional, physical, and genetic factors.'[260]

IS PMS ALL IN YOUR HEAD?

The complexity surrounding the potential causes of PMS was perhaps not considered in a meta-analysis study conducted by a team of Canadian researchers in 2013, which concluded that emotional symptoms of PMS do not in fact exist—that it's a myth and all in our heads![261] The research team concluded that that there was no clear evidence of a 'specific pre-menstrual negative mood syndrome.' It is not surprising that this theory has generated no small amount of controversy among other scientists, journalists and we women ourselves!

Jane Ussher, professor of women's health psychology at Western Sydney University, who, on the whole, subscribes to the results of the Canadian research review, qualifies it by saying that this does not strike out the existence of severe PMS, or the PMDD that a small percentage of women experience. She asserts that generally however, PMS is a 'myth', and the strong emotions women are said to experience close to their period actually just stem from the many stressors in a modern woman's life. She backs up her point by saying that premenstrual distress is more prevalent in women in their mid-30s onwards who have 'multiple responsibilities—juggling home, work and children, with little support.' In addition, Professor Ussher says that PMS is higher in women who are experiencing relationship difficulties, or lack understanding and support from their partner.[262] Journalist Jacqueline Maley also suggests that PMS needs to be viewed 'within the context of our times.' She says, 'Contemporary women face a great deal of stress as they manage work and family life. Much of it they internalise. It's little wonder they get the grumps from time to time.'[263]

---

260 Christiane Northrup, M.D., *Women's Bodies, Women's Wisdom*, p.129

261 The study was called, 'Mood and Menstrual Cycle: A review of prospective data studies'. See: http://www.sciencedirect.com/science/article/pii/ S1550857912001349#

262 Jane Ussher, 'The Myth of Premenstrual Moodiness.' See: https:// theconversation.com/the-myth-of-premenstrual-moodiness-10289

263 Jacqueline Maley, 'PMS may be gone but women are in no mood to lose anger', *Sydney Morning Herald*, 15/1/2013

Aha! I would suggest that herein lies a chicken-and-egg conundrum! It begs the question—which comes first: the PMS symptoms of exhaustion, irritability and even rage, or the stressors of the modern woman? In other words, do our daily stressors make us feel more premenstrual, or does PMS (assuming you believe it still exists) make these stressors more unbearable? Is it even possible to separate one from the other?

In my opinion, the best counter-argument to the claim that PMS does not exist is expressed by Jayashri Kulkarni, professor of psychiatry at Monash University.[264] Professor Kulkarni argues that this issue is coloured by 'personal philosophy and politics, rather than reason and good research.' She says that PMS needs to be viewed holistically and within its historical and cultural context. 'Over the centuries, women have had to cope with dismissive views about their anger, depression or capabilities, and being labelled "irrational" during "that time of the month",' writes Kulkarni. 'In the 1970s, feminists fought hard against the concept of hormone influences on women's behaviour in their struggle to achieve equality for women. It was important back then to dismiss women's biology as the only determining factor of her life.' However, Kularni says that we now need to move forward from these outdated ideas within the current context of a third wave approach to feminism: 'Today, we don't have to take the view that women's biology, including their hormone profiles, are unimportant. We can reclaim biology and integrate it with the psychological plus social contexts to see that PMS does exist and does cause real suffering for many women.'

Kulkarni also recommends that PMS be viewed in the light of new discoveries in neuroscience, refuting the Canadian study's findings, which were based on a one-size-fits-all approach. 'The Canadian study assumes that all women universally respond to cyclical hormone changes in the same way, and at the same time of each cycle,' she says. Kulkarni's approach is congruent with Brizendine's claim, mentioned above, that different women exhibit different levels of stress sensitivity in response to fluctuating hormones. Kulkarni says, 'There are vast differences in individual's mental health changes in response to shifts in the complex array of hormones. Some women are mentally sensitive to hormone changes, while others are not.' This notion of personalizing our approach to each woman's experience of PMS sits in alignment with the feminine approach to yoga represented by my Moving with the Moon philosophy.

---

264   Jayashri Kulkarni, 'PMS is Real and Denying its Existence Harms Women.' See: http://theconversation.com/ pms-is-real-and-denying-its-existence-harms-women-11714

Back to the case that PMS is all in our heads—Jane Ussher points out that PMS has been found to be restricted to modern, Western countries and does not occur in poorer, Asian countries. In response, Kulkarni asserts that it's not that it doesn't exist in these countries, it's just that 'non-threatening conditions, such as PMS, are given little consideration in some non-Western, undeveloped countries' since people are probably more focused on survival-issues.

This apparent prevalence of PMS in the West may also be related to a kind of insidious by-product of feminism—'the superwoman syndrome'—in which women are expected to seamlessly manage a household and a career. This then would explain why the stress of women's busy lives seems to exacerbate their PMS symptoms, causing a monthly blow-out, as Ussher writes:

> For three weeks of the month, such women silence their irritation and unhappiness, conforming to societal expectations of the "good woman". Premenstrually, this self-silencing is broken, but the expression of negative thoughts and feelings is invariably dismissed as PMS. This means that nothing changes in the circumstances of women's lives, and the cycle of self-silencing and frustration continues.[265]

Ussher seems to be saying here that the diagnosis of PMS is used as a 'cop out' to avoid positive change in overwrought women's lives. I would argue, to the contrary: by acknowledging PMS and its triggers, we recognise that our feminine bodies are very clever, and if we are only to listen to the messages they broadcast, in the form of PMS, we can vastly improve our relationships and circumstances, not to mention our health and wellbeing.

UNDERSTANDING CREATES HEALING

As I have already touched on, premenstrual distress can be worsened by a woman's external surroundings. Research in 2005 pointed to the interesting fact that PMS can be more extreme for women who are in a relationship with a man than those in a same-sex relationship. Judy Skatssoon in her article, 'Do men cause PMS?', interviewed Professor Jane Ussher, who conjectured that this may be related to men having very little understanding of how to respond to us when we are moody and 'on their case.'[266]

---

265   Ussher: http://theconversation.com/
      the-myth-of-premenstrual-moodiness-10289

266   See: http://www.abc.net.au/health/features/stories/2005/12/08/1836110.htm

This raises this proposition: if we better taught our men how to understand and support us during this challenging time of the month, perhaps we would not experience as much PMS. In fact, a recent study has shown that a woman's PMS symptoms decrease when she is able to discuss the negative effects with her male partner and when they engage in couple's therapy together.[267]

The foundation of educating those around us about the fluctuations of our bodies and emotions is to make sure we first understand them ourselves. It amazes me how regularly women tell me, when I lecture on this subject, that they tend to only come to the realisation that they are premenstrual after the fact—once they start bleeding. They breathe a big sigh of relief and say, 'Thank God! I was just premenstrual!'

Awareness of what you are experiencing *at the time*, as well as implementing strategies to minimise or even transform your premenstrual distress can make all the difference (read on for more information on this).

In addition, if the premenstrual upset seems to be centred around a woman's reaction to her partner, she may need to consider if her relationship is sustainably healthy and functional; together with her partner, she may need to investigate ways to repair the relationship or, if it's unfixable, to leave it. I know from personal experience, that in a past, unhappy relationship, my PMS was much worse each month than it is now that I am in a harmonious relationship with my husband.

THE PREMENSTRUAL 'TRUTH SERUM'

> *When we routinely block the information that is coming to us in the second half of our menstrual cycles, it has no choice but to come back as PMS or menopausal madness, in the same way that our other feelings and bodily symptoms, if ignored, often result in illness.*

> —CHRISTIANE NORTHRUP, M.D.[268]

---

267 The study is by Jane Ussher and Janette Perz. See: http://journals.plos.org/plosone/article?id=10.1371/journal.pone.0175068. Also see Jane Ussher's article—https://theconversation.com/men-can-help-women-deal-with-their-pms-76401, which concludes, 'In the couples-therapy group, 84% of women reported increased partner awareness and understanding of PMS, compared with 39% in the one-on-one therapy group and 19% in the wait-list group'.

268 Northrup, *Women's Bodies, Women's Wisdom*, p.107.

So far, I have discussed the potential negative impact of this premenstrual phase. But what if your tendency for emotional turmoil during your Waning Moon phase also carried some hidden blessings? Medical scientist and psychologist Joan Borysenko, Ph.D., suggests that the premenstrual phase is your optimum time for 'emotional housekeeping'. Borysenko writes, 'Things that may be bothering us, but that we are unable to confront, tend to come to light as if they are being flushed from the unconscious to the conscious so that we can attend to them.'[269]

The hormonal shift that characterises the luteal phase means that many women seem to magically swallow a 'truth serum', and in so doing, relinquish their attachment to niceness and politeness. Lucy Pearce, author of *Moon Time: A Guide to Celebrating your Menstruation*, writes, 'I strongly believe that a large amount of the anger and tearfulness we experience pre-menstrually, is our body's way of expressing the deep truths which we try to stifle.'[270]

The good news is that relieving some of those intense premenstrual emotions and symptoms can be as simple as developing the self-awareness to listen to the messages your body is sending you. Alexandra Pope posits, 'Premenstrual sensitivity, which often manifests as crankiness, could be nothing more than the desire to be left alone.'[271] From my own experience, I concur: I know my period is imminent when I suddenly have an incredibly strong urge for personal space. This can result in my son, who likes to snuggle with me when we watch television, being gently but firmly moved to his end of the sofa!

CONNECTING WITH YOUR CREATIVE SELF

Many menstrual-positive educators suggest that women can minimise their premenstrual distress by reframing their attitudes towards this part of their cycle to highlight the positive aspects. Miranda Gray calls the premenstrual phase the 'creative' phase, claiming that this is when women are more attuned to their creative and intuitive energies.[272] Gray says that in the lead-up to your menses, messages from your subconscious become more accessible. 'During the Creative phase we have the ability to readily

---

269   Joan Borysenko Ph.D., *A Woman's Book of Life: The Biology, Psychology, and Spirituality of the Feminine Life Cycle*, p.55

270   Lucy Pearce, *Moon Time*, 1139 (Kindle edition)

271   Alexandra Pope, *The Wild Genie*, p.89

272   'The Creative phase is not called "creative' for nothing. The subconscious has a powerful ability to imagine, extrapolate, and create reality,' writes Miranda Gray in, *The Optimized Woman*, p.42.

access the information that is processed outside of our conscious awareness. This means that what we have stored in our subconscious becomes more reachable, making us more likely to experience creative leaps and sudden shifts in perception and realization.'[273]

This ties in with research cited by Dr Christiane Northrup showing women's brain function shifts during the premenstrual phase to increased right hemisphere dominance (connected with creativity and intuition), and decreases in its left hemisphere abilities (rational, logical).[274] As mentioned in chapter four, research has also indicated that women tend to experience more vivid, intense and longer dreams during the later phase of their cycles, perhaps reflecting the idea that this is a heightened time of connection with the subconscious.[275] Indeed, it's even backed up by that Canadian research review—while discounting a specific occurrence of negative moods during the premenstrual phase, the researchers did verify that women can experience some positive mood changes that include a heightened creativity.[276]

Rather than bemoaning the highly emotional qualities of your Waning Moon (premenstrual) phase, you can embrace it as an excellent time for big-picture thinking, or just engaging in your favourite creative pursuit. Although a woman has less access to her rational thinking-processes, she has traded this off for enhanced creative capabilities. I find that if I can avoid niggly, analytical tasks during this phase, and instead make time to express myself creatively, which for me is writing, my PMS symptoms are lessened, and I am able to discover a new enjoyment of this much-ma-ligned, darker phase.

---

273 Miranda Gray, The *Optimized Woman*, p.42

274 Northrup, *Women's Bodies, Women's Wisdom*, p.108, referring to a study called 'Neuropshycological Correlates of Menstrual Mood Changes,' by Artemus, Wexler and Boulis, 1989

275 Ibid., p.107, Northrup cites studies that 'have shown that women's dreams are more frequent and often more vivid during the premenstrual and menstrual phases of their cycles', and this is footnoted with the references: Hartmann, 'Dreaming Sleep (the D State) and the Menstrual Cycle', *Journal of Nervous and Mental Disease*, and Swanson and Foulkes, 'Dream Content and the Menstrual Cycle,' *Journal of Nervous and Mental Disease*. Also, Shuttle and Redgrove in *The Wise Wound*, p.91–92 cite findings of Ernest Hartmann, M.D., who suggests that women's REM sleep increases towards the end of their cycle.

276 '...many studies reported positive changes in the premenstrual phase, including increased creativity, energy, and sexual drive,' writes Professor Ussher. See: https://theconversation.com/the-myth-of-premenstrual-moodiness-10289

WORKING WITH THE CLEANSING ENERGY OF THE WANING MOON

There is a dominant force of cleansing and reorientation.
The waning cycle offers ample opportunity to expend
energy, complete tasks, strengthen our breath power
and life force, detoxify and cleanse the organism,
and bring the fruits of our labor to completion

—MAYA TIWARI[277]

Your Waning Moon premenstrual phase equates to the autumn of your cycle. During this time there is a natural energy of clearing and preparation—a harvesting of your efforts from the past month, as your body begins the process of moving inwards towards the winter-like hibernation of your Dark Moon (menstrual) phase. You can support this cleansing and releasing process by tidying up any loose ends; like a squirrel gathering nuts for the winter, now is the time to finish any urgent tasks and projects so that you can afford yourself the time and space for uninterrupted rest during your upcoming menstrual (Dark Moon) phase.

Not only is this clearing of your to-do list beneficial, but you can also support yourself by emotionally detoxing during this phase. I recommend that you carve out some personal space for yourself and engage tools to facilitate emotional release (see the suggested strategies below) to help you come to terms with and work through any accumulated and unaddressed frustrations from the previous month. This process can be very healing and can progress you on your own path of personal growth.

---

277 Maya Tiwari, *Women's Power to heal through Inner Medicine*, p.65

STRATEGIES FOR MOVING THROUGH THE WANING MOON PHASE GRACEFULLY

During the waning cycle following the full moon, the body, mind and spirit also wane. A woman naturally yearns for quietude and resolve. At this time, you can do serene practices such as meditation, journaling, drawing, painting, fasting, and other heart-opening activities that build and strengthen your inner harmony.

—Maya Tiwari[278]

Instead of looking outward and interacting with others, your Waning Moon phase is an excellent time for solitary consolidation. Here are some guidelines for navigating this phase with enhanced ease and grace:

- While it's important to develop the self-awareness to recognise any issues behind emotions as they come up for you during your Waning Moon phase, Miranda Gray suggests you should save discussion or any attempt at solving these issues until later in your cycle.[279] Ideally, heart-to-heart sharing with your loved-ones is better suited to your Full Moon ('expressive' phase) when you will be better able to communicate your needs and desires for change, or deeper understanding, in a more loving and compassionate way.
- You will be most productive and harmonious during this phase by indulging your creative side—in whatever form that might take—and also working through any simple, repetitive tasks that will help 'clear the decks' for when you bleed.
- It is vital to find some alone-time so that you can work through any strong feelings that have arisen without the risk of unduly hurting those around you. Taking time out for yourself sets up a positive flow-on effect: the more time you have to yourself—to dream, to feel, to release powerful emotions, to be creative—the less likely you will be to express negative emotions to those around you. The savage PMS beast can be soothed and fed in this way.

---

278   Tiwari, *Women's Power to Heal*, pp.70–71

279   'This is not the time to sit down and battle out our relationship problems at work or at home, but rather it is the time to sit down, turn inwards and uncover the underlying cause of our reactions,' writes Gray in, *The Optimized Woman*, p.47.

Here are some other practical ways you can support yourself during your Waning Moon phase:

- **Take long baths.** Adding 1–4 cups of Epsom salts to your bath helps boost the magnesium levels that are often depleted in your premenstrual phase—causing those chocolate cravings![280] A warm Epsom salt bath will help you relax and sleep better, and may alleviate period cramping.

- **Indulge in high quality raw chocolate.** This will pacify those chocolate cravings in a healthy way. According to naturopathic health consultant Eileen Fedyna, 'Cocoa is loaded with magnesium and can positively impact our mental and emotional states, helping to relieve common PMS symptoms.'[281]

- **Take long walks in nature.** This can be especially beneficial in helping you find perspective when your 'monkey mind' spirals down into negative, unhelpful thoughts and you find yourself overreacting—'making a mountain out of a molehill'.[282]

- **Write in your journal.** This is a simple way to safely process strong emotions that tend to arise during your premenstrual phase.

- **Take some time to read, rest and daydream.** Respond sensitively to your declining energy levels, as you near your Dark Moon (menstruation) time, with contemplative rest. This is a time of heightened intuition so make sure you are available to listen to any messages coming from your subconscious.

- **Get more sleep.** According to dream researcher Dr Ernest Hartmann, a woman's REM (deep dreaming sleep) naturally increases during the later part of her menstrual cycle. Hartmann found that premenstrual symptoms are worse when women don't get enough sleep, and improve when they sleep more than usual. He concludes, 'treatment for premenstrual tension should include a prescription for more sleep.'[283]

---

280 Jerome Sarris and John Wardle in, *Clinical Naturopathy: An Evidence Based Guide to Practice*, p.352, write, 'Magnesium has been shown to reduce PMS mood and fluid retention symptoms'.

281 See: http://www.mindbodygreen.com/0-14765/beat-pms-5-ways-to-get-rid-of-bloating-mood-swings-food-cravings.html

282 Borysenko in, *A Woman's Book of Life, pp.57–58*, refers to a study— 'Neurophysiological Correlates of Menstrual Mood Changes', *Psychosomatic Medicine* 51, 1989—that showed that premenstrual women exhibited a greater tendency to *not* hear positive words when exposed to positive, negative and neutral words.

283 Cited by Shuttle and Redgrove in, *The Wise Wound*, pp.91–92

- **Give yourself a nurturing breast massage.** Breast massage may help with the common premenstrual symptom of breast pain and tenderness.[284] Massaging your breasts will increase circulation to the area and can also help with lymphatic drainage, which may relieve feelings of congestion in the breasts. See page 165 in chapter five for instructions on how to do breast self-massage.
- **Practise a soothing Waning Moon yoga practice.** Tailor your practice to suit your particular mood and energy levels. Waning Moon practice guidelines and sequences are following, and you will also find yoga tips for different types of PMS in chapter eight on page 364.
- **Exercise!** Studies show that women who regularly exercise report fewer PMS symptoms.[285] 'Exercise raises endorphins and serotonin boosting mood and reduces pain and inflammation. Exercise also helps burn fat for a healthy BMI (a higher level of obesity means a higher level of PMS symptoms),' writes fitness coach, Amber Larson.[286] If you follow the Moving with the Moon philosophy of tuning into how your energy feels each day throughout your cycle, you will be able to adjust the intensity of exercise accordingly. For example, if you feel you have the energy and are physically strong, you might enjoy a vigorous walk, run, session at the gym, dancing (a personal favourite!), or a more dynamic Waning Moon practice. This Waning Moon practice might involve flowing Lunar Salutes (for example—see the Classical Waning Moon Premenstrual Sequence) and Standing poses, or more Active Inversions.
- **Try herbal medicine or acupuncture.** In 2012, a systematic review of the research literature on the efficacy of complementary medicine on moderate PMS symptoms was conducted by a Korean research team, and they concluded that, 'Acupuncture and herbal medicine treatments for premenstrual syndrome and premenstrual dysphoric disorder showed a 50% or better reduction of symptoms compared to the initial state.'[287] So, it's worth a visit to your local acupuncturist or herbalist!

---

284 Jonathan S. Berek, in *Berek and Novak's Gynecology,* p.655, suggests management of cyclical mastalgia (breast pain) may be eased by heat and cold packs as well as 'light breast massage'.

285 One such study can be found at: https://www.ncbi.nlm.nih.gov/pmc/articles/PMC3748549/

286 See: https://breakingmuscle.com/learn/how-to-alleviate-the-symptoms-of-premenstrual-syndrome

287 See: https://bmccomplementalternmed.biomedcentral.com/articles/10.1186/1472-6882-14-11

YOGA FOR YOUR WANING MOON PHASE

*I am feeling completely out of sorts. Disconnected and
disaffected. Nothing pleases me at this time of the month.
At any given moment I am apt to cry or snap. I am brittle
around the edges. I am the definition of hormonal!*

*My partner asks innocently, 'How are you?' I feel
like he is talking to me from another world. Not my
world; my world is so disconnected from the everyday
world. I answer darkly, 'Not exceptional'.*

*I want to curl up in a ball. I am crying out for 'me-time'.
I cannot handle the demands of my family and my
business. I just want them all to go away!*

*Finally, I find the time to do my Waning Moon yoga
practice. I breathe a deep sigh of relief. At last! I
close the bedroom door, play some soothing music
and melt my sorrows into my mat and bolsters.*

*I invert, invert, invert. I need to do whatever it
takes to shift my perspective—that negative, stuck
energy needs to be shaken up and turned.*

*Sometimes I choose to move my stagnancy with
gentle, rhythmical Womb Salutes. Or, if I'm feeling
heavy with physical and nervous exhaustion, I just
allow myself to be still in sweet, supported poses.*

Oh, this sacred rest is a balm to my body and soul!

—ANA'S MENSTRUAL DIARY

The main intention behind a Waning Moon yoga practice is to soothe the nerves and calm the mind at this oft-challenging time. Escaping into your sacred yoga space also provides you with that precious alone-time, in which you can process any disturbing or distressing feelings. I cannot count the times during this phase when I have had a private weep upon my yoga mat that felt so cathartic and healing. Or at other times, I have enjoyed the release of shaking off my anger and tension to emerge from my Waning Moon practice a little softer around the edges.

An established and regular home practice really pays off during this phase of your cycle. When you retreat to your yoga mat, you will have the ready tools and experience to skilfully customise your practice according to how you're feeling— whether it's tiredness, sadness, anger, or just generally feeling out of sorts. It can therefore be much more beneficial to practise at home (on your own) during this phase, rather than attend a one-size-fits-all yoga class, which may end up aggravating your PMS symptoms.

Principles and guidelines for a Waning Moon Yoga Practice

Cool the fire

From an Ayurvedic perspective, the quality of *pitta* (see Appendix 1) tends to predominate during a woman's Waning Moon phase. Anger and irritability are both common emotional PMS symptoms and are considered to be manifestations of this excess of *pitta* or fire in the body.

This interpretation also makes sense from a Western physiological point of view when you consider that due to a surge in luteinising hormone (LH), precipitating ovulation, as well the predominance of the hormone progesterone, the body's basal temperature increases and stays a little higher throughout this whole luteal (Waning Moon) phase of your cycle.[288]

Therefore, a key focus in your Waning Moon yoga practice is on cooling the body and the mind, to pacify this fiery energy. This can be done by practising Supported Seated Forward Bending postures as well as Supported Standing Forward Bends (see Appendix 3, Cooling Restorative postures, p.451). You can also choose cooling Pranayama practices like the Feminine Nadi Shodhana (see p.105) and Sitali (see p.264).

Slow down, nourish and restore

A Moving with the Moon approach means we aim to practise yoga in an individualised way that supports the natural decline in our physical energy and emotional robustness during this luteal or premenstrual phase.

---

288   See: http://www.passmyexams.co.uk/GCSE/biology/menstrual-cycle-and-hormones.html . Also, reproductive endocrinologist Dr. Danzier says, 'Increased progesterone acts on the temperature-regulating area in the brain. It can rise about four-tenths of a degree in this phase, from 98.6 to about 99 degrees.' See: http://www.womansday.com/health-fitness/womens-health/a1605/a-month-in-the-life-of-your-hormones-107587/

The first step for many women is taking the time to fully acknowledge and respond to the natural downshift that occurs during this phase. Yoga teacher Donna Farhi recommends you start to tune in ten days before your period by 'spending a quiet time each day scanning the garden of the body and mind for disturbances.' A good time to do this is when you sit or lie on your yoga mat each day, before you begin your yoga practice. It's especially important during your Waning Moon phase to take this pause, connecting with your breath and the sensations within, and to 'check in', asking what your body-mind truly needs before you launch into your yoga practice. 'You may notice fatigue, nervous agitation, constipation, swelling in your breasts, or heaviness in the pelvis,' writes Farhi.[289] She suggests you respond sensitively by adjusting your diet and taking herbs and, of course, modifying your yoga practice.

Farhi recommends practising both Active and Supported Backbends if you notice that you're experiencing bloating, breast tenderness or pre-cramping sensations in the pelvis. If your energy is also quite low, I would add that it's best to stick to the *supported* variations of the Backbends, like Supported Bridge variations (see p.450).

Otherwise, if you're feeling sluggish (i.e., lethargy rather than fatigue) and sense you need to move 'stuck' energy in the body, opt for the more Active Backbends, like Bridge Pose (see Figure 16, p.92), the Bow Pose (see Figure 221) or even Urdvha Dhanurasana (see Figure 14, p.91).

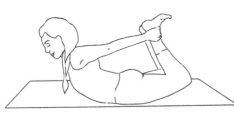

Figure 221

Farhi also recommends that you may want to include some 'cramp poses', to boost circulation in the lower belly, as you get closer to your period. You will find more information on these kind of postures on page 320 in chapter eight but, suffice it to say, the Classical Women's postures (see Appendix 2) like Baddha Konasana (see Figure 383, p.441) or Upavista Konasana (see Figure 384, p.442) are beneficial for relieving or preventing menstrual cramps. Personally, I love to practise Upavista Konasana just before my period when I notice that I feel very tight in the inner thigh and groin region. This pose feels like it opens me up and relieves that pressure.

---

289   Donna Farhi, 'Yoga for Menstrual Cramps', an article in *The Yoga Journal*, pp.7–10, May/June 1986

Overall, to support your waning energy levels during this phase, a gentle Restorative Yoga practice[290] can work beautifully to quiet your agitated mind and soothe your over-stimulated nervous system, particularly if you focus on Supported Forward Bends, which have a cooling effect on the body-mind (as we have seen above). Plus, these postures have the added benefit of helping to ease pre-menstrual headaches and migraines.

Balance the body and mind

Inversions are a must for this phase of your cycle, particularly the Supported Inversions (see Appendix 3, p.453). Inverted postures help balance your hormonal system, potentially alleviating PMS symptoms, and they also nourish and balance the nervous system which can help with those commonly experienced Waning Moon feelings of edginess, anxiety and irritability.

Another reason that I like to practise Inversions during my Waning Moon phase is that they literally and metaphorically turn my perspective upside down, which can help reverse those premenstrual-induced negative thoughts and feelings.

Postures that challenge your physical balance skills, such as the Tree Pose (see Figure 254, p.282) and Kneeling Toe Balance (see Figure 255, p.282) are also beneficial during this phase. The great thing about balance postures is that they require your full attention—if your mind wanders, you tend to lose your balance and fall out of the pose. In this way, not only do they work to strengthen your core muscles, but they also help reinstate much needed mental and emotional focus and balance during this potentially turbulent phase of your cycle.

Support the detox

Interestingly, both Western and Chinese medicine recognize the connection between liver health and PMS. In TCM (Traditional Chinese Medicine), PMS is thought to be caused by liver stagnation.[291] Dr Libby Weaver is a Nutritional Biochemist and author of *Rushing Woman's Syndrome*, and she says that PMS can be caused by a 'congested liver', and explains that in a

---

290   See Appendix 3 for an overview of some recommended Feminine Yoga Restorative postures.

291   According to TCM, some of the common symptoms of 'stuck liver-chi' are: depression, mood swings, irritability and frustration, irregular or painful periods, and PMS with irritability or swollen breasts. See: http://www.cycleharmony.com/remedies/pms-pmdd-moods/pms-and-liver-qi-stagnation

healthy cycle any excess oestrogen in your system is excreted by the liver. However, if the body has been under stress with too many 'liver loaders' like caffeine, alcohol and sugars, the oestrogen is reabsorbed and you may end up with an oestrogen-excess.[292]

To assist with the healthy function of your liver and the removal of excess oestrogen at the end of your cycle, it may be helpful to include some Twist poses and some deep Side Bends during your Waning Moon phase.

Postures like Halasana (the Plough Pose—see Figure 133, p.186) and Paschimottasana (Seated Forward Bend—p.451) are beneficial in toning the kidneys[293] and adrenals,[294] assisting this hormonal detoxification process and supporting hormonal balance.

Waning Moon contraindications and cautions

The overall Moving with the Moon approach encourages you to listen to your body, not your ego, when you get on your mat, and this definitely applies during this critical phase of your cycle. Make sure you always go *with*, not *against* your energy, particularly if you're experiencing any PMS symptoms. If you're feeling tired and strung-out, that's a clear signal from

---

292   Dr Libby Weaver, *Rushing Woman's Syndrome: The Impact of a Never Ending To-do List on our Health*, location 5357 (Kindle edition)

293   Linda Sparrowe, former editor of the *Yoga Journal* and author of an article entitled 'Menstrual Essentials', writes, 'The liver also plays a role in alleviating our PMS symptoms. If we keep the liver healthy through proper diet, exercise, and stress relief, it has no problem breaking down excess hormones and passing them along to the kidneys, which excrete them from the system.' See: https://www.yogajournal.com/lifestyle/menstrual-essentials

294   Medical journalist Helen Anderson explains that progesterone 'depends on DHEA, a steroid secreted in the adrenal gland, and low levels may possibly be affected by or contribute to adrenal fatigue,' See: https://www.livestrong.com/article/496026-adrenal-fatigue-low-progesterone/ Lara Briden, naturopathic doctor, concurs: 'Losing progesterone at the end of your cycle can destabilise your HPA axis and worsen symptoms of "adrenal fatigue",' location 3409, *Period Repair Manual*. Related to this idea of 'oestrogen dominance' is Michael Lam, M.D's assertion: 'Many women with estrogen dominance will see their symptoms improve by simply optimizing the adrenal gland function for the simple reasons that a properly functioning adrenal gland will put out the necessary progesterone needed to balance any excessive estrogen,' See: https://www.drlam.com/blog/estrogen-dominance-part-2/1781/ However you look at it, this all helps us appreciate the potential importance of taking care of the adrenal glands in the case of low progesterone or excessive oestrogen.

your body to do a gentle, Restorative practice, rather than a strong, dynamic practice. It's common sense, really! If you don't follow this principle, you're likely to learn the hard way; if you persist in practising in a way that is counter to your energy, you may find that you will pay the price physically and emotionally and feel worse at the end of your practice compared to when you started. Your aim should always be to adjust your practice—whether that means gently soothing or stimulating your energy—so you end up feeling better.

As we saw in chapter four, the hormone relaxin works to relax and soften the ligaments and joints in the body, often with particular effect on the pelvis and lower back, and is released in the body during the luteal phase of the menstrual cycle.[295] This means you need to be mindful of not overstretching in the latter part of your Waning Moon phase because there is a risk of injury.[296]

Finally, Donna Farhi counsels caution with the inclusion of Standing poses in your premenstrual practice. 'Continue to practise standing poses as long as they do not agitate the nervous system,' writes Farhi. She recommends that if you're suffering PMS, to avoid 'strenuous standing poses.'[297] These equate to the standing lunge Warrior postures, such as Virabhadrasana I (Figure 10, p.90) and II (see Figure 11, p.90).

---

295   'Relaxin levels in the circulation rise after ovulation, during the second half of the menstrual cycle'—according to this article: http://www.yourhormones.info/ hormones/relaxin.aspx

296   As mentioned in chapter four, see: BBC News article, 'Menstrual Cycle Injury Risk Link', (http://news.bbc.co.uk/2/hi/health/6354303.stm)2007, citing a research study by London's Portland Hospital that concluded women are more likely to injure themselves at specific times in their menstrual cycle: 'At the end of the cycle levels of (another) hormone, relaxin rise. This is to allow the cervix to open so that menstruation can occur, but it also means the ligaments in general are softened.' Another research study, 'Serum Levels of Relaxin during the Menstrual Cycle and Oral Contraceptive Use' found that, 'Women with posterior pelvic and lumbar pain had higher relaxin levels than did healthy women' See: https://www.ncbi.nlm.nih.gov/pubmed/7789917

297   Donna Farhi, 'Yoga for Menstrual Cramps', *The Yoga Journal*, pp.7–10, May/ June 1986

Waning Moon Pranayama

> *The Lord of the senses is the mind, the Lord of*
> *the mind is the breath; the master of the breath*
> *is the nervous system; quietness of the nerves and*
> *concentration depend solely on the steady, smooth,*
> *and rhythmic sound of inhalation and exhalation.*

—HATHAYOGA PRADIPIKA, IV, 29 [298]

General guidelines

The Waning Moon phase is the time in your cycle when you are most likely to be agitated or low-spirited, and can therefore benefit greatly from the calming and energising effects of Pranayama (breathing techniques) on the mind and nervous system. Maya Tiwari says that women are especially in need of 'rich prana to the body and mind' during this premenstrual phase.[299]

Depending on your premenstrual symptoms you may want to adjust the focus of your Pranayama. If you are feeling sluggish and a bit 'stuck' (a *kapha*-dominated cycle—see p.362 in chapter eight), you may want to practise a more stimulating Pranayama, like Kapalabahti (see p.268), or enjoy deep, full Ujjayi Breaths (see p.165) with a focus on the inhalation (see p.209), which help invite inspiration into your life.

If you are feeling overwrought and overwhelmed (a *vata*-dominated cycle—see p.362 in chapter eight), your focus will be on longer exhalations to ground and calm by engaging the calming, parasympathetic nervous system.[300] Pranayama such as the Falling-Out Breath (see p.104) and Brahmari (see p.267) will benefit you the most in this case.

If you are experiencing a fiery Waning Moon phase with symptoms of anger, irritability and overheating in the body (a *pitta*-dominated cycle— see p.362 in chapter eight), you will benefit most from the more cooling and pacifying Pranayama practices, like Sitali (and variation, Sitkari—see p.264) or Chandra Bhedana (see below).

---

298 As quoted in this article: https://www.ekhartyoga.com/articles/
finding-the-balance-between-effort-and-ease

299 Maya Tiwari , *Women's Power to Heal*, p.257

300 See Note 129 for an explanation of the two branches of the autonomic nervous system—the parasympathetic and sympathetic nervous systems.

Specific techniques

The Soft Belly Breath

This breathing technique can help if you find yourself too much in your head or are having difficulty sleeping—a common challenge during the Waning Moon phase. See page 100 for instructions.

The Falling-Out Breath

This simple breathing technique can facilitate deep release of emotional tension and stress, particularly if practised whilst in a Restorative posture. See page 104 for instructions.

Feminine Alternate Nostril Breath

Described by Bija Bennett, author of *Emotional Yoga*, as 'an exquisite technique for emotional balancing',[301] Nadi Shodhana helps balance the right and left sides of the brain, as well as the active (sympathetic) and passive (parasympathetic) aspects of the nervous system. See page 105 for instructions.

Chandra Bhedana

This practice means 'cooling with the moon', and takes the focus of Feminine Nadhi Shodhana—on the left, cooling, 'lunar' nostril—one stage deeper. According to Bija Bennett, Chandra Bhedana will help to calm your mind, relieve anger, ease insomnia, cool an overheated body, and reduce restlessness, anxiety and stress.[302] These are all symptoms of PMS that can be manifested during the Waning Moon phase!

How to do it

With your right hand in Deer Mudra (see Figure 29, p.106) close your right nostril and inhale slowly, smoothly and fully through your left nostril. Now close your left nostril and exhale deeply through your right nostril. That's one round. Repeat by inhaling through your left nostril and so on. Practise for 10–18 rounds.

In my Moving with the Moon, feminine approach, I like to practise Chandra Bhedana and Nadi Shodhana Pranayama with my left hand on my lower belly (womb-space), whilst the right hand is in the Deer Mudra (see Figure 225, p.265).

---

301   Bija Bennett, *Emotional Yoga*, p.130

302   Ibid., p.132

Sitali and Sitkari

Another excellent practice for the Waning Moon phase is Sitali (and Sitkari—a variation), which is a classic, cooling Pranayama.

This practice works to cool an over-heated mind and body, and is also good for alleviating anxiety and tension. 'As you cool down your breath you'll find unhealthy emotions such as anger, resentment, and jealousy instantly dissolving,' says Maya Tiwari.[303]

If you can naturally curl your tongue, practise Sitali, otherwise, you will need to practise Sitkari. Note that some people genetically can curl the tongue while others cannot.

How to do it

Sitali

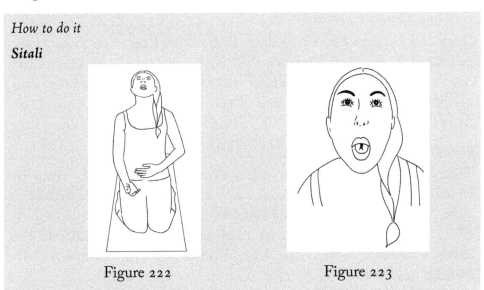

Figure 222   Figure 223

Sit comfortably and take a few slow, deep breaths down into the belly (Soft Belly Breath—see p.100). Then, begin Sitali by curling the tongue and raising the chin slightly as you breathe slowly and gently through the curled tongue (see Figure 222 and Figure 223). It is like you are sipping the breath through a straw. Feel the coolness of the breath as it fills the head, moves down the airways and all the way into the belly, cooling, soothing and balancing the reproductive organs. Pause for a moment with the chin lifted, throat open and the tongue gently pressed against the roof of the mouth. Then, lower the chin again so it is parallel to the floor and exhale smoothly and fully through the nostrils. Continue for 12 rounds.

---

303   Tiwari, *Women's Power to Heal*, p.260

Sitkari

Sit comfortably and take a few slow, deep breaths down into the belly (Soft Belly Breath—see page 100). Then, begin Sitkari by gently closing the teeth and opening the lips. The tongue lies flat along the bottom palate. Raise your chin gently and inhale strongly through the teeth to create a hissing sound. Pause for a moment with the chin lifted, throat open and the tongue gently pressed against the roof of the mouth. Then, lower the chin again so it is parallel to the floor and exhale smoothly and fully through the nostrils. Continue for 12 rounds.

Excellent PMS Variation: Sitali Pranayama with Nadi Shodhana Exhale

I first came across this wonderful variation in *Yoga for Wellness* by Viniyoga teacher Gary Kraftsow.[304] Kraftsow recommends this breathing practice for PMS, and I have personally found it very beneficial.

By combining two types of Pranayama—Sitali and Nadhi Shodhana— this variation doubles the calming and cooling effects. It is a little more complicated than practising each of these Pranayama on their own, so I suggest practising Nadi Shodhana and Sitali separately for a number of times before embarking on this variation. Once you're ready for it, the beauty of this variation is that because it is that little more complex, it helps keep the mind focused, which can be particularly beneficial during the Waning Moon phase when your mind is likely to snowball with negative thoughts.

How to do it

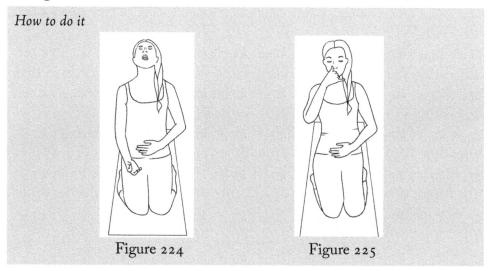

Figure 224   Figure 225

304   Gary Kraftsow, *Yoga for Wellness: Healing with Timeless Teachings of Viniyoga*, p.300

Sit comfortably and take a few slow, deep breaths down into the belly
(Soft Belly Breath—see p.100). When you are ready, inhale through the
curled tongue as you raise your chin slightly, sipping the breath (Sitali—
see Figure 224)—if you are unable to naturally curl your tongue, practise
Sitkari instead (see above). Then, release the tongue to touch it gently to
the roof of your mouth as you bring your chin back down towards the floor
and raise the right hand—there is a slight breath retention here. Now, bring
your right hand into Deer Mudra (see Figure 29, p.106) and gently close off
the right nostril as you exhale slowly and smoothly through the left nostril
(Figure 225). Lower the hand and inhale again through the curled tongue
(Sitali) or through the teeth and over the flat tongue (Sitkari) as you raise
your chin. Again, pause with the chin raised, throat open, releasing the
tongue to roof of the mouth. Now, as you lower your chin, raise your right
hand into Deer Mudra and close off the left nostril and gently and deeply
exhale through the right nostril. This completes one round. Continue for
another 8–9 rounds.

When you have finished sit quietly for some time just allowing yourself
to soak up the quietness and peace that this beautiful Pranayama offers.

Equanimity Breath (Sama Vritti Pranayama)

This Pranayama means 'equal wave' or 'movement' and is a balancing and
gently stimulating practice that helps if you are experiencing depression,
lethargy and are low in energy[305]—all classical premenstrual complaints.

How to do it

This practice is simple—it involves lengthening both the inhalation and
exhalation equally, and including a pause at the end of each breath that
is half the length of the inhale/exhale. For example, inhale for 8, hold for
4, exhale for 8, hold for 4. Repeat for 8–10 rounds. If you like, you can
progressively work on extending the inhale and exhale a further 2–4 counts
over. But always do one or two rounds at your original count (e.g. 8: 4: 8:
4) to bring balance and equanimity before you finish. Focus on keeping
the breath smooth and unforced and only maintain a count that is totally
easeful for you.

305 Bija Bennet, *Emotional Yoga*, p.123

Brahmari (Humming Bee Breath)

This Pranayama technique is said to be very good for pacifying anxiety[306] because of its calming effects on the nervous system. It involves making a long, humming 'mmm' sound, which naturally extends the exhalation in relation to the inhalation. This has the corresponding effect of engaging our parasympathetic nervous system ('rest, repair and digest) and disengaging our sympathetic nervous system (fight of flight).[307] Timothy McCall M.D., a board-certified specialist in internal medicine, says that Brahmari helps us maintain a healthy level of carbon dioxide in the blood and also facilitates relaxation.[308]

From a yogic physiology point of view, Brahmari is said to activate Ajna or the Third-Eye Chakra (energy centre), and has a profound effect on uniting personal consciousness with universal consciousness. From a Western physiological perspective, it activates the pituitary gland and hypothalamus, which are governing glands of our endocrine (hormonal) system. It is therefore a beneficial practice for regulating our hormones, and is especially beneficial during pregnancy.[309]

How to do it

Sit comfortably and take a few Soft Belly breaths (see p.100), allowing your body and mind to settle. Then, take a deep breath in and make a long, slow, deep 'mmmmmm' sound as you exhale, feeling it reverberate at your third eye-centre (Ajna Chakra—the point between the eyebrows and deep into the brain). Focus on elongating the 'mmm' sound as much as possible without straining. Continue for as long as you are comfortable.

Variation

Close off the ears by pressing the index fingers gently against the flaps of the ears as you hum (see Figure 226). This variation helps cultivate the practice of *pratyahara*, or withdrawal of the senses, as you listen to the humming sound reverberating inside your head, which serves as a powerful preparation for meditation.

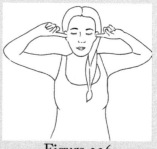

Figure 226

306   Timothy McCall, M.D., as quoted in *Yoga Journal* article: http://www. yogajournal.com/article/practice-section/buzz-away-the-buzzing-mind/

307   See: https://yogainternational.com/article/view/5-ways-to-practice-bhramari

308   See: https://www.yogajournal.com/practice/buzz-away-the-buzzing-mind

309   See: https://www.yogameditation.com/reading-room/bhramari-the-bumble-bee/

Kapalabhati

Kapalabhati is a cleansing, heating and stimulating breathing technique that is excellent for raising your energy and therefore beneficial for *kapha*-like PMS symptoms (see p.362)—when you are feeling sluggish and heavy during this phase.

Kapalbhati means 'skull shining breath'. As you practise it, you might like to visualise your head filling with white light, enjoying the purifying and rejuvenating effect of this breathing practice on the mind and body.

How to do it

Sit comfortably and take a few deep Soft Belly Breaths (see p.100). Take a deep cleansing inhalation and exhalation to prepare. Then, inhale deeply and do ten rapid exhalations. This involves gently but decisively pumping the belly—the abdominal wall draws back to the spine as you exhale and relaxes as you inhale.

At first, while you get used to this practice, you can place one or both hands on your belly around the navel to feel the sensation of the abdominal muscles moving. After your ten rapid exhalations, take a deep inhalation and exhale gently out of an open mouth (Falling-Out Breath). Take a few normal inhalations and exhalations through the nose, before repeating another round of 10 rapid Kapalabhati breaths. Do up to 5 rounds, but initially just stick with 2–3 rounds until you get used to the practice.

Cease or avoid the practice if you feel dizzy, anxious or uncomfortable in any way. And definitely do not practise this Pranayama if you're menstruating or pregnant.

Waning Moon Relaxation and Meditation Practices

Waning Moon Yoga Nidra

Enjoy this deep relaxation practice to rejuvenate your body, mind and nervous system.

How to do it

Lie down on to the floor, or even your bed, with a small cushion or folded blanket underneath your head and a bolster or pillow underneath the knees. Place an eye-bag on your eyes and cover yourself with a blanket or shawl if necessary so you can be warm and comfortable for the duration of the practice. Make sure you have created a space for yourself where you will not be disturbed for the next 15-20 minutes.

Position the arms so that they are a little way out from the sides of the body and not touching the body. The palms are uppermost, fingers lightly curling. The feet are at least hip distance apart and allow them to fall out to the sides so that your hips are loose and relaxed. Make any final adjustments to your posture so that you are as comfortable and supported as possible and so that you will not need to move for the remainder of the relaxation practice.

Now, feel your body settling in. Know that this is your time, just for you. Nowhere to go, nothing to do, nobody you have to be. Just *be*. Time to rest and take some precious time to connect with yourself, your inner self.

Take three slow, deep breaths. With each exhalation feel the weight of your body surrendering completely into the floor or bed beneath you.

Now, allow your breath to become natural, not trying to change the breath in any way, just let it be.

Now bring your awareness to your *sankalpa*. This is your positive resolution for change, your deepest heartfelt desire. You may already have a *sankalpa* that you are working with; if so, bring this to mind now. Or, you can create a new one—a short, positive affirmation in the present tense. If you like, you can cultivate a *sankalpa* directly related to your Waning Moon phase. Here's an example:

> ***My experience of my monthly cycle is easeful,***
> ***joyful and connected, as I trust that I can***
> ***take care of myself in so many ways.***

Mentally repeat your *sankalpa* three times, with conviction. 'Planted deep into the fertile soil of your unconscious, your *sankalpa* is a potent agent for positive change in your life.

Now, let go of your *sankalpa* and again become aware of your breath— the natural rise and fall of your breath through the nostrils. Feel your breath subtle and easeful, without any force or strain. Simply allow the breath to rise and fall of its own accord. Feel the slight coolness of the breath on the inhalation as it draws in through the nostrils and the warmth of the breath, gently heated by the airways, as you exhale.

Now we begin the rotation of awareness around the body that is a key element of Yoga Nidra. As I name each part of the body, sense into that part of the body—picturing it, feeling it letting go. If you find that your mind wanders or becomes sleepy, bring yourself back to the practice, even if you must do this many times.

Begin by becoming aware of your left hand thumb, first finger, second finger, third finger, fourth finger. Palm of the hand, back of the hand, left wrist, forearm, elbow, upper arm, armpit, shoulder. Left waist, left hip, upper left leg, knee, lower leg, left ankle, top of the foot, sole of the foot, big toe, second toe, third toe, fourth toe, fifth toe.

Now, move your awareness to your right hand thumb, first finger, second finger, third finger, fourth finger. Palm of the hand, back of the hand, right wrist, forearm, elbow, upper arm, armpit, shoulder. Right waist, right hip, upper right leg, knee, lower leg, right ankle, top of the foot, sole of the foot, big toe, second toe, third toe, fourth toe, fifth toe.

Now, moving up through the back of the body, become aware of the left heel, right heel, back of the left knee, back of the right knee. Left buttock, right buttock. Sacrum, the bones of your sacrum. The lower back—left kidney and adrenal, right kidney and adrenal. The upper back—left shoulder blade, right shoulder blade. Back of the neck. Back of the head. Crown of the head.

Moving your attention now to the front of the body. Left side of the forehead, right side of the forehead. Left temple, right temple. Left eyebrow, right eyebrow, eyebrow-centre. Left eye, right eye. Left cheek, right cheek. The nose—left nostril, right nostril, bridge of the nose. The mouth—upper lip, lower lip. Inside of the mouth. Left side of the jaw, right side of the jaw. The tongue. The chin. The throat—swallow and relax the inner walls of the throat.

Become aware of the chest—left side of the chest—left breast, right side of the chest—right breast. Centre of the chest, heart-centre. Now become aware of your abdomen—upper-abdomen (solar plexus), mid-abdomen (navel-centre), lower abdomen (womb-space). Stay here for a few breaths—feeling each inhalation creating a sense of space and ease in your belly and womb-space; each exhalation releasing any tension or gripping in the belly.

Finally, become aware of your left hip, right hip, the pelvis—the bones of the pelvis. And now the vagina—walls of the vagina.

Now, bring your consciousness into your whole body. Your whole body, resting on the floor in this moment. Whole body awareness.

Becoming aware of your breath again—of the sound and sensation of the in and out breath. On your next inhalation visualise the ocean and a cleansing wave washing up through the body from your feet to head. As you exhale, the wave moves back down the body from your head, back out through the soles of your feet, washing away anything you no longer want or need. Continue to work with this visualisation and sensation of a cooling, cleansing wave moving up through your body as you breathe in, and then out and away as you breathe out. Repeat this visualisation for a few more cycles of breath.

Letting go of the breath-visualisation practice now, become aware of the breath at the eyebrow-centre. Simply watch the breath, sensing, visualising it coming in and out of the point between your eyebrows. Stay here for several rounds of breath.

Now, letting go of eyebrow-centre breathing, and bring to mind again your *sankalpa*—your heartfelt prayer for positive transformation. And mentally repeat your *sankalpa* three times, with conviction, knowing that in time this will come to pass.

Bring your awareness now to your whole body, your *whole body*, resting on this floor (or bed) in this moment. Feel the sensations within and around your body. Feel the air against any uncovered skin, the clothing and coverings against your skin. Feel the floor (or bed) beneath you. Without yet opening your eyes, become aware of your surroundings, your position in the room (as if you were looking at yourself from above). Become aware of any sounds around you.

In a few moments you will be moving out of this Waning Moon Yoga Nidra practice, but before you do, just allow yourself to savour these last few moments of deep relaxation, deep rest, deep quiet and peace. And know that when you awaken from this practice you will feel refreshed and renewed, your nervous system nourished and your mind calm.

Begin now to bring movement into the body. Move the fingers and toes, wrists and ankles. Stretch and yawn, gradually awakening the energy in the body. And when you feel ready, without any sense of hurry, roll to the right hand side and rest there for a few breaths in a foetal position.

Always remembering to be gentle with yourself.

When you are ready, use your top left hand to press into the ground and roll yourself up to sitting. Finish this practice sitting quietly in a comfortable position for you—spine erect, shoulders relaxed back and down, and face and belly soft. With your eyes still closed, rub your palms together vigorously to create heat and friction there. After a few seconds place your warm palms over the closed eyes and feel the energy, the *prana*, from your palms, soothing and energising your eyes, the optic nerve, as you breathe in and out deeply. Then place your right hand on your low belly (womb-space) and your left palm over the centre of your chest (heart-centre) in the Heart-Womb Mudra (see Figure 154, p.222), coming home to yourself.

Finish by placing both palms over the heart in Hands to Heart Mudra (see Figure 152, p.212) and take a few moments to smile into your heart-centre, cultivating joy and contentedness there, and perhaps saying a little prayer of gratitude.

Namaste

Heart Cleansing Meditation

This is a beneficial meditation practice for the Waning Moon phase that helps drop you out of your head and into your heart. See page 214 in chapter six for instructions.

Waning Moon Detaching from the Emotions Meditation

This meditation is excellent for calming any premenstrual agitation that is worsened by the 'monkey mind' snowballing one negative thought into another.

It involves chanting the Mantra, '*so hum*', which means, 'I am that'. 'That' refers to universal consciousness, or all that is. It is a powerful mantra that helps detach us from our busy mind (*citta vrtti*) and from overly identifying with our negative thoughts and ideas, which take us away from *santosha* (contentment).

According to yoga teacher Swami Gurupremananda Saraswati, So Hum Mantra meditation stimulates the Heart Chakra and helps with balancing the emotions and is 'good for all relationship harmony'.[310]

I recommend you practise this meditation, with a timer on, for a minimum of 15 minutes.

How to do it

Begin by sitting in a comfortable position—kneeling, cross-legged or on a chair if you prefer. Allow the body and mind time to just settle and drop into stillness, especially if you have been busy caught up in a negative, premenstrual spiral.

Notice your breathing—notice its quality—is it shallow and broken, or is it already deep and full? Initially just notice without feeling the need to change anything about your breathing.

Now take some time to scan the awareness around the body, searching

---

310   Swami Gurupremananda Saraswati, *Mother as First Guru*, p.2170

for any areas of tension or disconnection in your physical body. When you find tightness, pause with your awareness in that part of your body, taking a deep breath into that part of the body, then exhale through an open mouth—consciously letting go of that tension as you release the breath out of an open, relaxed mouth. If it feels good, work with a sounded exhale through the mouth (Falling-Out Breath—see p.104), progressively allowing yourself to soften into your body and into this moment.

When you are ready, cease the Falling-Out, tension-relieving breath, and again notice the gentle, natural breath in and out through the nostrils. Gradually deepen the sound of the breath into Ujjayi Breath (see p.165)—in which you draw the breath over the back of the throat to create a deep, sibilant, ocean-sound to the breath.

Begin to hear the sound of the Mantra in the breath. As you inhale, hear the sound '*so*' and as you exhale, hear the sound '*hum*'.

Place the right palm on your lower belly, womb-space, and your left palm on the centre of chest, your heart-space (Heart-Womb Mudra—see Figure 154, p.222). Feel the breath, along with the '*so hum*' sound, travel up and down the subtle, energetic pathway between the womb and the heart. As you inhale, feel the breath travel up through your torso from the womb-space to the heart, with a rising, filling energy—continuing to hear the '*so*' sound. As you exhale, feel the breath travel back down from your heart to descend into your womb, feeling a grounding, descending energy with the out breath—continuing to hear the '*hum*' sound. And as you exhale and hear the sound '*hum*', let yourself soften right down into your womb-space, feel a letting go, and experience a beautiful pause, a moment or so of blissful release and emptiness, at the end of the out-breath, before the next ascending action of the '*so*', inhaling breath.

If your attention wanders, which it probably will do, especially if you're premenstrual and in the midst of a negative-thought-feeling spiral—taking you off into a whole imagined narrative that will involve replaying the past or projecting into the future—gently coax the mind back to the task at hand: focusing on the '*so-hum*' sound of the breath, and the subtle energetic, rising-falling pathway of the breath.

Continue this practice for as long as you are comfortable—for at least 10–15 rounds.

After a while, let go of the '*so hum*' breath and allow the breath to come back to gentle quietness again—just allowing it to be spontaneous, and no longer listening for the Mantra-sound.

Place both palms over the heart-centre (Hands to Heart Mudra—see Figure 152, p.212), sensing for any feelings, energy resonations, there at the heart-centre. Allow any feelings or thoughts to arise as you contemplate the energy of your heart-centre, there behind the palms. Try to simply watch these emotions or thoughts as if you were viewing them on a television screen.

Then, like peeling an onion, let go of those emotions, thoughts, images, and go deeper. Go into pure awareness. What is it like to connect with your self—the part that is *pure awareness?* That deep part of yourself that is always equanimous, that is always aware, that is always OK, not matter whatever is going on externally. If this is a difficult concept, try imagining that you were looking down on yourself, or stepping outside of yourself, watching yourself from the outside. Picture yourself sitting here in meditation. What do you look like from the outside? What do you look like when your Awareness views you through the lens of compassionate detachment?

Stay with this exploration of pure awareness for as long as you like, or until your timer sounds.

When you're ready, finish your meditation practice by placing your palms together into Anjali Mudra (Prayer gesture —see Figure 151, p.212).

With the hands still in prayer, finish by touching the fingers to the eyebrow-centre (third-eye point), symbolising purity of thought, then lightly touching the fingers to the lips, symbolising purity of speech, and lastly touching to the heart-centre, symbolising purity of heart.
Namaste.

Additional *Waning Moon* Meditations:

See page 358 in chapter eight, for a Mindfulness Meditation, and an Open Heart Meditation for PMS on page 360.

Waning Moon Yoga Sequences

POSTURES AND PRACTICES TO SUPPORT YOUR PREMENSTRUAL PHASE

CLASSICAL WANING MOON PREMENSTRUAL SEQUENCE

Best time to practise

Do this sequence at any time you need a holistic and supportive practice during your Waning Moon (premenstrual) phase. It's especially beneficial if you're experiencing symptoms of *pitta*-excess—anger, irritability, agitation. See Appendix 1 as well as page 362 for further explanation of *pitta*-excess.

Sequence duration

45-50 minutes

Sequence benefits

This sequence is designed to incorporate a number of postures that help bring balance to the body and mind during this challenging phase of your cycle. It will calm your mind and nervous system, gently stimulate your energy if you're feeling tired, and provide a rinse to your internal organs (liver, kidneys and adrenals) to support maximal hormonal health and balance.

Props for this sequence

A yoga mat, a chair, a yoga bolster, and a yoga block. You may also need a folded blanket for the seated poses if you have difficulty sitting up tall.

1. Chi kung horse pose

Benefits

Calming and grounding; helps you connect with your essential self—your quiet, sustaining inner resource—and draws your awareness away from busy thoughts in your head influenced by the outside world.

Props for this posture

Nothing! This simple Chi Kung-inspired centring practice can be done anywhere without any equipment—for example, outside in nature.

Recommended timing

Stay for several minutes (or as long as you like), or for approximately 5-10 deep breaths.

How to practise

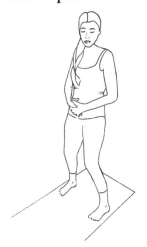

Figure 227

Step your feet apart a little wider than your hips, feet parallel to the outer edges of your mat. Have the knees softly bent, with about 60% of the weight into the heels, tailbone lengthening down towards the earth. Rest your right palm on your lower belly, left palm on top (see Figure 227).

Close your eyes and take a few moments to settle and quieten within yourself. Allow your shoulders to soften, melting like ice into water, and feel your connection with the earth through the soles of the feet, especially the heels. Begin to take some deep breaths down into your belly, your deep womb-space (Soft Belly Breaths—see p.100). Progress to some Falling-Out Breaths (see p.104) combined with Apana Breaths (see p.102)—inhaling deeply through the nose, breathing down into your belly, and as you exhale out of an open mouth feel that you are breathing away any tension and tiredness, any negative energy, out and down through the hips, legs, out of the soles of the feet, into the earth beneath you. Work with this cleansing, releasing breath for another 4-9 rounds.

2. 'Pulling down the heavens' clearing breath

Benefits

This is a clearing and energising practice that brings you quickly into a space of relaxation and centeredness, slowing you down

Props for this posture

Nothing! This simple Chi Kung breathing practice can be done anywhere without any equipment—for example, outside in nature.

Recommended timing

Do up to 10 repetitions.

How to practise

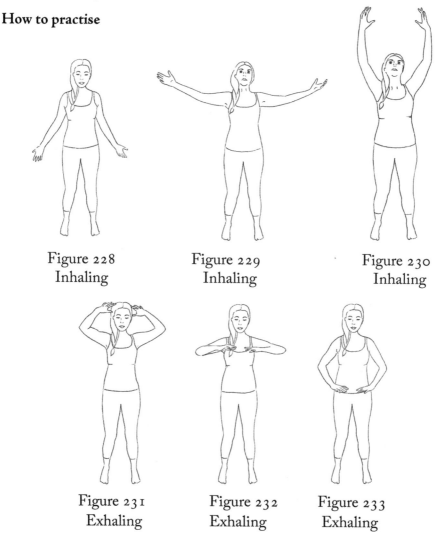

Figure 228
Inhaling

Figure 229
Inhaling

Figure 230
Inhaling

Figure 231
Exhaling

Figure 232
Exhaling

Figure 233
Exhaling

Still in the Chi Kung Horse stance, inhale as you sweep the arms to the side and overhead (see Figure 228, Figure 229 and Figure 230). Exhale as you bring the arms down through the front the body, palms gently pushing down as you pull the energy down from the heavens (see Figure 231, Figure 232 and Figure 233). Continue these slow, mindful movements synchronised with the breath.

As you inhale and raise the arms up gazing up to the heavens, imagine you are drawing in fresh energy (*chi/prana*), filling up your lungs; as you exhale and pass your hands down the front of the body, imagine you are clearing the whole body of toxins, of negativity. You can make a soft, gentle, long out-breath through your mouth, even making the healing sound that accompanies this practice—'heee'. Do up to 10 rounds of this breathing and centring practice.

3. Waning moon salutes

Benefits

- Warms up the body, stretching and strengthening the whole body.
- This salute sequence can be practised slowly and mindfully, pausing for several breaths during some/all of the poses (especially Down Dog Pose) in order to deeply calm the mind and nervous system. Alternatively it can be practised more briskly holding each pose just for a breath to stimulate a sluggish mind and body.

Props for this posture

Just your yoga mat.

Recommended timing

Do 4-10 rounds of this Lunar Salute depending on how much energy you have.

How to practise

Part 1: Basic Lunar Salute: Rounds 1 & 2

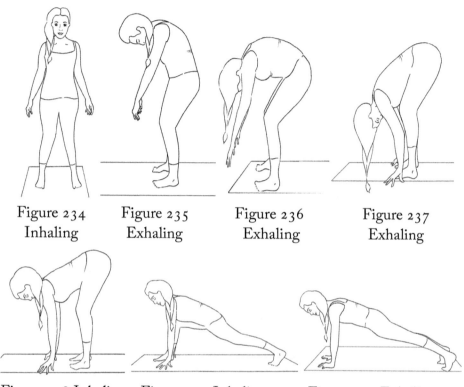

Figure 234
Inhaling

Figure 235
Exhaling

Figure 236
Exhaling

Figure 237
Exhaling

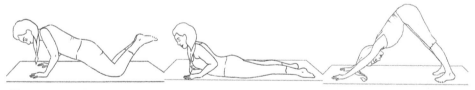

Figure 238 Inhaling   Figure 239 Inhaling   Figure 240 Exhaling

Figure 241 Exhaling   Figure 242 Inhaling   Figure 243 Exhaling

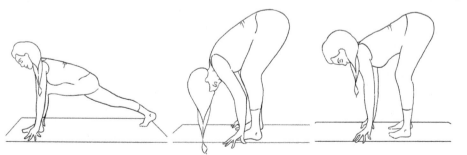

Figure 244 Inhaling   Figure 245 Exhaling   Figure 246 Inhaling

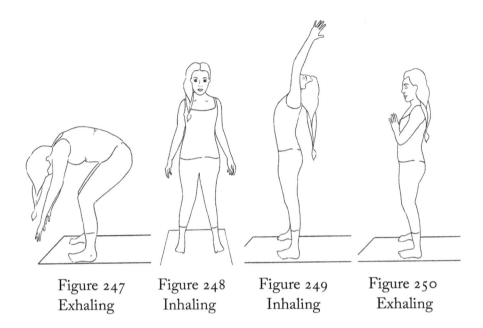

Figure 247   Figure 248   Figure 249   Figure 250
Exhaling   Inhaling   Inhaling   Exhaling

Start in Tadasana (Mountain Pose) with your feet hip-width apart and parallel—so from the Chi Kung Horse Stance narrow your feet a little. Have your hands by your side (see Figure 234). Take a deep breath in to prepare and as you exhale slowly roll down through your spine, vertebra by vertebra, head heavy, arms heavy, abdominal muscles pulling in and up towards the back-body (see Figure 235 and Figure 236). Once your hands reach the floor (see Figure 237)—bend your knees if you need to—inhale into Urvha Uttanasana with the chest lifted away from the thighs (see Figure 238). Then exhale and hang into Uttanasana again, head and arms heavy (see Figure 237).

Inhale as you step your left leg back into High Lunge Pose (see Figure 239), and as you exhale step your right foot back into Plank Pose (see Figure 240). Continuing to exhale, drop your knees to the mat and lower your chest and belly in one line down to the floor in the Half Push-Up Pose (see Figure 241). On your inhalation raise the head and chest into Baby Cobra (see Figure 242), then pressing your palms into the mat, turning the toes under and pushing back onto your knees, move into Down Dog, as you exhale (see Figure 243).

On your next inhalation step the left foot between the hands into High Lunge Pose (see Figure 244) and as you exhale step the right foot also to the front of the mat into Uttanasana (see Figure 245). On your inhalation lift the chest forward into Urdvha Uttanasana (see Figure 246), and as you exhale hang the head and roll up through the spine (see Figure 247), bone by bone, all the way up into Tadasana (see Figure 248). From here, inhale and sweep the arms to the side and overhead, bringing your palms together, gazing up (see Figure 249). And finally, exhale the hands down through the centre-line into Anjali (Prayer) position (see Figure 250).

Repeat the whole sequence, this time stepping back with the right foot into High Lunge, and stepping forward with the right foot into High Lunge after you've completed the Plank, Cobra and Down Dog Postures.

Safety and Comfort Notes

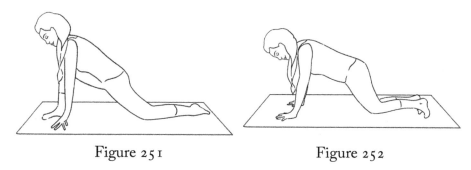

Figure 251   Figure 252

If you find the High Lunge Pose too challenging or you prefer a gentler practice, you can substitute the Low Lunge Pose with the back knee on the floor (see Figure 251). Likewise, if you find the Full Plank Pose too strong, you can substitute a Kneeling Plank Pose (see Figure 252) with the knees on the floor.

Part 2: Building on the Lunar Salute

After 2-4 rounds of the Basic Lunar Salute you can add the following poses as you continue a few more rounds of the Salute.

Twisting High Lunge Pose

Do this posture once you come into the High Lunge Pose (Figure 239). With the left foot back, place your left palm onto the floor underneath the line of the left shoulder (about 10 cm away from, and in line with, your right foot), and reach up towards the ceiling with the right arm as you twist around to the right, towards the frong, right leg (see Figure 253). Keep extending actively up through that

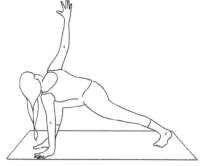

Figure 253

right arm to be light into the bottom left shoulder and twist the belly towards the front right thigh with each exhalation.

Hold the Twist for 3-5 deep breaths. Then, unwind and place the right hand on the outside of the right foot back into the High Lunge Pose, ready to continue on with the Salute Sequence.

Tree Pose

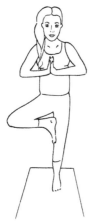

After a round of the Lunar Salutes do this pose from standing before starting again. From Tadasana (Figure 234), bring the feet together and shift your weight into your left foot as you place your right foot on the inside of the left thigh. Keep pressing the sole of the foot into the thigh and the thigh into the foot (engaging the inner thigh adductor muscles). Inhale and bring your hands overhead (upper arms beside the ears). Then, bring your hands into Prayer (Anjali) Mudra at the centre of the chest, elbows wide, chest broad and lifted, crown of the head lengthening to the sky (see Figure 254).

Figure 254

To help keep your balance, make sure you distribute the weight evenly across the standing foot (don't grip the toes), focusing particularly on pressing down through the base of the big toe. It also helps your balance to gaze at a spot on the wall or the floor in front of you. Balance and breathe evenly and smoothly for at least 5 breaths before changing legs.

Kneeling Toe Balance

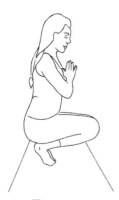

After stepping forward into Uttanasana (see Figure 245), bend your knees and bring your feet together and raise your heels off the floor as you sit your buttocks onto your heels. If you need to, have your hands on the floor but if you can, raise your hands at your chest into the Prayer (Anjali) Mudra (see Figure 255). Squeeze the thighs together and gaze at a spot on the wall or the floor in front of you to help keep your balance. Finally, make sure you don't hold your breath. Breathe steadily and evenly here for 3-5 breaths.

Figure 255

4. Supported prasarita padottanasana (standing wide-legged forward bend) with a chair

Benefits

See page 446 for some key benefits for this supported Classical Women's Restorative pose.

Props for this posture

A yoga mat, a chair, and possibly additional propping to put on top of the chair such as a folded blanket and/or a bolster.

Recommended timing

Stay here for as long as you're comfortable—anywhere between 2-5 minutes.

How to practise

Setting up

Stand on your yoga mat, facing its long edge, and step the feet wide apart, at least a leg length. The feet are parallel or even a little pigeon-toed and make sure the heels are in one line—you can even have the heels on the back edge of the mat to ensure this. Have your chair in front of you. Place your hands on your hips. Inhale and draw the elbows towards each other, opening the

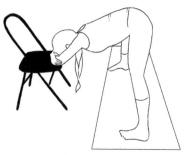

Figure 256

chest. As you exhale, fold forward from the hips (pelvis rolling forward) into the Forward Bend and place your hands on the top of the chair. As you inhale again, lengthen the sternum forward, towards the chair, creating more length through the front and sides of the torso. Then as you exhale, fold more deeply into the Forward Bend, coming to rest your forehead onto your folded forearms on top of the seat of the chair (see Figure 256).

If you find that your spine rounds or you can't comfortably straighten the legs you may need to add additional height to the chair, adding a folded blanket and/or bolster, and then resting on top of this to make sure you feel as comfortable and as supported as possible in this Restorative pose. Remember, the golden rule with Restorative Yoga is to provide yourself with adequate propping so that the props meet you, rather than you trying to meet the props.

Being there

Take a few breaths to settle in and open into the pose, allowing the body to become still and quiet after the more dynamic salutes you've just done. Let the breath slow down and deepen as the mind begins to move inwards in this restful, cooling Forward Bend. Feel the lift and tone of the belly and length and space in the lower back and sacrum. As you exhale you can work with grounding Apana Breaths: sending the breath down through the legs into the earth; letting go of tension, holding and anything that's not serving you in your body, in your life.

It's up to you as to how dynamically you work the legs; you can lift the knee-caps and engage the quadriceps, or you can keep the legs soft, even bending the knees a little, particularly if you find the stretch in the hamstrings and inner thighs very strong.

Coming out

Heel-toe your feet closer to about hip width distance, or a bit wider, and then bend your knees and slowly roll up through the spine. Stand quietly with your feet hip-width for a few breaths before continuing your practice. You can even try a few gentle, hip circles (Womb Circles—Figure 187, p.230) in both directions to release the lower back and free up the energy after this static pose.

5. Mermaid pose with side stretch and bharavadjasana (sage pose twist)

Benefits

- Limbers up the spine and releases tightness through the spinal muscles.
- Brings circulation and nourishment to the liver, kidneys and adrenals—detoxing and cleansing.
- Opens up the hips, and stretches the groins.

Props for this posture

A small cushion or a folded blanket to put under one buttock to balance out the hips if necessary.

Recommended timing

Do 2-4 rounds of the dynamic side-to-side breath and then hold the static stretch for 3-5 breaths and the more advanced stretch (Figure 258) for a further 5-10 slow breaths, or up to 1 minute.

How to practise

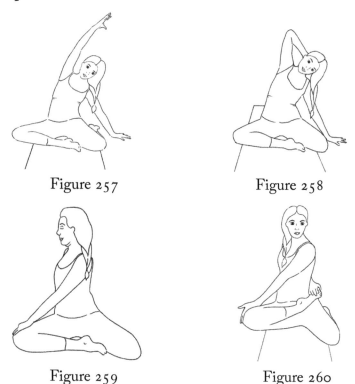

Figure 257   Figure 258

Figure 259   Figure 260

Bend up your right leg in front and your left leg behind to form a 'figure 4' shape—right foot in front of left thigh, left foot near left buttock. See if you can allow the left sitting bone to sink towards the floor (which releases the inner thigh and pelvic floor muscles). If you find that the hips are very uneven, place a folded blanket or small cushion underneath the left buttock to even up the hips.

Begin by dynamically moving in and out of the side stretch. Inhale and sweep the right arm up and over so you are curving your spine towards the left (see Figure 257); exhale as you press both sitting bones towards the floor and use your core muscles (in particular the pelvic floor) to bring your spine back to upright. Repeat to the left. Continue with this dynamic stretching for another 1–3 rounds (both left and right side is a round). Then hold the side stretch statically, curving the spine to the left with the right arm up. Focus on sending you inhalations into the right ribs, opening up the right lung and the whole right side of the body. Stay for 2–5 breaths.

For an even deeper Lateral Stretch you can try a variation[311] in which you bend up the top right arm and place the hand behind the head (see Figure 258). You can hold this for up to 1 minute (about 10 breaths), feeling the stretch radiating all the way into the right kidney and adrenal gland, nourishing these organs.

When you're ready to come out, move out of the pose slowly as the after-effects (flushing and detoxing) are powerful. Before you change legs and sides, come into a Twist pose by placing your left hand on the right knee, right hand behind you (see Figure 259). Or for a more advanced variation try the Half-Lotus variation of Bharvadjasana (Sage Pose—Figure 260). Hold the Twist Pose for 3-5 breaths before bending up the legs the other way and doing the whole side-stretching sequence on the other side.

6. Supported cross legged forward bend

Benefits
- Soothes the nervous system, relieving stress, fatigue and anxiety.
- Relieves migraine and stress-related headaches.
- Stretches the hips (rotator muscles) which can help relieve lower back pain and hip stiffness.
- Relaxes the belly, encouraging deeper breaths.

Props for this posture
Depending on your flexibility and comfort you can rest your forehead on a yoga block (on its tallest, side or flattest edge) or even a chair for a more modified version. If you have difficulty sitting up tall in the cross-legged position, you may also need to sit on a folded blanket (good for beginners or those who have tight hips).

Recommended timing
Stay for 2-5 breaths on each side.

---

311   I learnt this simple but powerful variation of the Mermaid Side Stretch from Yin Yoga Teacher Tara Fitzgibbon. Find out more about her work here: https://www.facebook.com/TerrafirmaYoga/?timeline_context_item_type=intro_card_work&timeline_context_item_source=747805732&pnref=lhc

How to practise

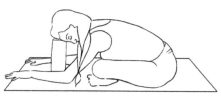

Figure 261

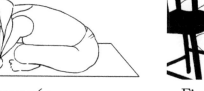

Figure 262

Come into a seated cross-legged position—on a folded blanket if you like to help support you to sit more upright and facilitate the pelvic tilt for the Forward Bend (sit-bones perched on the very edge of the folded blanket). The correct cross-legged position (Sukhasana) should be with the legs in a wide, cross-legged position—crossing at the shins, the shins almost parallel, feet well away from the groin, so there's a large triangle when you look down between your legs (see Figure 91, p.152). Have your chair or block in front of you. Inhale, and raise the arms overhead, lengthening out of the waist at the same time as grounding down through the sit-bones. As you exhale, tip the pelvis forward so that you come into the Forward Bend, still with the spine long. Then either fold your forearms onto the chair and rest your forehead onto the top forearm (see Figure 262) or, rest your forehead onto your block (see Figure 261).

Allow the shoulders to release down away from the ears and soften into the belly. Breathe deeply and enjoy this nourishing, Supported Forward Bend. If you like, you can work with some sighing, Falling-Out Breaths here.

When you are ready to come out, come up slowly and stretch the legs out in front in Dandasana (Staff Pose—Figure 123, p.182) before changing the cross-leg and repeating the Forward Bend on the other side.

Safety Notes

Avoid or do a modified version of this Forward Bend with a chair if you have sacroiliac pain (SIJ) flare-up. Alternatively, do the Supported Child pose (see p. 134).

If your knees are high off the ground in this position support them by placing yoga blocks or cushions underneath the knees.

7. Prone savasana with transverse bolster under pelvis

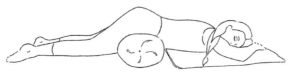

Figure 263

For benefits and instructions see the Alternative from Posture 3 in the Busy Days Nurturing Waxing Moon Sequence, page 194.

8. Sitali/ Sitkari Pranayama

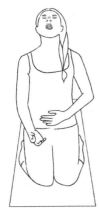

See page 264 for instructions on how to practise this cooling, calming Pranayama (breathing practice).

Figure 264

WANING MOON SEQUENCE FOR EXHAUSTION

Best time to practise

Practise this special Restorative sequence when you are feeling physically and/or emotionally exhausted, a condition that can arise if you're depleted during your premenstrual (Waning Moon phase), as well as during your perimenopausal years. It's also beneficial if you've been suffering from insomnia and feel too tired to do a standard, non-restorative practice.

Sequence duration

About 40 minutes, depending on how long you choose to relax in each Restorative pose.

Sequence benefits

A rejuvenating, Restorative Yoga sequence that will revive and gently lift your physical and emotional energy levels.

Props for this sequence

A yoga mat, 1-2 yoga bolsters, a wall space, a folded blanket, a yoga strap, and a yoga block.

1. Viparita Karani (legs up the wall) with a bolster

Benefits

- Calms the nervous system and good for relieving fatigue.
- Boosts circulation—increases blood flow to the abdominal and pelvic region.
- Balances the hormonal system.
- Facilitates deeper breathing.

Props for this posture

A yoga mat, a bolster, a yoga strap, and an eye-bag (if you like).

Recommended timing

Stay here for as long as you're comfortable—an optimum time is 10 minutes.

How to practise

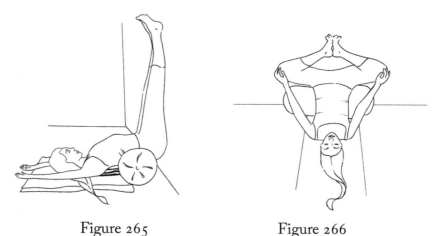

Figure 265   Figure 266

Setting up

Place your bolster parallel to the wall, about an inch or so away from the wall. Sit on the middle of your bolster, side on, with the right hip into the wall. Then, lie back as you swing your legs up the wall. Lift your bottom and walk your shoulders in to move yourself as close as you can get to the wall. In the final position, your sit-bones drop down a little in the space between the bolster and the wall, the bolster supports the lower back, and the pelvis is in neutral. Your hips are level, sit bones equidistant from the wall, and your spine is in a straight line (see Figure 265). Buckle a strap around your thighs, just above your knees, to hold the legs together. This simple prop will deepen the relaxation of the hips and lower back in the position.

Being there

Take some deeper breaths as you settle in here. This is a wonderful pose that you can't help but relax in! Allow the facial features to soften, and swallow and relax the throat. Feel the shoulder blades spreading into the floor and relax your buttocks and lower back. Feel your belly relaxing as your abdominal wall softens back towards the spine, particularly as you exhale. During the timing here you can just breathe naturally or you can work with Ujjayi Breathing (see p.165) or Falling-Out Breaths (see p. 104).

Coming out

When you are ready to come out, untie your belt and bend up the legs. To transition, bend up your legs into Baddha Konasana—the soles of the feet together, little toe edge of the feet into the wall, heels towards the groin, and knees opening to the wall (see Figure 266). Take some deep breaths visualising energising *prana* filling your pelvic area, nourishing your reproductive organs and genitals. After a few breaths, draw your knees towards each other and roll to the side and come gently up to sitting.

2. Supported pigeon pose with a bolster

Benefits

- Opens the hips—specifically the buttock/piriformis muscles; stretches the psoas muscle and hip-flexors.
- Brings circulation to the pelvic area (blood circulation and *shakti prana*), boosting your reproductive health and feminine vitality. Dr Sara Gottfried recommends Pigeon Pose as her 'go to' pose for PMS.[312]
- This Restorative version of this posture in which you rest on a bolster increases the calming and restful effects on the nervous system and enables you to stay in the pose for longer, enhancing its therapeutic benefits for your hormonal system.

---

312   See this video by Dr Gottfried: https://www.youtube.com/watch?v=uKNtKZn5Kq8

Props for this posture

A yoga bolster. And I recommend you place a folded blanket under the hip (sitting bone) of the leg that is bent up in front (see Figure 149, p.208). Propping the front hip helps prevent knee injury and torqueing in the sacrum, protecting the SIJ (sacroiliac joint).

Recommended timing

Stay for at least 3 minutes on each side

How to practise

Place your bolster in front of you on your mat, the long end parallel with the long end of your mat, and place a folded blanket to the left side of your

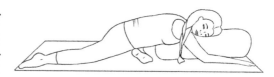

Figure 267

mat. Come into Down Dog or all-fours, and step your left leg through so that your left knee comes just behind and to the outside of your left wrist and your foot is in front of your right groin. Place the folded blanket underneath your left sitting bone so that your hips are level and you are not dropping down to your left side.

Extend your right leg behind you, directly in line with the hip and rest the top of the right foot into the floor, toes pointing behind you. Inhale as you walk your hands on either side of the bolster and get as much length as you can through the front and sides of your torso. Exhale, and rest your torso down onto the bolster. Turn your head to rest onto one cheek and let your forearms relax into the floor, your elbows slightly further forward of the shoulder-line (see Figure 267).

Take a few releasing, or Falling-Out Breaths to begin as you surrender yourself forward into the support. Breathe out and away any tightness in the front, left hip (piriformis) and also into the right groin/hip flexors. This pose is completely about surrender and deep rest—lap it up!

When you are ready to come out, either step your left leg back into Down Dog Pose, or just come into the all-fours kneeling position, to prepare to change sides.

3. Supported bridge pose: t-bolster (variation b)

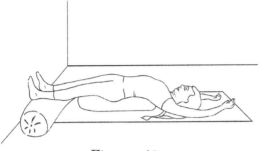

Figure 268

See Posture 9, Variation B, in the Classical Dark Moon Menstrual sequence, page 137 for benefits and instructions on how to practise this posture. If you only have one bolster you can always do the Variation A pose.

4. Supported bolster shoulderstand with variations

Benefits

- See the benefits for Half Shoulderstand on page 186.
- An additional benefit of this posture is that it may help relieve insomnia, a common premenstrual (and perimenopausal) symptom.

Props for this posture

A bolster and your yoga mat in case the bolster slips on a hard floor.

Recommended timing

Hold the Shoulderstand variation (Figure 269) for around 10 slow breaths or up to 4 minutes; hold the Happy Baby variation (Figure 270) for a further 5-10 breaths; do 8-10 repetitions of the Supported Bolster Twist (Figure 271); and hold the Bolster Psoas Stretch (Figure 272) on a bolster for approximately 5 breaths on each side.

How to practise

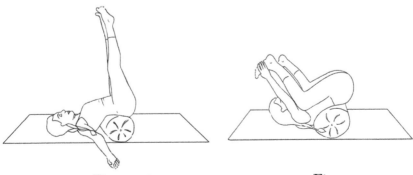

Figure 269   Figure 270

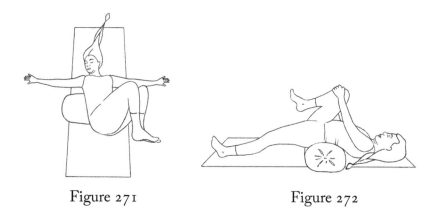

Figure 271   Figure 272

Lie down with the bolster next to your mat. Lift your hips and slide the bolster under your lower back so that the long edge of the bolster is parallel to the short end of your mat. Your buttock bones should be just dropping over the far side of your bolster. Then, raise your legs up to approximately 90 degrees (see Figure 269). The pose should feel quite effortless. If you do feel that you are strongly engaging your leg, back or abdominal muscles to hold the position you'll need to adjust your position on the bolster—forward or backwards; usually moving your buttocks a little further over the edge of the bolster (towards the far end of your mat) brings ease.

Once you're comfortable, gently swing the legs overhead and behind you (towards your head), and then back to the start position. Do this a few times to loosen up the lower back and settle yourself into the position. Then, come into stillness and stay here and breathe gently and evenly.

After several minutes, bend up your legs and lower them on either side of your head into Happy Baby Pose—taking the instep of each foot in each hand as you draw each knee in towards each armpit (see Figure 270). Stay here for a minute or so.

Then, move on to do the other variations. Firstly, the Supported Bolster Twist: release your hands and bring them out shoulder-height onto the floor, palms down. Draw your knees together into the chest. Keeping the knees bent up, exhale as you lower your knees over towards the left armpit (see Figure 271), inhale as you draw the knees back to centre, trying to keep them together the whole time. Repeat on the other side. Then do 7-9 more rounds, moving slowly and with control.

The final variation—the Bolster Psoas Stretch—involves bringing your knees back to centre and keeping the right leg bent up. Extend the left leg slowly away from you. Interlace your hands around the outside of the right shin as you draw that knee in towards the right side of your chest. Take several breaths to gradually straighten out the left leg fully, breathing into the stretch into the front of the left hip and thigh and into the left side of the belly (see Figure 272). After a few breaths, change sides, bending up the left leg and extending the right leg.

To come out, bring your feet onto the floor (on the far side of the bolster) and raise your hips into the Bridge position to slide out the bolster. Once you've removed the bolster, roll your buttocks down to rest onto the floor.

5. Simple savasana

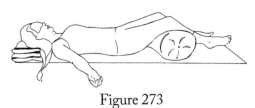

See Posture 18 in the Waxing Moon Post-Menstrual Sequence, page 189. You can simply rest and relax here, or you may wish to practise the Waning Moon Yoga Nidra (see p.268).

Figure 273

WANING MOON SEQUENCE FOR NOURISHING THE NERVOUS SYSTEM

Best time to practise

This is a calming and grounding sequence for when you are experiencing an excess in *vata* during your premenstrual (or perimenopausal) phase. These symptoms may include anxiety, mental agitation and insomnia. See Appendix 1 for more information on how to balance *vata*-excess.

Sequence duration

30-40 minutes depending on how long you stay in the Restorative postures.

Sequence benefits

A calming and grounding sequence to relax the body and mind, nourishing the nervous system. After completing this sequence your body should feel more relaxed and your mind more spacious.

Props for this sequence

A yoga mat, 1-2 yoga straps, a wall space (optional), a folded blanket, a yoga bolster, and a chair.

1. Rolling bridge vinyasa

Benefits

- Warms up the body—legs, spinal muscles (upper and lower back); opens the hips and pelvic area.
- The ab-curl up movement (Figure 279) tones the abdominals; the Bridge pose strengthens and tones the buttocks and hamstring muscles.
- The synchronising of breath with movement is calming and grounding.

Props for this posture

Just your yoga mat.

Recommended Timing

Repeat this sequence 5 times, slowly and mindfully

How to practise

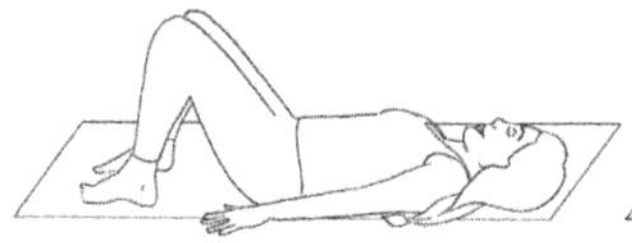

Figure 274
Inhaling and exhaling

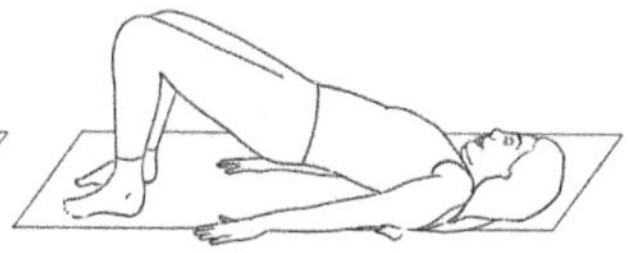

Figure 275
Exhaling

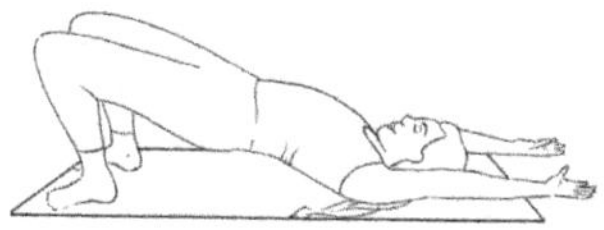

Figure 276
Inhaling and exhaling

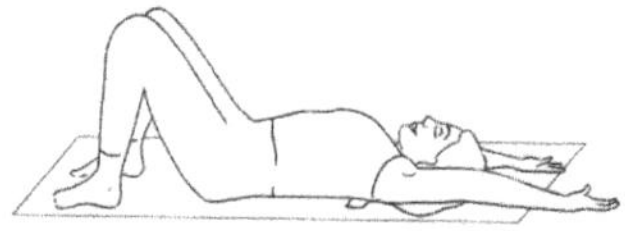

Figure 277 Exhaling

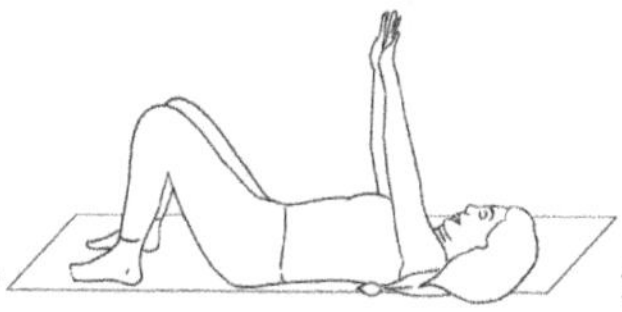

Figure 278 Inhaling

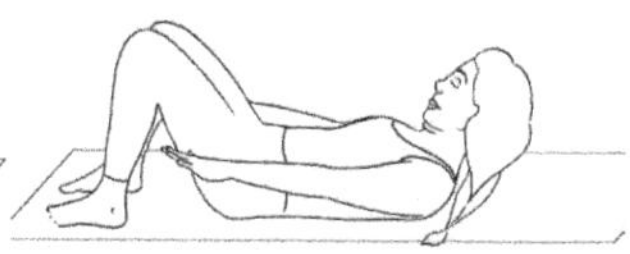

Figure 279 Exhaling

Start in Constructive Rest Position with arms by the side, palms down (see Figure 274) and take some deep Soft Belly Breaths (see p.100) to centre and prepare yourself for the practice. Then begin by working with some simple warm ups for the deep core muscles and pelvic floor by doing some simple Pelvic Tilts—see Posture 2 from the Waxing Moon Post-Menstrual Sequence, page 171. From here, evolve into the Baby Bridge out of the Pelvic Tilts—do this by exhaling and coming into posterior pelvic tilt (see Figure 105, p.171) and then continue exhaling to roll the sacrum, lower back and mid back off the floor into Baby Bridge (see Figure 275). Hold the Bridge Pose—pelvis and thighs lifting—as you inhale and bring the arms up and overhead behind you (see Figure 276). On your exhalation, keep your arms overhead and roll your spine back into the ground, vertebra by vertebra, as you reach actively through your arms to the wall behind you.

Once you've placed the sacrum back into the floor, inhale and raise the arms up to 90 degrees, fingers to the ceiling (see Figure 278). As you exhale, curl your head and shoulders off the mat and bring your hands down on the outsides of your thighs (see Figure 279); reach towards your feet as you flatten your navel to the spine. Finally, inhale and lower your head and shoulders down, and rest your arms, so you are back in the starting CRP position (see Figure 274).

Repeat the whole sequence another 2-4 times beginning from the Baby Bridge Pose (Figure 275).

2. Head in a hammock pose (supported supta padangusthasana)

Benefits

- Gently stretches the hamstrings of the raised leg and the hip flexors of the leg that is on the floor; remedial for the lower back.
- Relaxes shoulders, and releases tension in the neck.
- Very relaxing and calming for the nervous system

Props for this posture

1 or 2 yoga straps; a block to rest your head on initially can be helpful in transitioning into the pose, but not necessary. And, a wall-space—although this is optional as you can also do this posture without a wall.

Recommended timing

Stay for 2–3 minutes on each leg

How to practise

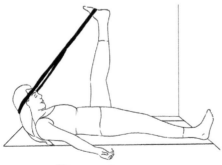

Loop two straps together into a big loop, or if you're more flexible, you may be fine to use just one strap looped onto itself. Come to lie onto your back with your head resting on the block and your legs extended, heels into the wall.

Figure 280

Bend up your left leg and bring one end of the looped strap(s) around the ball of your foot and the other end of the loop goes round the back of your head, at the top of the occiput (base of the skull)—see Figure 280). Adjust the size of your loop to make it smaller or bigger depending on your comfort. You should feel like the head can rest comfortably back into the support of the strap, while the leg should be at a bearable (mild) stretch without hiking up the left hip and torqueing or unbalancing the pelvis. There should be a gentle stretch at the back of the neck caused by it being placed into flexion and you should feel totally relaxed in the shoulders and the whole torso. At the same time extend that other right leg actively, the heel pressing into the wall.

It's the counter-weight of the head and leg moving in opposite directions that makes this pose beautifully effortless and therefore restorative. Stay here and breathe gently, enjoying this floating, hammock-like support and traction for your head, neck and spine, as your arms just rest on the floor in a relaxed way.

When you're ready to come out, release your head and leg from the strap loop and rest the leg down and the head back onto the block before changing sides.

Safety Note

Take care or avoid this pose if you have a neck injury.

3. Forward virasana (forward facing 'heroine' pose)—down dog pose (against the wall)—child pose

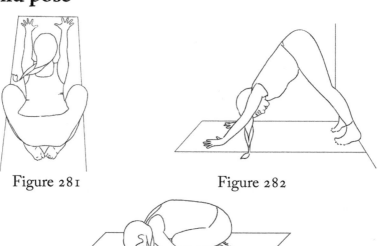

Figure 281   Figure 282

Figure 283

See Posture 6 in the Classical Dark Moon Menstrual Sequence on page 130 for a description of the benefits and how to practise Forward Virasana. And for details on the Down Dog Pose see Posture 6 in the Waxing Moon Post-Menstrual Sequence on page 175.

Note that the benefit of this particular version of Down Dog enables beginners to deepen into the pose more easefully (by having the heels higher up the wall) and for more experienced students, helps you open up the calve and Achilles muscles (by having the heels lower down the wall).

How to practise

Come into Forward Virasana (see Figure 281) with your feet facing a wall and your head to the centre of the room. Hold for 5-8 breaths before pushing up into Down Dog Pose (see Figure 282). Do this version of Down Dog by turning the toes under and extending your legs so your heels push against the wall (as pictured). You can have your heels higher up the wall for less of a stretch and lower down for a more intense stretch through the calves, Achilles and hamstring muscles.

Hold Down Dog for 5-10 slow breaths before coming down and resting in Child Pose (see Figure 283) for a minute or two.

4. Gentle dynamic paschimottanasana— supported restorative paschimottanasana

Benefits

- Calms the mind and relaxes the body.
- Beneficial for digestion.
- Stimulates the liver, kidneys and adrenals.
- Stretches the spinal muscles and hamstrings.
- This flowing way of moving in and out of the posture helps move stagnant energy in the body-mind, and synchronising the breath with the movement is calming and soothing. It also warms up the body for the static version of the pose—Supported Restorative Paschimottanasana.

Props for this posture

A folded blanket—if you need to help you sit up tall through the spine. And for the supported Restorative version of Paschimottanasana you will need a folded blanket and/or a bolster, or a chair.

Recommended timing

Do 5 repetitions of the dynamic movements (Vinyasa) from Figure 284 to Figure 291. Then hold the supported, Restorative version (Figure 292) for 2-3 minutes.

How to practise

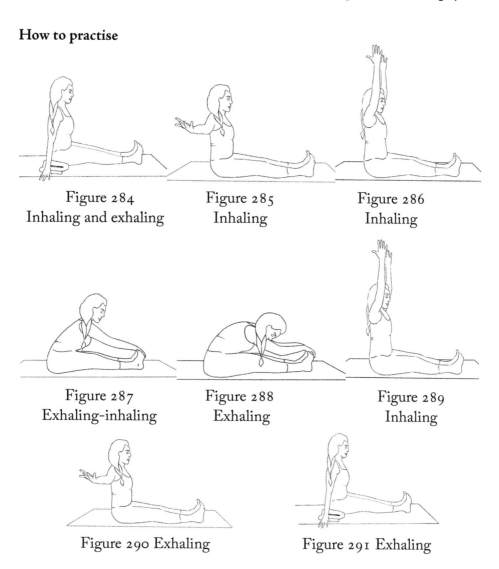

Figure 284
Inhaling and exhaling

Figure 285
Inhaling

Figure 286
Inhaling

Figure 287
Exhaling-inhaling

Figure 288
Exhaling

Figure 289
Inhaling

Figure 290 Exhaling

Figure 291 Exhaling

Come to sit in Dandasana (see Figure 284) with the legs out in front of you. If you find that you slump through the spine sit up on a folded blanket, your sitting bones perched on the edge of the blanket fold—as pictured. Inhale as you raise the arms to the side and overhead (see Figure 285 and Figure 286) lifting up tall through the spine, drawing the lower back in. Exhale as you fold forward into Paschimottanasana bringing the hands out in front of you and onto the tops of the feet (see Figure 287). If you can't easily reach the feet or you find your spine is bowing, bend your knees enough so that your spine stays long. With your hands on your feet, inhale as you lift your chest forward and up, flattening your back, drawing your shoulder blades into the back ribs, looking forward and up. Exhale as you fold a little deeper into the pose, looking down to your legs, crown of the head extending forward towards your feet (see Figure 288). Inhale as you raise your arms forward and up overhead and bring your torso to upright (see Figure 289). Exhale as you float your arms back to the sides (Figure 290), back into Dandasana, the starting position (Figure 291). Repeat the whole sequence up to 4 more times.

Supported Restorative Paschimottanasana

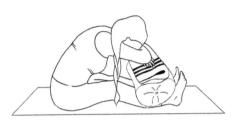

Figure 292

After doing the flowing Vinyasa into-out-of Paschimottanasna (as detailed above), take your props(s)— a folded blanket/and or a bolster— place them across your shins and rest your folded forearms on the support, your forehead resting on the top forearm (see Figure 292).

Note, if you need more height because your hamstrings are tight or your back is rounding, use a chair instead and rest your forearms onto the seat of chair (see Figure 403, p.451). Stay here for anywhere from 2-3 minutes softening into the Forward Bend, breath by breath.

5. Chair shoulderstand

Benefits

- Relaxing and rejuvenating: relieves stress and nervous disorders.
- Can relieve insomnia.
- Balances and nourishes the hormonal system including improving the functioning of the thyroid and parathyroid glands.
- Good for adrenal fatigue.
- Good for aching legs during PMS (fluid retention).
- Can boost the immune system.

Props for this posture

A chair, a yoga bolster, a folded blanket (may need an additional thin-fold blanket to rest the head and shoulders on if the floor is hard), and a yoga mat (if working on a hard floor to stop the chair and bolster sliding).

Recommended timing

5–10 mins

How to practise

Place a folded blanket on the seat of the chair and a bolster in front of the chair so that the long end of the bolster is parallel with the front of the seat. Sit on the bolster, lie back, and rest your calves on the chair. Your sacrum should be supported on

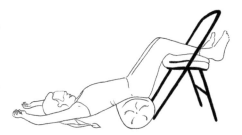

Figure 293

the bolster and the chair comes right up to the backs of your knees. (see Figure 293).

In the final pose there will be a cascading effect where the blood is able to flow down the legs into the belly nourishing the abdominal organs, then continuing to flow into the chest to nourish the heart and lungs and thyroid glands.

Stay here as long as you are comfortable, softening and breathing gently and naturally, allowing your body and mind (and emotions!) to rest deeply.

To come out, lift the bolster out from underneath you and rest with you sacrum on the floor before drawing your knees into your chest and rolling to the side.

6. **Sitali pranayama with nadi shodhana exhale**

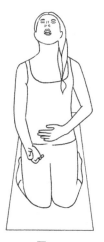

Figure 294

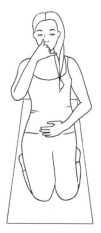

Figure 295

To finish practice this wonderfully calming, cooling and balancing breathing practice. See page 265 for detailed instructions.

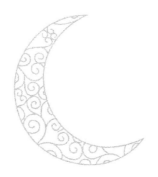

Part Four
Broadening the knowledge

CHAPTER EIGHT
MENSTRUAL MEDICINE: YOGA FOR MENSTRUAL DISORDERS

We're not meant to suffer when we bleed. Our menstrual suffering that's so often passed off as 'normal', is neither normal nor our lot. The menstrual cycle is the stress sensitive system in women. When we experience distressing symptoms, it's a signal to attend to our overall health and place in the world. Illness and physical symptoms are like signals leading us to new ground: under ground, above ground, into the world, lots of places. Illness opens the way.

—ALEXANDRA POPE[313]

When something is wrong with your menstrual cycle it's usually an indication of a larger health or personal issue at play. Menstrual irregularities such as heavy or painful periods, absent or irregular periods, and PMS may be caused by any number of things, including: lifestyle factors (diet and smoking), body-weight (being underweight or overweight), underlying health conditions, and genetic causes.[314] For many women who suffer menstrual disorders, a significant contributing factor may be stress.

---

313   Alexandra Pope, *The Wild Genie*, p.23

314   See: https://www.nichd.nih.gov/health/topics/menstruation/conditioninfo/ Pages/causes.aspx

THE STRESS CONNECTION: A FINE BALANCE

I find it fascinating to observe how much my experience of menstruation changes according to my stress levels in the preceding month. When I am on holiday and have been enjoying the luxury of letting go of my daily responsibilities and the faster pace of life, I am surprised to find my bleeding time arrives with absolutely no fuss! There is no build-up of heaviness and cramping in my womb, my pre-menstrual moods are relatively equanimous, and my flow is lighter and more easeful.

- ANA'S MENSTRUAL DIARY

A woman's hormonal system operates within a delicate balance that can be upset by the negative impact of stress causing either an excess or deficiency in the key female hormones—oestrogen and progesterone. If your body is in chronic 'fight or flight', induced by an overstimulation of your sympathetic nervous system, the non-essential body functions may shut down, reproduction being one of them.[315] In this case, an undersupply of oestrogen means we may not ovulate, resulting in menstrual anomalies like irregular, delayed or missed periods, or no menstruation at all—what's known as amenorrhea.[316]

For other women, ongoing stress can cause a reduction in their progesterone levels, essentially causing what has been called an 'oestrogen dominance'.[317] This can lead to PMS symptoms such as anxiety, insomnia,

---

315   See: http://www.ladycarehealth.com/relationship-between-stress-and-menstruation/#sthash.6aaa6DDn.dpuf

316   See Sara Gottfried, M.D., *The Hormone Cure*, regarding the effects of low oestrogen levels and how it causes a range of menopausal symptoms in addition to amenorrhea—location 3239 (Kindle edition)

317   Lara Briden prefers to call it 'oestrogen excess' and says: 'Estrogen excess causes heavy periods, breast pain, fibroids, and premenstrual irritability. It also suppresses thyroid and increases the risk of breast cancer.' Briden points to a number of potential causes for oestrogen excess including hormonal birth control, perimenopause, obesity, exposure to 'xenoestrogens' like plastics and pesticides, and alcohol consumption. See: https://www.larabriden.com/the-ups-and-downs-of-estrogen-part-2-estrogen-excess/

fatigue, bloating and breast tenderness. Disproportionately high oestrogen can also cause irregular or heavy periods, headaches, rage and cysts.[318]

A study by the National Institutes of Health (NIH) in 2010 concluded women who experienced stress up to two weeks prior to menstruation were more likely to suffer from exacerbated premenstrual and menstrual symptoms. These symptoms included psychological symptoms like depression, sadness, crying spells, anger, irritability connected with their period, as well as physical symptoms like body aches, abdominal bloating, lower back pain, fatigue, menstrual cramping, headache and food cravings. 'Overall, women reporting high stress levels were two to four times more likely to report moderate to severe psychological and physical symptoms during menstruation than were women who did not report high stress levels,' say the authors of this study.[319]

Another Chinese research trial that studied 388 women to ascertain the connection between stress and the occurrence of dysmenorrhea (menstrual cramps) found that 'the risk of dysmenorrhoea was more than twice as great among women with high stress compared to those with low stress in the preceding cycle'. This study concluded there was 'a significant association between stress and the incidence of dysmenorrhoea, which is even stronger among women with a history of dysmenorrhoea.'[320]

How does stress affect the menstrual cycle?

As mentioned in chapter four, the hypothalamus, an important governing gland of the female endocrine (hormonal) system, can be affected by emotional stress in the limbic (emotional) brain. In turn, the brain sends out faulty messages to the pituitary gland, resulting in the body producing too much or too little oestrogen or progesterone.

Stress can also create hormonal havoc when your body's demand for the stress hormone, cortisol, exceeds what the adrenals can produce, thus causing the body to 'steal' from the pre-hormone pregnenolone, which can rob you of your requisite progesterone levels. 'Cortosol can block your

---

318   See Gottfried in *The Hormone Cure*, chapter five (location 2175, Kindle edition) for an overview of the symptoms and treatments for abnormally low progesterone / high oestrogen.

319   See: http://www.nih.gov/news-events/news-releases/ prior-stress-could-worsen-premenstrual-symptoms-nih-study-finds

320   See: https://www.ncbi.nlm.nih.gov/pmc/articles/PMC1740691/

progesterone receptors—can make your body create more hormones at the expense of progesterone,' expands Sara Gottfried, M.D.[321]

Stress can also cause your muscles to clench and tighten. Tension in the abdomen and pelvic area can be a contributing factor towards menstrual cramps[322] and may also have an undesirable impact on the healthy functioning of your reproductive organs—your uterus, ovaries and fallopian tubes—because it reduces optimal blood flow to these organs. Timothy McCall M.D. in, *Yoga as Medicine* explains that when your body is stressed, the circulation to your abdominal organs is compromised and the stress hormone, epinephrine, causes constriction of the blood vessels there.[323] This is also supported by Rahul Sachdev M.D., specialist in reproductive endocrinology and infertility, who says, 'constriction may also occur in the uterus interfering with conception.'[324]

Another stress-related impediment to optimal menstrual health is a chronically tight iliopsoas muscle.[325] According to psoas expert, Liz Koch, the psoas muscle is your fight/flight/freeze muscle that contracts in response to trauma and perceived threat. While connecting the legs to the trunk, a branch of the psoas, the iliacus, passes through the pelvic bowl, and if it is overly tight, pain and restriction in the reproductive organs may result. The psoas can become tight and short due to deep-held, old fears and nervous tension. 'Fears associated with menstruating, reproduction and sexuality need to be understood and addressed,'[326] Koch says. She concludes, 'Because the Psoas muscle is a messenger of the central nervous system, regaining a healthy Psoas, in combination with nourishing the nervous system, really does play an important role in facilitating a healthy menstrual cycle.'[327]

---

321 From a YouTube talk by Sara Gottffried, M.D., https://www.youtube.com/watch?v=aqnzEGluXig

322 See: Bobby Clennell, *The Women's Yoga Book*, p.198

323 Timothy McCall M.D., *Yoga as Medicine: The yogic prescription for health and healing*, p.50

324 As quoted in an article by Judith Lasater at: http://www.yogajournal.com/article/lifestyle/when-you-want-to-have-a-baby-but-can-t/

325 See p.96 in chapter four for an explanation of the psoas muscle.

326 Liz Koch, *The Psoas Book*, p.61

327 See: http://coreawareness.com/menstrulcycles/

YOGA FOR STRESS RELIEF

It's clear that stress is not a good thing for women's cyclical bodies and psyches. As Gottfried says, 'stress relief is essential for more than regulating high or low cortisol. That's why I put a big focus on ways for harried women to manage stress.'[328]

So, what can a woman do to bring her body back into balance? The NIH study suggests, 'It may be possible to lessen or prevent the severity of these symptoms with techniques that help women to cope more effectively with stress, such as biofeedback, exercise, or relaxation techniques.'[329]

Enter, centre stage: yoga!

Numerous studies show that yoga, especially 'integrated yoga' (incorporating not just the postures but also meditation and yoga philosophy), can help reduce your stress levels.[330] The various practices of yoga—postures, breathing, meditation and relaxation—help balance your nervous system, de-activating the sympathetic nervous system (stress response) and inducing the parasympathetic nervous system (relaxation response). Mel Robin, author of, *A Physiological Handbook for Teachers of Yogasana* writes, 'The parasympathetic dominance that is necessary for this reversal can be attained through *yogasana* practice, most especially through the control of the breath and tension in the muscles.'[331] Dr Gottfried agrees, suggesting 'Yoga teaches how to release muscle tension and this helps lower cortisol.' Dr Northrup also recommends relaxation practices to help lower the levels of the stress hormones—cortisol and epinephrine—in your blood supply, which can help balance your biochemistry and reduce inflammatory chemicals.[332]

Yoga also promotes vagal tone by activating the vagus nerve, the longest nerve in the body that connects the brain with the heart, lungs and digestive system and communicates with the parasympathetic nervous system.

---

328 Gottfried, *The Hormone Cure*, location 2312 (Kindle edition)

329 See note 319.

330 One such study can be found at: https://www.ncbi.nlm.nih.gov/pubmed/15352751 and two recent systematic reviews can be found at: http://www.ncbi.nlm.nih.gov/pubmed/22164809 http://www.ncbi.nlm.nih.gov/pubmed/22502620 and at: http://www.ncbi.nlm.nih.gov/pubmed/21614942

331 Mel Robin, *A Physiological Handbook for Teachers of Yogasana*, p.157

332 Christiane Northrup, M.D., *Women's Bodies, Women's Wisdom*, pp.135-136

According to women's health and fertility specialist, Dr Shawna Dauro, higher vagal tone can enhance your mood, decrease anxiety and build greater stress resilience.[333] Diaphragmatic breathing, chanting, meditation, certain Restorative Yoga postures and Inversions can all help promote vagal tone.

The evidence supporting yoga for a healthy menstrual cycle

While the general stress-relieving health benefits of yoga are now well known, there are not as many studies proving the specific benefits of yoga for the menstrual cycle. Still, there are sufficient to make one consider the potential benefits of an integrated yoga practice for alleviating and even, in some cases, correcting menstrual imbalances.

One study published in the IOSR Journal of Dental and Medical Sciences involved a yoga intervention (with a series of yoga postures) for medical students who suffered primary dysmenorrhoea (menstrual cramps). Of the women surveyed, 88% reported complete pain relief (with 82% reporting complete stress relief) and 12% reported mild relief. The authors of the study concluded, 'Yoga lessens psychosocial stress levels, so it should be implemented among college students to augment their menstrual well-being.'[334]

Another research study looked at the benefits of practising the classical yoga deep relaxation technique of Yoga Nidra over 6 months, and contends, 'The results indicate that somatoform symptoms in patients with menstrual disorder can be decreased by learning and applying a program based on Yogic intervention (Yoga Nidra).'[335]

Robin Monro Ph.D., from the Yoga Biomedical Trust, surveyed 2,700 people, and 68% self-reported that their menstrual problems had improved after regular yoga, while 77% self-reported that their PMS symptoms improved.[336]

Alice Domar, Ph.D., is the executive director of the Domar Centre for Mind/Body Health and has pioneered mind-body programs that offer complementary support to women suffering from infertility, PMS,

333   See: http://healthycures.org/6-ways-to-instantly-stimulate-your-vagus-nerve-to-relieve-inflammation-depression-migraines-and-more/

334   See: http://www.iosrjournals.org/iosr-jdms/papers/Vol4-issue1/P0416973.pdf

335   See: http://www.ncbi.nlm.nih.gov/pmc/articles/PMC3530296/

336   McCall, *Yoga as Medicine*, p.5

abdominal pain, menopausal symptoms, and breast or gynaecological cancer. Domar says that her programs always include yoga, and explains, 'Yoga uses the mind-body connection in a healthy way. It allows my patients to become more in touch with their bodies and to see that their bodies can lead them to relaxation and fitness. The gentle movements and poses they learn help them to use their bodies to their benefit and, for many of my patients, this is an enormous revelation.'[337]

MENSTRUAL MEDICINE: GUIDELINES FOR HEALING

Before exploring the specific yoga practices used to address menstrual imbalances, it's helpful to gain an understanding of the broader natural health guidelines that underpin the Moving with the Moon, feminine approach to yoga and our lives.

Take a menstrual health break

If you can cancel all your activities for the first few days of heavy flow, so much the better; if not, at least re-schedule any impending activity that may be stress-inducing. Reduce your normal level of exercise during those days to a minimum; a brief walk is optional. Avoid cooking—now is the time to get your spouse and kids into the kitchen!

- ROVERT SVOBODA[338]

An overarching guideline to support your menstrual health is to listen to your body and rest during your Dark Moon, bleeding time.[339] As discussed, stress can be detrimental to your hormonal balance, and if you push yourself too hard, you may generate unhealthy levels of stress within your body and mind, and find that the healthy balance of your menstrual cycle is compromised.

---

337   As cited by Linda Sparrowe, *Yoga for a Healthy Menstrual Cycle*, Foreword, p.viii

338   Dr Robert E. Svoboda, *Ayurveda for Women: A Guide to Vitality and Health* p.78

339   The idea of resting during menstruation is explored in its historical context in chapter one and is also discussed in chapter four with specific reference to how yoga can support your monthly, menstrual retreat.

I always say to my students if you're suffering from a menstrual imbalance—whether it be heavy bleeding, painful periods, irregular or delayed periods, or extreme PMS—the *first* thing you need to institute in your life is the practice of resting and retreating when you bleed. As explored in chapter four, there are many health benefits in taking a little retreat-time during your period—the most delicate phase of your cycle.

I recommend you try some of the suggestions for honouring your bleeding time detailed in chapter four (see p.80) including using the Dark Moon yoga practices (also in chapter four) as a wonderful way to consciously rest during your menses.

> *Give up trying to get your leg straighter and your back*
> *more open, and focus on caring for yourself and purifying*
> *each cell of your body by bathing it in breath.*

> – LINDA SPARROWE[340]

Cultivate balance throughout the month

> *Vata and apana dominate during the days of the flow,*
> *during which the body appends to the flow all the ama and*
> *other filth which has collected in the blood over the course*
> *of the month. ... Any previously unnoticed disharmony*
> *that may have developed during the month will come into*
> *sharp focus just as apana mobilizes to begin its work,*
> *which is why you may first notice symptoms of imbalances*
> *only when your period begins, or is about to begin.*

> —DR. ROBERT E. SVOBODA[341]

I hope that, at this point, you truly recognise the need to slow down during your Dark Moon, bleeding time. I also trust that the idea of treating yourself compassionately throughout the *whole* of the month, throughout your four menstrual phases, has landed. In terms of healing menstrual anomalies, this is a vital take-home message: if you don't eat a healthy diet, don't get enough rest, and don't employ appropriate stress management strategies to

---

340   Linda Sparrowe, *Yoga for a Healthy Menstrual Cycle*, p.43

341   Ibid., p.71

support your holistic health throughout all stages of your monthly cycle, you may find that, come your menstruation, your body has to work doubly hard to expel the accumulated *ama* (physical, mental and emotional toxins) during the natural cleansing process of this phase.[342] This may result in exacerbated menstrual cramps and heavy bleeding as the body strives to try to reset after an unbalanced preceding month.

Throughout your cycle, practise *ahimsa* (self care and compassion)[343] in how you eat, work, rest and play so that there is moderation and mindfulness in all that you do. Indulge regularly in light exercise and activities that nourish your nervous system and ultimately give you joy. These joy-elevating practices are unique to everyone. In addition to yoga and meditation, you could take a walk in nature, read a good novel, take a long bath, get a massage, garden, dance, play a musical instrument, play your favourite sports, just sit and 'be' with a cup of tea, or socialise with family and friends. These are just a few ideas.

'The problem is with the entire cycle, not just the portion of it during which you may be miserable, and the remedy lies in returning the entire cycle to harmony,' reminds Dr Svoboda.[344] The key then, from the Ayurvedic perspective, is to understand which *dosha*, or constitution is governing your menstrual cycle imbalance. If you have an excess of *vata*, you are more likely to suffer from irregular cycles, or regular cycles with longer spacing into between. You will also be prone to suffering pain and cramps during your menstruation (due to tension and blockage in the abdominal area), and your premenstrual symptoms will tend towards insomnia and nervous tension. If you are dominated by the *pitta dosha*, you may experience shorter cycles and heavy bleeding that lasts for longer periods of time; your premenstrual symptoms are more likely to manifest as irritability, acne flare-ups and headaches. For those with an excess of *kapha*, your periods will be regular, and you may experience dull pain or cramps when you bleed. You may also be prone to water retention, swollen breasts and bloating.[345]

As part of an overall holistic approach, you can use this Ayurvedic template to help you understand the root causes for your menstrual imbalance and build a healthier menstrual cycle. See Appendix 1 for some tips on balancing an excess of any of these three *doshas*.

---

342 See: Sparrowe, *Yoga for a Healthy Menstrual Cycle*, p.9

343 See p.50 in chapter three for more information on the important Feminine Yoga principle of *ahimsa*.

344 Svoboda, *Ayurveda for Women*, p.72

345 Reference: Svoboda pp.73-74

Take an integrated approach

If you have a long-standing and deep-seated menstrual problem that is distressing you and impeding your lifestyle, it may take some time and a concerted effort to come to a place of healing. You may need to try several techniques and modalities to form an integrated, multi-pronged approach that will facilitate recovery. In this case, yoga may comprise just one prong. Other prongs might include: seeking medical attention that may involve medication, surgery, or hormonal therapy; being treated by an acupuncturist or herbalist; and seeking counselling. You may also find that adjusting your diet and taking specific nutritional supplements (vitamins and minerals) can help.[346]

According to Dr Christiane Northrup, many of the gynaecological issues women can experience are caused by cellular inflammation. Dr Northrup recommends a low GI diet that is high in protein and healthy fats, and she also suggests reducing or eliminating your intake of inflammatory foods like dairy, refined white flour, sugar, caffeine and alcohol in order to address many menstrual imbalances. 'A nutrient-poor diet that contains too many refined foods that raise blood sugar too quickly (known as high glycemic index foods) favors the production of inflammatory chemicals through-out the body that result in pain and tissue damage,' she writes.[347] And stress can compound the problem. 'When high glycemic index foods are consumed in an individual who also has high circulating levels of stress hormones, the production of inflammatory chemicals is made even worse,'

---

346   In *Clinical Naturopathy: An Evidence Based Guide to Practice*, the authors, Jerome Sarris and John Wardle suggest that dietary factors may play a significant role in menstrual irregularities: 'Women with PMS typically consume more dairy products, refined sugar and high sodium foods than women without PMS. Fish, eggs and fruit have been associated with less dysmenorrhoea, while wine is associated with more. Women following a low-fat, vegetarian diet also had lower incidence of dysmenorrhoea.' See pp.350–351. The authors also note that calcium, magnesium, vitamins E, A and zinc have been shown to help in the reduction of PMS and menstrual pain.

347   Christiane Northrup, M.D., *Women's Bodies Women's Wisdom*, p.121. And in an article on fibroids, Northrup writes, 'White foods like sugar and starch increase insulin, which changes the way estrogen is metabolized, creating compounds that are more likely to cause cellular inflammation and fibroid symptoms, including enhanced growth of existing fibroids...' See: http://www.drnorthrup.com/fibroids/#sthash.7cZNg52t.dpuf

writes Dr Nothrup. She goes on to say, 'Menstrual cramps are just one manifestation of this vicious cycle. Others include fluid retention, headaches, insomnia, and muscle aches and pains. In fact, all of the symptoms of PMS are caused, in part, by cellular inflammation from the overproduction of inflammatory chemicals.'[348]

For more information on diet and nutritional support for hormonal imbalances, I recommend Dr Christiane Northrup's wonderful tome, *Women's Bodies, Women's Wisdom*, as well as Dr Sara Gottfried's comprehensive, integrated approach in her book, *The Hormone Cure*.

Acknowledge the mind-body connection

If your menstrual imbalance is chronic and intractable and you have exhausted all of the standard healing avenues, you may benefit from approaching it from a mind-body angle: be open to the idea that your health dilemma may not be just 'physical'. By being willing to journey into self-enquiry (which may include meditative enquiry and journaling), or even seeking counselling, you may contribute towards your healing by uncovering any potential mind-body causes for 'dis-ease' in your body.

Dr Northrup claims that emotional factors can very often be the root cause of issues in your reproductive system. While Dr Northrup is quick to suggest a middle-ground in which a woman also considers 'medical treatments as a bridge across the river to true health,' she also asserts that your thoughts and beliefs, fashioned from your past-conditioning, can manifest as physical imbalances. 'The science of the mind/body connection, or psychoneuroimmunology (PNI), helps explain how the circumstances of our lives can affect our bodies,' she explains. 'PNI and related research show that the hormonal and neurological events within the body and the subtle electromagnetic fields around and within the body form a crucial link between cultural wounding, which we think of as "psychological" and "emotional", and the gynaecological or other problems women have, which we think of as "physical".'[349]

Dr Northrup cites numerous case studies of women she has treated who only achieved healing once they recognised and transformed negative attitudes towards their bodies and ultimately their femininity. This includes

---

348 Ibid., pp.121–22. Dr Northrup explains that these 'inflammatory chemicals' include cytokines, bradykinins, interleukins, and prostaglandins (including PGF2 alpha) and prostacyclins.

349 Northrup, p.31

working with the disconnection and disassociation that can result from trauma. 'Many women who've survived sexual abuse, for example, divorce themselves from their bodies. Some experience themselves in their bodies only from the neck up,' writes Northrup.[350]

MENSTRUAL MEDICINE: YOGA FOR BALANCING YOUR CYCLE

Following are the yoga guidelines for balancing your hormones and bringing your cycle back to balance. For more specific 'yoga prescriptions', see under the relevant menstrual disorder in the remainder of this chapter, where I consecutively investigate: dysmenorrhea (menstrual cramps), menorrhagia (heavy bleeding), uterine fibroids, endometriosis, polycystic ovary syndrome, amenorrhea (absent periods), and PMS (Premenstrual Syndrome). The menstrual medicine 'go-to postures' at the end of this chapter can also serve as a handy resource for adapting yoga to specific menstrual symptoms.

Move with *your* Moon

The idea of Moving with the Moon—practising the most appropriate yoga for each phase of your menstrual cycle—forms the very premise of this book, and supports the goal of *ahimsa* (gentleness) as an overriding principle in how you live both on and off the mat. By practising your yoga in this way, you are able to make a positive impact on your menstrual health and overall wellbeing.

Yoga teacher and author of *The Women's Yoga Book*, Bobby Clennell agrees, saying, 'Different poses produce different responses within the system. You can nurture a state of good health by doing the right pose at the right time of your cycle. This will influence your short-term and long-term reproductive health, supporting fertility and healthy menstruation and a smooth transition into menopause.'[351]

If you want to balance and nourish your hormonal system, a key starting point is to follow the suggested guidelines for practice for each of the four phases detailed in this book (see Part Three: chapters four to seven). I also encourage you to follow your own intuition and self-knowledge along the way—qualities that are so important in the process of healing.

---

350 Ibid

351 Bobby Clennel, *The Women's Yoga Book: Asana and Pranayama for all Phases of the Menstrual Cycle*, p.17

Honour *apana*

An important ingredient in promoting the healthy functioning of your menstrual cycle is *apana*. As already mentioned, *apana*—the downward movement of energy that resides in the pelvis—is responsible for removal of all of the toxins, or *ama*, from the body.[352] Fostering *apana* is especially important during menstruation as this is your monthly opportunity to purge your body of *ama*. As Maya Tiwari writes, 'At the physical level, metabolic activity during the menstrual cycle increases ama, metabolic toxicity, which may manifest as menstrual cramps, physical pain, diarrhoea, nausea, nervous tension, and emotional distress. For this reason, most women experience a feeling of incredible lightness after the cycle is over.'[353]

Inverting the body and practising strong exercises that contract the abdominals and pelvic floor when you are menstruating can all potentially interfere with *apana*. According to Dr Robert Svoboda, if the menstrual flow is obstructed, *ama* can quickly 'perfuse the body'. He suggests that this can cause endometriosis and other reproductive imbalances like vaginitis, ovarian cysts and uterine fibroids.[354]

Nourish and heal with the Classical Women's postures

> ...all reproductive disorders relate to Shakti energy. When this
> energy is out of balance with the lunar cycles it influences
> the doshas, which in turn impacts the menstrual cycle.

—MAYA TIWARI[355]

In the overview of the principles of a feminine approach to yoga in chapter three, I explored how the healthy circulation of energy (*shakti prana*) within the pelvic bowl is essential for our health and vitality as women. All of the Classical Women's poses (see Appendix 2) promote the circulation of energy and blood flow within the pelvic region because they open the hips and pelvis, stretch and tone the pelvic floor and soften or gently stretch the lower belly.

---

352   For more on *apana* as an important and beneficial Feminine Yoga principle, see p.60 in chapter three, and p.84 in chapter four.

353   Maya Tiwari, *Women's Power to Heal*, p.107

354   Dr Robert E. Svoboda, *Ayurveda for Women* p.71

355   Maya Tiwari, *Women's Power to Heal*, p.105

Variously, the Classical Women's postures tone, nourish and stimulate the reproductive organs, soothe the nervous system and ground your energy, which is helpful for engendering the *apana* energy that is so balancing for your cycle, and makes them an important ally when working to correct menstrual anomalies.

Invert, invert, invert!

If you suffer from a menstrual imbalance, a particular focus in your yoga practice, outside of your Dark Moon menstrual phase, should be to regularly practise Inversions.

Inversions help pacify the nervous system because they tone the vagus nerve that is connected with the parasympathetic (calming) nervous system. The vagus nerve passes through the neck and can be activated due to the pressure caused by the position of the head in postures like Shoulderstand (see Figure 132, p.186) which involves the Jalandhara Bandha (throat lock) and compresses the throat and stretches the back of the neck.[356]

Shoulderstand, often called the 'queen of all yoga postures', is a quint-essential Feminine Yoga posture. 'Sarvangasana (Shoulderstand) develops the feminine qualities of patience and emotional stability,' writes Geeta Iyengar. Iyengar goes on to claim that Shoulderstand can correct urinary disorders, uterine displacement, and menstrual disorders. Likewise, she says that Halasana (the Plow Pose—see Figure 133, p.186) soothes the brain and the nervous system and can cure menstrual and urinary disorders.[357] Medical doctor and yoga therapist, Dr Krishna Raman concurs, suggesting that Inversions, 'lift the floor of the pelvic organs, strengthening them... regulating any disorder of blood flow'.[358]

Even simple Legs up the Wall (Viparita Karani—see Figure 410, p.453) can have a positive effect on your nervous system, and by association your hormonal system. Sara Gottfried, M.D., says that whenever you put your feet above the level of your heart, you activate the parasympathetic (rest and digest) nervous system.[359]

In addition to calming the nervous system, Inversions can have a direct beneficial effect on the organs of the hormonal system. They promote

---

356 Mel Robin, *A Physiological Handbook for Teachers of Yogasana*, p.152

357 Geeta S. Iyengar, *Yoga, A Gem for Women*, p.179

358 Dr Krishna Raman, *A Matter of Health: Integration of Yoga and Western Medicine for Prevention and Cure*, location 1739 (Kindle edition)

359 See this online article by Gottfried: http://www.healthylivingmagazine.us/Articles/574/

increased blood circulation to the endocrine glands throughout the body[360] and in the brain.[361] Dr Krishna Raman says that Inversions 'drain the stagnated uterine blood and secretions and irrigate the organs with fresh blood'.[362]

The last word on Inversions goes to Geeta Iyengar, who suggests that they are a 'veritable boon to women and should on no account be missed'.[363]

COMMON MENSTRUAL DISORDERS

Menstrual cramps: dysmenorrhea

Menstrual cramps, or dysmenorrhea, occur just before or during menstruation and may be experienced as sharp colicky twinges, spasmodic contractions in the belly, or dull, achy cramping in the lower back, inner thighs and groins. Dysmenorrhea can also be associated with headaches, nausea and vomiting, diarrhea and light-headedness.[364]

Approximately 60% of all women suffer from menstrual cramps[365] although some studies suggest as many as 90% of women experience pain and discomfort when they bleed.[366] A smaller percentage are unable to function for one or more days each month because of the severity of their pain.[367]

---

360   See: Geeta Iyengar, *Yoga, A Gem for Women*, p.192

361   John Friend, an American yoga teacher, explains, 'the blood circulation affects the glands of the endocrine system. Each gland pulsates just like every cell in our body pulsates; so as blood flow diminishes, the pulsation of the actual gland diminishes too. In fact, if circulation to the particular gland is either excessive or restricted, he says, you won't get an optimal level of health for that gland.' Cited by Linda Sparrowe here: https://www.yogajournal.com/lifestyle/menstrual-essentials

362   *Yoga and Medical Science FAQ*, Dr Krishna Raman and Dr S Suresh, location 3766 (Kindle edition)

363   Iyengar, *Yoga a Gem for Women*, p.192

364   See: https://www.betterhealth.vic.gov.au/health/conditionsandtreatments/menstruation-pain-dysmenorrhoea

365   According to Northrup in *Women's Bodies, Women's Wisdom*, p.120

366   See: http://www.nhs.uk/conditions/Periods-painful/Pages/Introduction.aspx

367   See: http://www.nhs.uk/conditions/Periods-painful/Pages/Introduction.aspx where a study is cited stating that up to 14% of women reported frequently being unable to go to work due to menstrual pain.

Menstrual cramping can be divided into two types: primary or secondary dysmenorrhea. Primary dysmenorrhea is 'the garden variety' of menstrual cramping and tends to be more common in teenagers and younger women and to decrease when a woman has children. Primary dysmenorrhea is thought to be caused by the excessive release of prostaglandins, a hormone that also occurs in childbirth and causes contractions in the uterus. If the uterus contracts too strongly it can press against nearby blood vessels cutting off the oxygen supply to the muscle tissue of the uterus triggering pain.[368] Secondary dysmenorrhea can be more serious, and the pain can last longer, reflecting an underlying problem such as endometriosis, pelvic inflammatory disease, fibroids or ovarian cysts.

If your doctor has established that your cramping is of the secondary dysmenorrhea-type, in addition to trying the suggestions that follow for alleviating cramps with yoga, you may want to skip forward to the appropriate section in this chapter that relates to your particular underlying menstrual anomaly. For example, if you have ascertained that your menstrual cramps are caused by endometriosis, you can read more on page 339, or if they are related to fibroids, you will find more information on page 335.

Yoga for Menstrual Cramps

Stretch the areas that are cramping

According to Mel Robin, stretching the area where pain is occurring can help alleviate cramping and in fact will work as a preventative.[369] To clarify how this works, you only need to consider a beginning yoga student who is frequently struck down with uncomfortable cramping in the calf or foot when attempting to stay in kneeling positions in yoga class, and to juxtapose that with the experienced yogini who has become more accustomed to the yoga positions that stretch these muscles, and she is able to sit serenely without any cramping sensations.

Therefore, the Classical Women's postures like Baddha Konasana (see Figure 383, p.441) or Upavista Konasana (see Figure 384, p.442) that stretch the pelvic area may reduce or eliminate menstrual cramping pain. Supta Virasana (see Figure 397, p.450) may also help as it is a posture that stretches the front of the thighs and groins, which can be affected by referred cramping pain.[370]

---

368   See: http://www.webmd.com/women/menstrual-cramps

369   Robin, *A Physiological Handbook for Teachers of Yogasana*, p.231

370   Ibid., p.231

Soothe and soften with Restorative postures

A number of Restorative Yoga postures are wonderfully therapeutic for menstrual pain and discomfort: they help to dispel fatigue, calm the nervous system, and provide an opportunity to breathe and relax into any cramping pain.

One of the most effective poses for easing menstrual cramps is Supported Adho Mukha Virasana (Child Pose— see Figure 296). This pose is extremely soothing due to the gentle counter pressure of the belly into the bolster, as

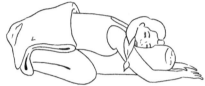

Figure 296

well as the quietening effects on the nervous system. For added menstrual pain relief and to enhance its soothing effect, try placing a heat pack or hot water bottle on your sacrum. Or, simply placing a folded blanket on the lower back can provide warmth, comfort and nurturing (as pictured in Figure 296).

Providing a similar soothing, massaging effect on the belly is the Prone Savasana with Towel Roll (see Figure 297). Roll up a bath towel so it is about 30 cm wide and at least 10 cm thick. Come to lie in a prone position, resting your lower belly onto the towel, and have your arms bent up over-head, head to one side. Let the feet and arms relax, to release deeply from the hips and the lower back.

Another favourite for soothing men-strual pain is Supta Baddha Konasana

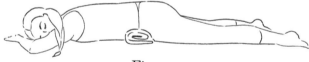

Figure 297

(see Figure 395, p.449). This Restorative, Classical Women's posture can alleviate congestion in the abdominal and pelvic areas. As always, when you practise this reclining, supported posture, it's important to support the knees with a blanket wrapped around the legs, or blocks or bolsters or cushions under the knees (see Figure 20, p.96 and Figure 21, p.97) so that you can enjoy maximum relaxation through the inner thighs and pelvic floor muscles and the belly remains soft.

It should be noted that it's very individual what works for each woman. For some women suffering menstrual pain they instinctively feel the need to get into a kind of foetal position; this is when the Supported Child Pose is most effective. Other women find that they need the opposite—to create openness and space for the belly—and this is where Supta Baddha

Konasana, Supta Virasana and Supported Bridge Pose (see Figure 399, p.450) are more beneficial. If the pain is severe and the woman is experiencing relief in her chosen posture—whether it be in a Forward Bending movement like the Child Pose, or a supported Backbending position like Supta Baddha Konasana—she can stay there as long as she feels good and experiences relief; this may be for as long as 10–15 minutes.

A replenishing pose that may also alleviate or even prevent menstrual cramping is the Constructive Rest Position (see Figure 418, p.456). This simple yet profound resting posture offers a passive release of the psoas muscle, which runs through the very core of the body.[371] As mentioned, there may be a connection between a tight psoas and menstrual pain. Liz Koch says that her clients who had been taking pain medication for severe cramps found that by releasing this deep muscle—that passes through the pelvic bowl—they have been able to become pain and drug free. She writes, 'Rather than the cramps occurring from within the uterus it is often a contracted psoas muscle that presses on the reproductive organs; constricting blood circulation and impeding, possibly irritating the nerves that innervate both the muscle and the specific organs.'[372]

Also, see the 'Menstrual Medicine Go-To Postures and Practices' at the end of this chapter for a summary list of beneficial postures for menstrual cramps.

Putting it all together: creating a sequence for menstrual pain

When suffering menstrual, cramping pain, you can practise any of the above-mentioned therapeutic postures individually. Or you can put together a complete sequence, combining a few of these postures. If you're not confident in creating your own sequence, try the Classical Dark Moon Menstrual Sequence in chapter four, which involves a full, yet gentle, range of movement for the spine—Supported Backbends counter-posed with Supported Forward Bends (and vice versa)—to help increase the circulation into the pelvic area, relieving pelvic congestion and discomfort. The combination of these postures also alternately stretches and releases the lower back to relieve lower back tightness, pain and general achiness.

---

371   See p.96, chapter four, for more information on the psoas muscle.

372   Liz Koch, *The Psoas Book*, p.61

Harness the healing power of deep relaxation

Manisha was a student of mine who suffered from severe endometriosis (see page 339, for an explanation of this condition) that caused debilitating menstrual cramps. On some days of her period she was forced to take time off work, doubled up in pain, despite taking strong painkillers. Manisha found the relaxation practices of yoga beneficial. 'I loved the relaxation time at the start of our class, when you are encouraged to check in with your body,' she remembers. 'It helped me move from one space to another, like a "circuit-breaker".'

As she lay there in a supported Restorative pose, or in Savasana (the re-laxation at the end of the class), Manisha was able to reflect, 'I'm in pain, but I'm in control'. Relaxing and breathing in this way provided Manisha with an opportunity to focus in on the pain, but not in a negative way. 'Rather than fight the pain and feel I had to push through it, yoga taught me to simply set the intention: "Now I'm going to heal my body",' she explains.

Geeta Iyengar suggests that dysmenorrhea may be the result of not just a physical imbalance but also a psychological one. She says a 'nervous temperament' as well as 'fear, disharmony, anxiety and neurosis' are all fac-tors.[373] Perhaps Iyengar is intuiting the proven connection between stress and dysmenorrhea. Restorative Yoga as well as relaxation practices like Yoga Nidra[374] can therefore be beneficial for menstrual cramps by calming your mind and nervous system, and balancing out the stress response.

There are three different Yoga Nidra practices to choose from in this book—each one tailored to a different phase in your cycle. When you are menstruating, try the Dark Moon Yoga Nidra in chapter four (see p.116); leading up to your period, try the Waning Moon Yoga Nidra in chapter seven (see p.268); and around your ovulation phase, try the 'Full Moon Yoga Nidra' in chapter six (see p.214). If your self-awareness allows you to recognize that you are a person of 'nervous temperament'—in other words you are easily stressed, anxious or overwhelmed—make a prescription for yourself of practising one of these Yoga Nidras at least several times a week.

373 Geeta Iyengar, *Yoga a Gem for Women*, p.47

374 See Note 335 referencing a 6-month research trial that showed that regular practice of Yoga Nidra can lessen the psychological symptoms of menstrual disorders. The results showed, 'There was significant improvement in pain symptoms ($P<0.006$), gastrointestinal symptoms ($P<0.04$), cardiovascular symptoms ($P<0.02$) and urogenital symptoms ($P<0.005$) after 6 months of Yoga Nidra therapy in Intervention group in comparison to control group.'

Like Manisha, you may find that the practice of deep, conscious relaxation helps you move through the pain and discomfort of severe menstrual cramps.

Set a clear, positive intention

The Yoga Nidra practice includes a ritual called *sankalpa*—a positive, heartfelt intention or resolution that you repeat three times to yourself at the beginning and then again at the end of the Yoga Nidra. By working with *sankalpa*, specifically one around your menstrual health, you can promote a more positive attitude towards your body and your cycle, which can feed into your menstrual cycle healing.

Note that a *sankalpa* is most effective when it is framed as a short, positive statement in the *present* tense.[375] I have suggested these sample *sankalpas* in the three Moving with the Moon Yoga Nidras in this book:

- *My bleeding time is easeful and joyful—I honour myself during this sacred time and I am completely connected to my body and my inner self.*
- *My experience of my monthly cycle is easeful, joyful and connected as I trust that I am able to take care of myself in so many ways.*
- *I am joyful, grateful and deeply connected to my feminine self.*

You can also create a *sankalpa* of your own—whatever arises spontaneously from your deepest intuition. For example, you may conceive a *sankalpa* that is specifically connected with your dysmenorrhea such as:

- *I am healthy, whole and healed and now enjoy an easeful period.*
- *My womb releases my moon-blood easefully and joyfully.*

The main thing is to stick with a primary *sankalpa* that feels right until it comes to fruition—avoid 'chopping and changing'.

---

375   Richard Miller, Ph.D, a clinical psychologist and expert in Yoga Nidra writes, 'When we position our prayers in the future, we strive for something that will never arrive. So we always phrase prayers in the present tense. Instead of saying "I will be healthy," I will feel loved," or "My friend will be cured of a disease", we affirm "I am whole, healed and healthy," "My True Nature is love, which I am in this moment," or "My friend is healed, whole and healthy." When the future arrives, it will be now. So we acknowledge this fact by making the future reality of our prayers the actuality of this moment and set our prayers in the language and reality that they are true, now.' From *Yoga Nidra: The Meditative Heart of Yoga*, pp.35–36

The power of *sankalpa* is not be underestimated. Swami Satyananda Saraswati, a major proponent of Yoga Nidra, writes, '...when you withdraw your mind a little bit, and enter into a state where you are neither in deep sleep nor completely awake, whatever impressions enter the mind at that time become powerful, and they remain there'.[376]

While *sankalpa* is particularly potent when practised within the context of the deep relaxation of Yoga Nidra, you can also use it as an affirmation that you repeat to yourself throughout your day. I like to repeat my various *sankalpa* or positive affirmations (applying to different aspects of my life—my health, family, work, etc.) when I take a solitary walk along the beach, and I also repeat them as I sit quietly at the end of my yoga practice.

Breathe through the pain

A beneficial Pranayama (yoga breathing technique) to help relax the body and manage menstrual pain is the Soft Belly Breath (see p.100). This feminine breathing technique will help you consciously breathe into the spasms in your womb and also to relax the abdominal muscles that tend to harden when you are stressed or in pain. Focus on really allowing the abdomen to soften and relax in response to your deep, healing belly breaths. It may also be helpful to imagine a calming colour, or a feeling of comforting heat, entering and soothing your womb with each deep abdominal breath. Donna Farhi offers this simple imagery:

> Visualise the uterus as calm and relaxed, as the os of the cervix opens to allow the blood to flow unrestricted.[377]

After a few rounds of Soft Belly Breath, you can evolve into lengthening the exhalations, which will engage the parasympathetic (relax and repair) aspect of the nervous system, helping instil a sense of calm that can positively influence your experience of menstrual cramping. I agree with prenatal yoga teacher and doula Katie Manitsas who uses this breathing practice to help her pregnant students with pain management and anxiety and says, 'If I had one "technique" that I could share with all pregnant women for labour it would be learning the practice of extending the exhale to manage pain.'[378] As I have mentioned, menstruation is like a 'mini-birth' so this is an appropriate breathing technique to support pain management during this phase of your menstrual cycle.

---

376   Swami Satyananda Saraswati, *Yoga Nidra*, p.5

377   Donna Farhi, 'Yoga for Menstrual Cramps', *Yoga Journal*, pp.7–10, May/June 1986

378   Katie Manitsas, *The Yoga of Birth*, p.66

Extending the exhalation

To begin this practice, count what your natural, easy exhalation is—for example, five counts. Then, progressively, every second breath, see if you can lengthen the exhalation by one count until you can no longer extend the breath without risk of strain or building tension. Just allow the in-breath to take care of itself—no need to count the duration of your inhalation. You may find that by the end you have managed to double the length of your exhalation so that if it started out at 5 counts it has evolved into 10 counts by the end of the practice.

As always, never strain or force, and cease the practice if you are uncomfortable in any way. Allow the breath to return to a completely natural, uncontrolled pace again, before you come out of the practice.

Another feminine breathing technique that can help with menstrual cramping-pain is the Falling-Out Breath (see p.104). As you exhale through an open, relaxed mouth, visualize that you are breathing pain and discomfort out and away from your body. You can enhance the benefits if you practise sounding with this releasing, Falling-Out Breath. Try working with low, deep sounds like 'ahhh' and 'uhhh' that come from deep within your belly, from your womb. Sound is a very effective tool for pain management when we are in labour[379] and you can also use this tool to help you with your monthly 'mini-birth' when your uterus is contracting during menstruation.

Mudras for menstrual pain

Three Mudras that are said to alleviate menstrual cramping are the Shakti Mudra, Maha Sacral Mudra and Yoni Mudra. They are best performed at the beginning or end of your yoga practice when you are sitting quietly in meditation.

---

379   The efficacy of sound as a pain management tool has long been acknowledged in natural birthing circles. Using sound to help manage labour pain was perhaps first posited by well known midwife Ina May Gaskin. Obstetric physiotherapist Juju Sundin writes in her book, *Birth Skills: Proven Pain Management Techniques for your Labour and Birth*, 'If you work off excess adrenalin with sound and activity your oxytocin (a hormone that increases the efficiency of contractions during labour) will flow more proficiently', p.7. She also writes that vocalizing helps build our endorphins (our natural opiate hormones) and produces a 'wonderful non-painful rhythmic focus to concentrate on', p.59

Shakti Mudra

This Mudra brings pleasant relaxation to the pelvic and lower intestinal area. It may help settle menstrual cramping and is also good if you're suffering from insomnia.[380]

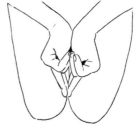

Figure 298

How to do it

Place the tips of the little fingers and ring fingers together and tuck the thumbs into the palms loosely wrapping the index and middle fingers around the thumbs (see Figure 298). Place the hands in front of your belly and take a few deep Soft Belly Breaths (see p.100). Focus on feeling the breath (and therefore the energy) circulating around the pelvic area. Stay for up to 15 minutes. Practise several times a day to help with menstrual cramps.

Yoni Mudra

Yoni Mudra helps with menstrual cramps, menopausal imbalances[381] and with aligning your menstruation to the new moon ('white moon cycle'). It also induces a sense of calmness.[382]

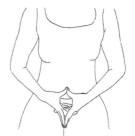

Figure 299

How to do it

The simplest version of this Mudra involves interlacing your hands, then extending just your index and thumbs so that the index fingers touch each other and the thumbs touch each other, to form a diamond (*yoni*) shape (see Figure 299). Position the hands in front of the naval with the index fingers pointing down, thumbs pointing up. Sit quietly for up to 10 minutes, focusing on smooth, even breathing and feeling calm energy pervading the whole body.

---

380   See: Gertrud Hirschi, *Mudras: Yoga in your Hands*, p.124

381   See: https://www.youtube.com/watch?v=7IO_jNpJNCY

382   See: Maya Tiwari, *Women's Power to Heal*, p.155

Maha Sacral Mudra

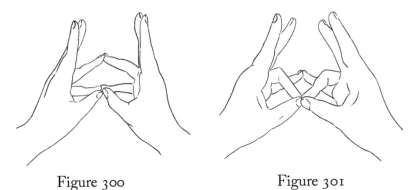

Figure 300   Figure 301

This Mudra has a relaxing and balancing effect and, like Shakti Mudra helps settle spasms of the pelvic and intestinal organs, and is particularly good for soothing menstrual cramps. It is also good for bladder and prostate problems and if you combine it with Mula Bandha (pelvic floor lift) you may help with incontinence and haemorrhoids.[383]

How to do it

There are two stages to this mudra. The first stage is to place the tips of your ring fingers together, and the tips of the little fingers and thumbs together—creating a rounded 'figure 8' shape with the little fingers and thumbs (emulating the shape of the bones of the two sides of the pelvis—see Figure 300). Stay here for 10 deep breaths. Then, move to the second stage, extending the little fingers and bringing their tips together and rounding the tips of the ring fingers and thumbs together (see Figure 301). Again, stay here for 10 deep breaths.

What to do the rest of the month

In addition to practising menstrual-friendly Restorative Yoga, relaxation practices, breathing and Mudras when you bleed and are experiencing the cramping, I recommend that you also pay attention to practising therapeutically throughout the whole month. This means following all the principles of Moving with the Moon—adjusting your yoga practice to suit each phase of your menstrual cycle (as detailed in chapters four through seven).

An emphasis on Inversions—practised when you're not bleeding, of course—can also be beneficial, helping to balance and regulate the hormonal system, which may result in the reduction of menstrual cramps.

383   See: Gertrud Hirschi, *Mudras: Yoga in your Hands*, p.126

According to B.K.S. Iyengar, Shoulderstand, in particular, can reduce menstrual cramps and help regulate the menstrual flow.[384]

Iyengar also suggests a regular practice of Backbends to 'create elasticity and strength in the pelvic muscles', which may also help prevent or alleviate menstrual cramping.[385] Again, only Backbends that are supported and menstrual-friendly should be practised during your period.

Finally, as I touched on chapter seven, it's a good idea to practise some of the Classical Women's postures like Upavista Konasana, Baddha Konasana, Trikonasana and Ardha Chandrasana (see Appendix 2) just before you bleed, as preventative, 'anti-cramp' movements.

Heavy periods: menorrhagia

Menorrhagia refers to heavy, excessive or prolonged bleeding, and is one of the most common gynaecological disorders around the world, affecting 20% of women in Australia[386] and more than 10 million women in America every year.[387]

How heavy is 'heavy bleeding'? One definition states that your flow is heavy if you need to change your pad or tampon every two hours or less, while another defines it as the loss of more than 60-80 mls of blood over your period.[388] 'The best guide is to decide whether your period is impacting on your quality of life, causing you to be housebound, interrupting your daily activities or causing you stress and anxiety,' concludes the Jean Hailes women's health organization.[389]

And how prolonged is 'prolonged bleeding'? This is defined as bleeding continuously for more than seven days.[390] The colour of normal, healthy

---

384   B.K.S. Iyengar, *Yoga: The Path to Holistic Health*, p.125

385   Cited by Bobby Clennell in *The Women's Yoga Book*, p.198

386   See: http://www.racgp.org.au/afp/2015/july/
      obstetric-and-gynaecological-problems-in-australian-general-practice/

387   See: http://www.medicalnewstoday.com/articles/295202.php

388   According to an article on Medical News Today, 'Average blood loss during menstruation is around 30 to 40 milliliters, or 2 to 3 tablespoons, over a period of 4 to 5 days. Officially, menorrhagia is a loss of over 80 milliliters of blood in one cycle, or twice the normal amount.' See: https://www.medicalnewstoday.com/articles/295202.php

389   See: https://jeanhailes.org.au/health-a-z/periods/heavy-bleeding

390   See: http://www.medicalnewstoday.com/articles/295202.php

menstrual bleeding is bright red. In a condition like menorrhagia there may be clotting, heavy cramps and the woman may feel 'wiped out' due to the excessive loss of blood.

If menorrhagia continues cycle after cycle, a woman may suffer from iron deficiency or anaemia (low red-blood cell count), especially if she is not getting enough iron in her diet or taking supplements to replace the blood loss.[391]

The heavy bleeding can be caused by underlying conditions like: endometriosis; fibroids; adenomyosis (a condition in which the glands that normally grow in only the lining of the uterus grow deeply into the walls of the uterus); Pelvic Inflammatory Disease (PID); or even uterine, ovarian or cervical cancers.

Menorrhagia can also simply be the result of an imbalance in the hormones that is more common during adolescence when women's bodies are finding a regular cyclical pattern, as well as later in life when they move closer to menopause. Heavy bleeding can be a symptom of the perimenopause (the lead up to menopause) as it can be related to a deficiency in progesterone that may cause oestrogen dominance, which is common during this transitional phase of women's lives.[392]

The mind-body connection may also play its part, with Christiane Northrup, M.D., suggesting that menorrhagia can be related to Second Chakra issues that include concerns around creativity, relationships, money and need to control others.[393] If you can make time to carve out creative space and listen to the messages your body is sending you as it 'weeps' with heavy bleeding, you may be able to resolve the imbalance within your body.

Yoga for Menorrhagia

Honour your lower energy levels

Heavy or prolonged bleeding can really sap your energy. In addition to seeking medical help if the problem is chronic and debilitating, you need to make sure you're allowing yourself the time and space to rest when you bleed. As I keep reiterating, the cornerstone of the Moving with the Moon, Feminine Yoga approach is to rest and conserve your energy during your bleeding time. Treating your menses with the respect that it requires—as

---

391   See: Northrup, *Women's Bodies, Women's Wisdom*, p.153

392   See: Northrup—http://www.drnorthrup.com/
heavy-menstrual-bleeding-menorrhagia/

393   See: Northrup, *Women's Bodies, Women's Wisdom*, p.153

a sacred time of rest and renewal—is even more important in the case of menorrhagia. With the excessive bleeding, your body is expressing 'dis-ease', and rather than ignore your body's cry for help, this is an opportunity to take the time to listen inwards for clues to your healing.

Heed your body's signal by resting, sleeping and meditating. If you feel the urge to do yoga, practise a gentle menstrual practice such as the Classical Dark Moon Menstrual Sequence and if you want to put your own practice together, ensure you follow all of the yoga guidelines for the Dark Moon menstrual phase (see chapter four). When you are bleeding, particularly if it's heavy or prolonged, your yoga practice needs to be very gentle and nurturing, with the focus on conserving your energy.

Note that the only Standing poses that are recommended for menorrhagia (during your menses) are: Trikonasana (Figure 24, p.100) against a wall, and Ardha Chandrasana (Figure 25, p.100) against a wall. Performing these postures while supported by the wall ensures you don't over-strain your abdominal and uterine regions, and instead create maximum opening and softening there. It is also beneficial to practise these postures at other phases in your cycle, when you're not bleeding.

If you have been suffering menorrhagia for some time and have developed an iron deficiency or anaemia, you will also need to go gently in your practice throughout the rest of the month, at least until you have stabilised the condition—which may include taking an iron supplement—and your energy levels have returned.

Cool and calm with Restorative postures

Supine Restorative postures like Supta Baddha Konasana (see Figure 395, p.449), Reclining Cross-legged Pose (see Figure 396, p.449), Supta Padangustasna II (supported with a bolster—see Figure 387, p.444) and Supported Bridge Pose (see p. 450) are all helpful for this condition as they provide deep relaxation, space and ease in the abdominal area. This, in turn, can help relieve throbbing in the belly, uterus and pelvic floor.

Forward Bending postures, like supported Pascimottanasana (see p.451), are also helpful because of their cooling and restful qualities and, according to B.K.S. Iyengar, they can also regulate and reduce bleeding.[394]

Additionally, the seated Classical Women's postures—such as Baddha Konasana (see Figure 383, p. 441) and Upavista Konasana (see Figure 384, p.442) are beneficial for softening and opening the abdominal and pelvic

---

394   B.K.S. Iyengar writes: 'Forward bends control the flow of blood and check excess bleeding'—*Yoga, The Path to Holistic Healing*, p.356

areas. For enhanced support, comfort and 'lushness' try practising these two postures (see Figure 302) with a vertical bolster standing on its end and resting on the wall behind you.

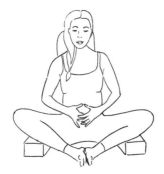

See the Menstrual Medicine Go-to Postures and Practices section at the end of this chapter for some additional postures that may be beneficial for menorrhagia.

Figure 302

Enquiry Meditation for menorrhagia

If you have been unable to find an obvious cause for your menorrhagia, try the following Enquiry Meditation to see if this helps you uncover any mind-body roots for your menstrual imbalance.

How to do it

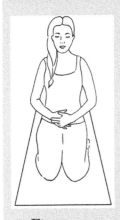

Sit or lie in a comfortable position. If you are very tired, adopt a supported supine position such as the Reclining Goddess Pose (see Figure 421, p.457) or Constructive Rest Position (see Figure 418, p.456). Otherwise you can sit upright in Vajrasana, straddling a bolster (see Figure 303). Sometimes, I've even done enquiry meditations like this one in the bath!

Close your eyes and place your palms over your lower belly, your womb-space—a gesture of nurturing and self-connection. Take a little time to just relax your physical body. Start by relaxing the muscles around and behind the eyes, across the forehead and around the

Figure 303

jaw. Then, move your awareness down your body to allow the shoulders to soften, the muscles in the chest and solar plexus to relax, and finally, consciously let go of any holding or gripping in the lower belly, pelvic floor and deep into your womb.

When you're ready, take some deep Soft Belly Breaths (see p.100). Fill up your lower belly, your womb-space with full, relaxing breaths. Breathe in and... *relax*... Breathe out and... *let go*... Allow the breath to massage the whole of your internal belly, right down to your pelvic floor. As you exhale, you may also want to practise some Falling-Out Breaths, allowing the breath to be relinquished from an open, relaxed mouth—perhaps even making some deep sounds as you do.

With each deep, Soft Belly Breath feel that your awareness is dropping more deeply into your body, your inner wisdom, your intuition and out of your head. Continue this breathing and dropping down into your deep, feminine self for as long as you like.

Once you feel like you are really connected with your internal space, your feeling-sense, allow your mind to form these enquiry questions:

What is my body telling me?
What are you telling me, my womb, as you bleed and bleed?

Then, simply wait. Wait to see if an answer spontaneously arises from within. Try not to force an answer to come, to pre-empt anything from the space of your logical, rational, thinking mind. Instead, wait and be open and receptive to whatever answer may arise from your deep wisdom-body, from your womb-space. It may take some time for anything to come. Just continue to wait, breathe and soften into your belly, into your womb-space.

If it feels right, repeat the enquiry question, and again wait.

The answer may come to you as a single word, a sentence, an idea, an image or a symbol. Be open to the answer coming to you in any form that your wisdom-body might offer.

Once an answer arises, sit with it a little while, holding the answer in your belly, deep into your womb-space. Breathe this answer in and out. Feel gratitude for the wisdom of your body and its remarkable ability to heal itself by knowing exactly what it needs at any given point.

If no answer comes to you no matter how long you wait, that's fine. Simply thank your body and move onto this next and final phase of the meditation. Know that you can practise this enquiry meditation again another time and an answer might come then. Know that the answer may come spontaneously, when you least expect it. In the meantime, you have opened the door to your subconscious. You can feel confident that this whole meditation and visualisation practice is very healing for your body and your womb. And all is well with the world.

Now, visualise your womb is a room. It's a room with a lot of light. It's a light, breezy room. Your womb is a beautiful room, flooded with natural light. This beautiful room has soft breezes blowing through the windows. In the windows there are light, filmy curtains moving gently in the breeze.

It's light and airy here. See and feel this light, airy, beautiful room that is your womb-space for the next few moments, be completely absorbed by the image and feel of this beautiful space. Know that the breezes and light are flooding this space and drying up the blood, allowing your womb to function more easefully, more gently.

Silently say to your womb:

> *That is enough, thank you. I don't need any more bleeding.*
> *Let go of the bleeding. Let it go!*

Then, let go of the visualisation and take a few more Soft Belly Breaths.

Still with your eyes closed, finish this meditation by placing your right palm on your lower belly, your womb-space, and your left palm over the centre of your chest, your heart-centre (Heart-Womb Mudra—see Figure 154, p.222). Feel love overflowing from your heart-centre, like golden rain. And feel that love from your heart flowing down into your womb, nourishing and healing your hard-working, over-worked womb.

Lastly, place both palms together into the prayer gesture, Anjali Mudra (see Figure 151, p.212), in front of the heart-centre and say a little silent prayer of gratitude:

> *My heart is filled with gratitude for...*

Insert whatever (or whoever) it is you are feeling grateful for in your life right now.

Namaste.

Take your time coming out of the meditation before you transition back into the world. You may want to make yourself a soothing cup of herbal tea. You may want to sit quietly and write in your journal, recording any feelings, thoughts, ideas, insights that may have arisen for you during this meditation. Journaling is particularly pertinent if you received a really clear message, image or action from the Enquiry Meditation—it's a way to document while it's fresh, and you can then refer back to your journal at a later time to support you on your healing journey.

Fibroids

Fibroids are benign tumours that grow in the walls of the uterus. They can be as small as an apple seed, and can grow right up to the size of a large grapefruit.[395] Approximately 20–50% of women[396] have fibroids, with most women not even aware of them because they are often asymptomatic. Women with fibroids that are growing in the uterine lining itself (submucosal) may experience painful periods with heavy bleeding (menorrhagia). Other symptoms may include painful intercourse, frequent urination and enlargement of the lower abdomen.[397]

In addition to painful symptoms, fibroids can cause complications during pregnancy and are the number one reason for hysterectomy amongst women aged 45–54 in the U.S.A.[398]

Medical professionals think that fibroids can be caused by hormonal imbalance—generally an excess of oestrogen—and they can also be hereditary. Fibroids tend to shrink after menopause because they are fed by oestrogen.

Ayurveda teachings suggest that fibroids are caused by a blockage in the release of *ama* (toxins).[399] This idea aligns with the mind-body perspective on the causes of fibroids, as described by Dr Christiane Northrup:

> The uterus and ovaries are the major organs in the second chakra. This area is both literally and figuratively creative space, out of which women can produce babies, relationships, careers, novels, insights, and other creative or artistic works. When our energy is not flowing smoothly in this area of the body, gynaecological problems, such as fibroid tumors, can result.[400]

Dr Northrup suggests that fibroids are 'often associated with conflicts about creativity, reproduction, and relationships'. She goes on to cite a case study of one of her patients who succeeded in shrinking her extremely large fibroid by a combination of 'reflective inner work', massages, therapeutic

---

395   See: https://www.womenshealth.gov/a-z-topics/uterine-fibroids

396   See: Northrup, *Women's Bodies, Women's Wisdom*, p.182

397   See: http://www.womenshealth.gov/publications/our-publications/fact-sheet/uterine-fibroids.html

398   See: Northrup, *Women's Bodies, Women's Wisdom*, p.182

399   Dr. Robert E. Svoboda, *Ayurveda for Women*, p.71

400   Northrup, *Women's Bodies, Women's Wisdom*, p.86

sound and dietary changes. Another of her patients successfully used prayer to shrink her fibroid and avoid a scheduled hysterectomy.[401]

According to Linda Sparrowe, author of *Yoga for a Healthy Menstrual Cycle*, women who take the time for inner reflection and then instigate healthy changes in their life choices—for example, ending a 'dead-end' relationship or finding ways to express themselves in the world—can support their healing from fibroids. She suggests, '…fibroids can often represent those nonphysical aspects of your being that you can't let go of, that you have trouble releasing into the world'.[402]

Yoga for Fibroids

There is no firm evidence that yoga can heal fibroids, however Dr. Krishna Raman claims that if a yoga program is instituted early when the fibroid is still small, after six months, the pain and heavy menstrual flow will diminish. He goes on to say, 'If the patient perseveres in her practice, the effects are long lasting and surgery can be avoided'.[403] Linda Sparrowe suggests that yoga can be one part of the treatment protocol that should also include dietary and lifestyle changes.[404]

Dry out the fibroid with Inversions

Dr Raman suggests that postures that alternatively starve then refresh the circulation of blood to the fibroid(s) are beneficial. He recommends daily practice of Inversions, particularly Headstand and Shoulderstand, because 'they drain the uterus of blood, and thus "dry" the fibroid which usually has a profuse blood supply'. He goes on to explain that the 'flushing and drying effect' caused by regular Inversion practice helps the circulation remain in a 'dynamic state'. 'The vaso-constrictive mechanism of the bleeding vessels during menstruation is better, owing to relief given to the nerves. The cells lining the arteries also join together better in reducing the blood flow,' writes Raman.[405]

---

401 Ibid., pp.182–187

402 Sparrowe, *Yoga for Healthy Menstrual Cycle*, p.100

403 Dr Krishna Raman, *A Matter of Health*, location 10694 (Kindle edition). Note, Dr Raman does not provide any clinical evidence for his claims regarding yoga for fibroids, and qualifies, saying: 'surgery may be needed for some patients'.

404 Sparrowe, *Yoga for a Health Menstrual Cycle*, pp.100–101

405 Dr Raman, *A Matter of Health*, location 10672 (Kindle edition)

Of course, Inversions are not to be practised when you are actually bleeding, but at any other time of the month, these postures may help in the treatment of fibroids because they also nourish and balance your endocrine system. By turning yourself upside down, you are providing the governing endocrine glands, the hypothalamus and the pituitary gland with fresh blood supply to help regulate the supply of hormones (ultimately oestrogen and progesterone), which, as we have seen, may be imbalanced, causing the fibroids.

Because fibroids can cause heavy bleeding and may lead to the condition of menorrhagia, a woman may be weak and exhausted from bleeding very heavily each menses. This, in turn, may flow into her energy levels for the rest of the month. Therefore, it may be more beneficial for her to practise supported, Restorative versions of the Inversions in order to not deplete her energy further. See Appendix 3 for some options for Supported Inversions.

Squeeze and soak with Twists

Dr Raman also recommends Twists, due to the internal action they create of alternately squeezing of the blood from the uterus and ovaries and then soaking with fresh circulation after coming out of the posture. 'This action is essential to regulate the growth of a cell and its behaviour,' he writes. 'Thus the size of the fibroid does not increase."[406]

Note that you need to avoid Closed Twists when you are menstruating; practising them the rest of the month however is fine. A good option for a gentle, Open Twist that is appropriate for your bleeding time is Bharadvajasana (Sage Twist—see Figure 8, p.87). According to B.K.S. Iyengar, this posture tones the muscles of the uterus.[407]

Create space in the pelvic area

Seated versions of Baddha Konasana (Figure 383, p.441) and especially Upavista Konasana (Figure 384, p.442) are also helpful because they create space in the pelvic area and can help tone the reproductive organs and regulate menstrual flow, which is beneficial if you experience heavy bleeding with your fibroids.

Some Standing poses—Trikonasana and Ardha Chandrasana (best done supported with hand your on a brick and back to the wall (see Figure 24 and Figure 25, p.100)—as well as the reclining, Restorative posture, Supta Baddha Konasana (see Figure 395, p.449) can help with the condition of fibroids as they gently stretch the pelvic area, relieving congestion there.

---

406   Ibid., location 10,687 (Kindle edition)

407   B.K.S. Iyengar, *Yoga, The Path to Holistic Health*, p.206

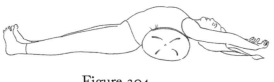

Figure 304

Dr Raman also recommends Backbends for fibroids as they 'help to thin down the lining of the uterus and prevent tissue thickening'.[408] As we know from the guidelines in chapter four, we should avoid Dynamic Backbends when we bleed, but we can safely practise gentle, Supported Backbends, such as Supported Bridge Pose (see p.450), as well as simple Supported Bolster Backbend (see Figure 304).

Additional notes

Sometimes, fibroids can cause the uterus to expand to the size of a 6–7 month pregnancy.[409] In this case, a woman can create more comfort and ease for her swollen belly by practising as if she were pregnant. This means for Supported Supine postures like Supta Baddha Konasana (see Figure 305) and Supta Virasana (see Figure 306) it will be best to prop up one end the end of the bolster with a brick or another bolster—as pictured—and also favour wide-legged Forward Bends like Upavista Konasana (see Figure 389, p.445).

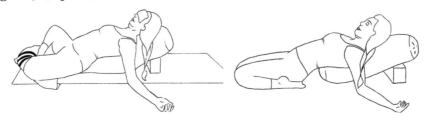

Figure 305   Figure 306

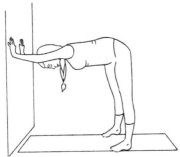

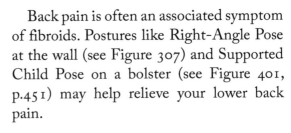

Back pain is often an associated symptom of fibroids. Postures like Right-Angle Pose at the wall (see Figure 307) and Supported Child Pose on a bolster (see Figure 401, p.451) may help relieve your lower back pain.

Figure 307

---

408   Dr Raman, *A Matter of Health*, location 10,643 (Kindle edition)

409   See: http://www.uterine-fibroids.org/questions-to-ask-about-uterine-fibroids/
      It should be noted that any yoga (or mind-body) practice for fibroids is merely complementary, and you should always seek medical attention as surgery or other intervention may be necessary.

Rest, reflect and engage *apana*

As we have seen, a possible cause for fibroids is a restriction in the flow of *ama*. It may therefore help to do practices that foster *apana* (downward moving energy) and therefore support the removal of *ama*. All of the seated Classical Women's postures (see Appendix 2) promote *apana*, and the Apana Breath (see p.102) may be helpful because it involves consciously using the breath to move the internal energy down and out, facilitating the release of internal holding.

It's also important that women with fibroids take some conscious time out. Sparrowe says the deep relaxation offered by supported poses such as Supta Baddha Konasana or Savasana ('Corpse Pose'—final relaxation pose) 'move the healing beyond the physical and allow you to spend pressure-free time with your body and mind'.[410]

Enquiry Meditation for fibroids

An Enquiry Meditation can help you connect with a deep, inner root-cause for your fibroids. Proceed as for the Enquiry Meditation for menorrhagia on page 332 and substitute the enquiry questions for these ones:

What is my body telling me?

What feels congested and stuck inside of me?

What do I need to let go of or express?

Endometriosis

> *One Jungian analyst has referred to endometriosis as "a blood sacrifice to the Goddess." It is our bodies trying not to let us forget our feminine nature, our need for self-nurturance, and our connection with other women.*

—CHRISTIANE NORTHRUP M.D.[411]

Endometriosis affects approximately 600,000 women in Australia and 176 million women worldwide[412] and, according to Endometriosis Australia, as many as 1 in 10 women suffer from this disease.[413]

---

410 Sparrowe, *Yoga for a Healthy Menstrual Cycle*, p.101

411 Northrup, *Women's Bodies, Women's Wisdom*, p.170

412 See: https://www.theguardian.com/commentisfree/2017/may/31/a-study-about-how-endometriosis-affects-mens-sex-lives-thats-enraging?CMP=Share_AndroidApp_MailDroid

413 See: https://www.endometriosisaustralia.org

So, what is it? Endometriosis occurs when endometrium-like tissue shows up outside the uterus, most often on the pelvic organs, the side walls of the pelvis, the outside surface of the uterus, the bowel, the ovaries, the fallopian tubes, the area between the vagina and the rectum, and sometimes the bladder. These 'endometrial' growths have even been known to appear on the lungs, thighs, arms, and just about anywhere in the body, except for the spleen.[414]

These stray bits of endometrial tissue or 'lesions' can behave like real endometrial tissue and bleed during menstruation, and they cause irritation and inflammation to the tissue and organs that surround them. Scar tissue forming around the lesions can result in adhesions that stick the pelvic organs together. This scar tissue may become even worse after surgery to remove the lesions. Due to the adhesions, the 'fused' organs are unable to move freely, making ovulation, sexual intercourse or going to the toilet painful. Over time, the endometrial lesions on the ovaries may enlarge and form cysts. These cysts are called 'chocolate cysts' because they are filled with old blood that is chocolate-like in colour.[415]

Symptoms of endometriosis include painful periods (often involving intense cramps that may continue beyond the first day of bleeding), heavy bleeding, irregular periods and spotting, pelvic pain outside of menstruation, painful intercourse, and lower back, thigh or leg pain. Endometriosis can also cause infertility.[416]

Women with severe endometriosis suffer emotionally due to anticipation of the pain, the ongoing nature of this pain and discomfort, and related difficulty in falling pregnant. 'The pain can be totally horrific, sometimes to the point where you have to vomit. I even had a nurse recently tell me that is it considered worse than child birth,' writes nutritionist Alexandra Middleton.[417] For many women with this condition it can take up to

---

414   See: Sparrowe, *Yoga for a Healthy Menstrual Cycle*, p.77. And see: http://alexandramiddleton.com.au/treating-endometriosis-a-multi-modality-approach/ in which Nutritionist Alexandra Middleton writes of the 'wandering' endometrial tissue: 'It can literally wander and proliferate anywhere. I have even heard stories from other practitioners of it being found in the lungs, heart and eyes.'

415   See: http://www.womhealth.org.au/conditions-and-treatments/endometriosis-fact-sheet

416   Ibid

417   See: http://alexandramiddleton.com.au/treating-endometriosis-a-multi-modality-approach/

seven years to get a correct diagnosis. It's hardly surprising therefore that women with endometriosis report feeling depressed, stressed, angry, anxious and hopeless.[418]

What causes endometriosis?

Doctors are not entirely clear what causes endometriosis. One theory is that it is due to 'retrograde menstruation' in which the endometrial tissue migrates the wrong way back up through the fallopian tubes into the pelvic cavity.[419] Another theory is that, like fibroids, it is due to oestrogen dominance.[420] Yet another theory posits that it is genetic and passed on from mother to daughter. Research sponsored by The Endometriosis Association suggests that endometriosis might also be connected to exposure to environmental toxins, like dioxins (present in rayon tampons).[421]

Then there's the possible stress connection. Joel Evans, M.D., author of a paper in the IMCJ (Integrative Medicine: A Clinician's Journal) called, 'An Integrative Approach to Fibroids, Endometriosis and Breast Cancer Prevention', goes so far as to suggest that 'stress and spiritual uncertainty or discomfort' are contributing factors. Evans further recommends an 'integrative treatment plan' involving 'normalizing estrogen production', 'enhancing estrogen elimination', 'decreasing inflammation and dysglycemia' and 'reducing as many life stressors as possible.[422]

Research shows that women with endometriosis are stressed, but the question remains whether their stress is caused by dealing with the disease, or if it has created the conditions for the occurrence of it in the first place. This is something the authors of a comparative research study on rats speculate:

---

418   See: http://www.womhealth.org.au/conditions-and-treatments/endometriosis-fact-sheet

419   See: Sparrowe, *Yoga for Healthy Menstruation,* p.78, and Middleton—http://alexandramiddleton.com.au/treating-endometriosis-a-multi-modality-approach/ Also, see note 156 from chapter four for a discussion on the theory of retrograde menstruation.

420   See this paper by Joel M. Evans M.D.: http://www.imjournal.com/resources/web_pdfs/popular/1008_evans.pdf

421   As cited by Sparrowe, *Yoga for Healthy Menstruation,* p.78

422   See: http://www.imjournal.com/resources/web_pdfs/popular/1008_evans.pdf

Taken together, data from both animal models and human studies strongly suggest that stress does play a role in endometriosis. Whether stress is a causal or exacerbating factor in disease is still unknown. Our results fill an important gap in knowledge of the endometriosis field, by providing evidence supporting the involvement of stress-activated neuroinflammatory mechanisms in this chronic, painful disease.[423]

Endometriosis is on the increase[424] and has sometimes been dubbed a 'career-woman's disease'.[425] Some sources attribute this to the fact that contemporary women tend to delay motherhood and have fewer children. Dr Svoboda writes:

The modern woman, [however,] goes through menarche earlier (thanks to better nutrition and artificial light) and commonly delivers only one or two children, whom she is usually able to nurse for a few months at best. She therefore has many more menstrual cycles, during which wide hormone swings dramatically affect the tissues of her ovaries, uterus, and breasts. Each of the swings acts as an opportunity for an imbalance to occur, or for an imbalance that already exists to be exacerbated.[426]

---

423   From a study called 'Stress Exacerbates Endometriosis Manifestations and Inflammatory Parameters in an Animal Model' found at: http://www.ncbi.nlm.nih.gov/pmc/articles/PMC4046310/#bibr73-1933719112438443.
The researchers also cite another study in which patients that eventually were diagnosed with endometriosis were significantly more anxious (Low, Edelmann, Sutton—'A psychological profile of endometriosis patients in comparison to patients with pelvic pain of other origins'). And, they point out, studies that have shown that women with endometriosis exhibit a greater degree of stress due to the negative effects of the condition. 'In fact, patients with endometriosis have reported to have high levels of stress due to the negative impact of the symptoms in all aspects of life, including work, relationships, and fertility.'

424   See: https://www.womentowomen.com/sex-fertility/endometriosis-start-with-a-natural-approach/

425   See: Peveler R, Edwards J, Daddow J, Thomas E. 'Psychosocial factors and chronic pelvic pain: a comparison of women with endometriosis and with unexplained pain', Psychosom Res. 1996;40(3):305–315

426   Svoboda, *Ayurveda for Women*, pp.70–71

Dr Northrup says that endometriosis is similar to fibroids in that it is associated with dietary factors, immunity, hormone levels, and blocked pelvic energy. She also suggests that there is a strong mind-body connection and that sufferers of endometriosis are likely to be the kind of women who 'drive themselves relentlessly in the outer world, rarely resting, rarely tuning in to their innermost needs and deepest desires'.[427]

From an Ayurvedic perspective, endometriosis represents a disruption in the natural downward energy (*apana*) required to efficiently remove accumulated *ama* (toxins) from the body. 'When apana moves upward it can [also] create endometriosis, which can produce severe pain during menses,' explains Dr Svoboda.[428]

Treatment for endometriosis

Allopathic treatment options for endometriosis include surgery[429] and hormonal treatments (e.g. the pill). A woman with endometriosis might also seek out alternative therapy like TCM (Traditional Chinese Medicine) and naturopathy, as well making changes in her diet.[430]

Since the connection between endometriosis and stress seems to act as a kind of negative feedback loop, it may also help this condition if a woman's stress levels are managed.

Yoga for Endometriosis

Emphasise rest and relaxation

As for all menstrual imbalances, the first thing you need to ensure is that you are resting as much as possible when you menstruate. This will help to reduce stress upon the body during this more delicate phase of your cycle, as well as to support you with managing the menstrual pain that is usually connected with endometriosis. You will also need to assess your

---

427   Northrup, *Women's Bodies, Women's Wisdom* pp.169–170

428   Svoboda, *Ayurveda for Women*, p.70

429   Conservative surgery for women with mild endometriosis has been shown to help women's chances of getting pregnant. See: https://www.thewomens.org.au/ health-information/periods/endometriosis/treating-endometriosis/

430   See: http://alexandramiddleton.com.au/treating-endometriosis-a-multi-modality-approach/ This website by nutritionist Alexandra Middleton offers comprehensive advice on modifying your diet to help with endometriosis. Middleton's suggestion is that this condition is actually an autoimmune disease and therefore must be managed by reducing inflammation by treating a 'leaky gut', stabilising blood sugar levels and eliminating dietary and environmental toxins.

overall lifestyle throughout your whole menstrual month and see if you can establish (or strengthen) a routine of supportive stress management techniques.

Yoga can play a significant role in managing stress and therefore give you a greater sense of control over your endometriosis symptoms. See the subsection, 'Harness the healing power of relaxation', on page 323 in the 'Yoga for Menstrual Cramps' section of this chapter, for tips on integrating the deep relaxation practice of Yoga Nidra into your life. I also recommend you incorporate a regular practice of the Restorative postures (see Appendix 3) as well as the relevant Pranayama practices for each phase of your cycle that are detailed in Part Three (chapters four to seven) of this book.

Create space: postures to help during menstruation

When you are bleeding, practise gentle Dark Moon Restorative postures (detailed in chapter four), and in particular, focus on those postures that create maximum space in the belly and pelvic area—gentle, heart-opening and belly-opening postures (see the Heart-Opening Restorative postures in Appendix 3). These postures will help ease cramping pain and provide space for the uterus and pelvic organs that can be constrained by the endometrial scar tissue. The Classical Women's postures (see Appendix 2) like Upavista Konasana and Baddha Konasana, in both their seated and supine versions, are also therapeutic.

Additionally, I recommend what I call 'endo-variations' (see Figure 308 and Figure 309) of the above-mentioned postures because they lift and elongate the abdominal and solar plexus region, creating even more space in the lower belly and pelvic area.

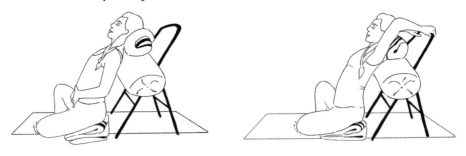

Figure 308   Figure 309

The T-Bolster variation of the Supported Bridge Pose (Figure 57, p.138) is also another beneficial posture for endometriosis. In this extremely restful variation, the feet are hip-width apart and raised, supported on a bolster, which provides a beneficial spreading action in the lower belly and pelvic area and boosts circulation there. You can also try the Simple Supported Backbend (see Figure 304, p.338) that offers an effective gentle stretch and opening and to the belly area.

Postures to avoid during menstruation

As always, you need to avoid Inversions during your period. This contraindication is perhaps even more critical for someone who has endometriosis because of the Ayurvedic belief that this disease is caused by an energetic backlog of *apana*. We also don't want to encourage the physical reversal of the blood flow due to the possibility that this may cause or exacerbate endometriosis—i.e., due to 'retrograde menstruation'.

If you have endometriosis, you will also need to avoid Forward Bends when you are bleeding. Dr Krishna Raman says this is because Forward Bends reduce the space in the belly when it

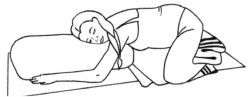

Figure 310

is already constricted due to the errant endometrial tissue jamming-up around the abdominal organs (and therefore causing the menstrual pain).[431] That said, the simple Supported Child Pose (see Figure 401, p.451)—a gentle, modified Forward Bend—can be practised, and for many women feels wonderful in easing the menstrual pain that is associated with endometriosis. If you find it uncomfortable to rest your belly on a bolster in this pose, try the pregnancy variation, in which you have a space between your pelvis and the bolster so that the belly is not resting on the bolster, only your chest (see Figure 310).

For the rest of the month

For the rest of the month when you are not menstruating, it can be helpful to practise Inversions regularly because these poses can regulate your hormones and have a calming effect on your nervous system.

Viparita Karani (Legs up the Wall—Figure 410, p.453) is a wonderful Restorative Inversion, especially with the following variations: legs apart in Upavista Konasana (see Figure 311), legs in the Baddha Konasana (groin stretch position—see Figure 266, p.289), and legs in cross-leg (see Figure 312). All of these variations relax the belly and pelvic areas, whilst boosting circulation to the heart, lungs, throat and brain (bathing the endocrine organs in the brain with fresh blood supply).

---

431   See: Dr Raman, *Yoga and Medical Science FAQ*, location 3808 (Kindle edition)

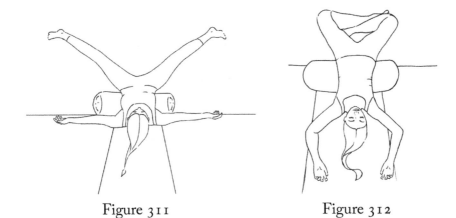

Figure 311   Figure 312

Pranayama for endometriosis

Regular practice of the Constructive Rest Position (see Figure 19, p.95) is beneficial because of its restful and rejuvenating qualities, and because it quite naturally relaxes the abdominal area by gently releasing the deep, core psoas muscle. It's a good posture in which to practise the Soft Belly Breath (see p.100)—with your hands lightly resting on the belly—as well as the Apana Breath (see p.102), which are both beneficial for endometriosis.

Polycystic Ovary Syndrome

Polycystic ovary syndrome (PCOS) is a common condition that affects up to 21% of women in Australia[432] and is the top reason for infertility in the United States.[433] PCOS manifests as a hormonal imbalance in the sex hormones, oestrogen and progesterone that seems to cause the woman's body to produce an excess of the male hormones, or androgens.

The symptoms of PSOS include irregular or absent periods, pelvic pain, infertility (caused by anovulatory cycles), cysts on the ovaries (caused by eggs that do not mature), excess body hair, acne, tendency to be overweight, and blood sugar imbalances (caused by the production of excess insulin). A woman with PCOS will also very often exhibit emotional symptoms such as depression, anxiety and poor self-esteem.[434]

---

432   http://www.racgp.org.au/afp/2012/october/polycystic-ovary-syndrome/ Note, the actual definition of PCOS has been contested and specialist women's health naturopath Lara Briden points out that there can be many different types of PCOS. See: *Period Repair Manual*, location 2295-2502 (Kindle edition).

433   See: Sara Gottfried, M.D.,— http://www.healthylivingmagazine.us/Articles/574/

434   See: http://www.racgp.org.au/afp/2012/october/polycystic-ovary-syndrome/#1 and http://www.healthline.com/health/polycystic-ovary-disease#Causes2

Since allopathic medicine is unsure about the exact cause of PCOS, treatment is limited to addressing the symptoms rather than the cause. Treatment may therefore include prescription of the contraceptive pill to regulate the cycle, drugs that decrease the levels of androgens, and fertility drugs to stimulate ovulation.[435] Doctors also recommend making healthy lifestyle choices to address weight gain.

From a holistic perspective, in addition to dietary changes and exercise, PCOS needs to be addressed by reducing stress. According to Dr Northrup, whenever there is a problem with ovulation it means that the root cause is hypothalamic dysfunction. The hypothalamus is the regulatory gland in the brain for the menstrual cycle, and as we have discovered, it can be affected by stress, precipitating imbalances in the hormonal flow. Furthermore, Dr Northrup points out that the stress hormone cortisol increases insulin levels, which is another negative symptom of PCOS. She suggests that there is a specific kind of emotional stress—'negative feelings about being female and also feeling subordinate or inferior'—that may be at the heart of PCOS. 'In some women, these negative feelings may work in the body to cause it to stop ovulating and become more "androgynous",' writes Dr Northrup.[436]

Sara Gottfried, M.D., concurs that stress may be a contributing factor because it can throw your adrenal glands into overdrive, increasing the level of androgens. 'Women with metabolic syndrome and insulin resistance have a higher tone to their sympathetic nervous system,' writes Gottfried. 'The coveted balance between the sympathetic nervous system, activated by the stress into fight or flight, dominates over the parasympathetic nervous system, also known as rest and digest. This may show up as increased diastolic blood pressure (the lower number of the blood pressure fraction).'[437]

Yoga for PCOS

Research shows that yoga can be helpful for PCOS. There are several studies[438] of adolescent girls that point to it being more beneficial than other forms of exercise—particularly so in reducing the physical and emotional symptoms caused by PCOS.

---

435 See: Northrup, *Women's Bodies, Women's Wisdom*, pp.218–219

436 Ibid., pp.217–218

437 Gottfried, *The Hormone Cure*, location 3737 and 3955 (Kindle edition)

438 These studies are:
http://www.ncbi.nlm.nih.gov/pubmed/22507264 and
http://www.ncbi.nlm.nih.gov/pubmed/22869994
http://www.ncbi.nlm.nih.gov/pubmed/22808940

Open the heart

Restorative Yoga postures allow a woman with PCOS to feel relaxed, supported and uplifted, especially if she focuses on the Heart-Opening Restorative postures like Supta Baddha Konasana and Reclining Goddess Pose (see Appendix 3). These postures not only help to release stress and tension in your body, but they also counteract depression, a common emotional symptom of this condition.

While the Restorative Heart-Opening postures are good to practise regularly, particularly when you are bleeding and at any time when your energy is low, the active Heart-Opening postures can also be helpful when you're feeling more energetic, outside of your Dark Moon (menstrual) phase. Dr Pooja Madella, a yoga therapist and clinician specialising in women's health[439] recommends the Standing Goddess Pose (see Figure 394, p.447) with the arms in a right-angle position, which combines heart-opening benefits with stamina-building, producing an energising and grounding effect on the body-mind. And Dr Madella suggests that women with PCOS need to work on reducing their *vata* (see Appendix 1), so the grounding effect of this Standing Squat makes it an excellent choice.

The Bow Pose (see Figure 221, p.258) is another active Heart-Opening posture that is beneficial for PCOS. Like any Backbend, it engenders feelings of positivity and vitality, plus, this pose massages the abdominal area, which can help with associated digestive symptoms of PCOS. Geeta Iyengar says Backbends, along with Twists and Inversions, are beneficial for kickstarting your menstrual cycle if ovulation has ceased due to emotional distress.[440]

Align with the moon

Dr Northrup recommends a woman with PCOS start to notice the phases of the moon so that she can work on syncing her cycle up with the moon. Often, just paying attention to the lunar cycle will create a shift in your body's cycle, and you can enhance this by sleeping with a night light on for three days a month to trigger ovulation.[441]

---

439 I attended a very informative talk on yoga for PCOS by Dr Madella at a Yoga Australia Conference in Brisbane, March 2016. See more of Dr Pooja Madella's work here: www.doctorpooja.com

440 Cited by Boby Clennell in *The Women's Yoga Book*, p.220

441 Northrup, *Women's Bodies, Women's Wisdom*, p.219, and also see: http://www.drnorthrup.com/audio/pcos-polycystic-ovarian-syndrome/

A Moving with the Moon yoga practice that responds to the changing energies of the lunar cycle (and your body's cycle) is a practical way you can align with the moon to help regulate your cycle, and therefore begin to heal PCOS. This means following my suggestions for adapting your yoga practice for the four phases of your cycle (and the moon) detailed in Part Three (chapters four through to seven) in this book.

Reduce *vata*

Dr Madella explains that, from an Ayurvedic perspective, the ovarian cysts that are characteristic of PCOS are like 'air bubbles' in your ovaries, and represent an excess of the elements of air and ether, which manifests as an imbalance in the *vata* dosha (see Appendix 1). A good practice for reducing your *vata* levels is the 'joint freeing sequence'—the Women's Pawanmuktasana Sequence—which is detailed at the end of chapter nine.

The simple movements involved in the Supine Single Knee to Chest Pawanmuktasana movement (see below) also help by facilitating *apana* (downward movement of energy) and stoking the 'digestive fire', which are necessary to address an excess in *vata*.

Supine Single Knee to Chest Pawanmuktasana

How to do it

Come to lie onto your back and bend up your right leg, drawing the knee into the right side of your chest, with your hands interlaced around the outside of the shin, just below

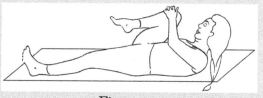

Figure 313

the knee. Extend the opposite left leg along the floor, dorsi-flexing the ankle (drawing the toes back towards you). As you exhale, curl your head and shoulders off the floor and draw your knee towards your forehead and your forehead towards you knee (see Figure 313). As you inhale, lower your head and shoulders again and move your knee away from you so that your elbows are extended. Repeat 3-5 more times. Then do it on the other leg.

Break the *kapha*

Some of the key symptoms of PCOS such as depression and weight gain can also represent an excess of *kapha* (see Appendix 1). Too much *kapha* causes sluggishness and stagnation, so Dr Madella recommends a woman with PCOS also adopt yoga postures and practices to help 'break the *kapha*'.

This means you should regularly practise Salute to the Sun Sequences (see the Full Moon Salutes, p.225) to shift any lethargy and stagnancy, and also to help with weight gain.

The Chopping Wood pose (see below) is also good for 'breaking *kapha*' and especially beneficial as a stimulating, morning practice.

Chopping Wood

How to do it

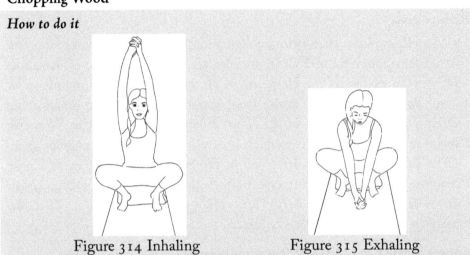

Figure 314 Inhaling   Figure 315 Exhaling

Come into a squatting position—feet a little wider than hip-width apart, toes turned out slightly. If you cannot easily rest your heels on the ground, place a folded blanket or cushion underneath the heels (as pictured). Interlace your hands and extend your arms in front of your, between your legs. As you inhale raise the arms overhead (see Figure 314), lengthening the spine, opening the chest, and rising onto the balls of your feet if you need to. With a vigorous exhalation, blowing the air out of your mouth, pursing your lips a little to make a 'phoo!' sound, rapidly and strongly bring your arms back down between your legs—like you are chopping wood with an axe (see Figure 315). Repeat 10-12 more times.

Pranayama for PCOS

The dynamic Kapalabhati breathing technique is another beneficial '*kapha* breaking' practice to stimulate sluggish energy. See page 268 for instructions.

Other Pranayama that are helpful for PCOS is the Soft Belly Breath (see p.100) to help relax the whole abdominal and pelvic area, and Bhramari 'Humming Bee Breath' (see p.267) because of its calming effect on the nervous system. And, the Feminine Alternate Nostril Breath (see p.105) not only nourishes the nervous system, but may also balance the hormonal system by harmonizing the masculine and feminine energy within the body-mind.

Affirmations and Mudras for PCOS

Dr Madella recommends Shakti Mudra (see p.327) as being helpful for PCOS. This Mudra is said to ease menstrual complaints as well as the intestinal spasms and slow digestion that can be symptoms of PCOS.

Shivalinga Mudra

Shivalinga Mudra helps to balance our masculine and feminine energies and is therefore beneficial for PCOS since it's a manifestation of excess male hormones (androgens).

This Mudra is also beneficial because it counteracts tiredness, dissatisfaction, listlessness and depression. According to Gertrud Hirschi, author of a wonderfully comprehensive book called, *Mudras: Yoga in your Hands*, Shivalinga Mudra is an extremely healing gesture, and she suggests you practise it along with the following affirmation, which I think is particularly relevant to the condition of PCOS:

Healing light illuminates every cell of my body, dissolves everything that should be dissolved, and builds up what must be built up again. Thank you![442]

How to do it

Place the right hand on top of the left palm. The fingers of the right hand are curled into the right palm with the thumb pointing up (see Figure 316). The right hand represents the dynamic masculine principle (*Shiva*) and the left open palm represents the receptive feminine principle (*Shakti*).

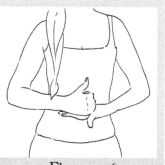

Figure 316

Enquiry Meditation for PCOS

Because there is a potentially strong mind-body connection with PCOS, it's recommended that in addition to consulting your doctor, keeping your weight and your diet in check, and practising the above-mentioned yoga practices, it may also be helpful to try an Enquiry Meditation similar to the one I suggested for menorrhagia (see p.332). Substitute these enquiry questions:

---

442   Gertrud Hirschi, *Mudras: Yoga in your Hands*, p.137

What is my body telling me?
What are you telling me, my ovaries, my adrenals?
Where am I stuck?
What do I need to embrace?

Finish the meditation with a positive affirmation like this beautiful one that Christiane Northrup, M.D., suggests:

I now give thanks to my fertility and my femininity. I am completely safe to be all of who I am.[443]

Amenorrhea

Amenorrhea means the absence of the menstrual period for a woman who is of normal reproductive age, and can be divided into primary and secondary amenorrhea.

The diagnosis of primary amenorrhea is given when a woman has never menstruated—for example, if a woman hasn't reached menarche by the time she is 16 years old.[444] This is usually due to structural problems in the reproductive organs or endocrine glands,[445] or due to birth defects or genetic factors.[446] Secondary amenorrhea is defined as the absence of menstruation for three or more consecutive menstrual periods, or for a period of six months or more, for a woman who has previously menstruated.

It should be noted that secondary amenorrhea is not to be confused with oligomenorrhea, which refers to infrequent periods (i.e., fewer than eight periods a year). Oligomenorrhea is common in perimenopausal women and adolescent girls who can experience natural disruption in their cycles. For adolescent girls, if they wait, their cycles will usually settle. This is preferable to taking the contraceptive pill, which is often recommended by doctors to regulate the hormones, but doesn't actually cause the girl to ovulate. As Linda Sparrowe suggests, 'birth control pills will only prolong the problem.'[447] Along with these times of transition (menarche and menopause), pregnancy and breastfeeding are also times in a woman's life when she may experience 'natural amenorrhea'.[448]

---

443   Northrup, *Women's Bodies, Women's Wisdom*, p.219

444   See: http://www.medicinenet.com/amenorrhea/article.htm

445   See: http://www.mayoclinic.org/diseases-conditions/amenorrhea/basics/causes/con-20031561

446   See: http://www.ayurvedacollege.com/book/export/html/22

447   Sparrowe, *The Women's Book of Yoga and Health*, p.92

448   See: http://www.mayoclinic.org/diseases-conditions/amenorrhea/basics/causes/con-20031561

There are numerous potential causes for secondary amenorrhea. It can be precipitated by certain medications, or when a woman stops taking the contraceptive pill. Amenorrhea can also be caused by lifestyle factors such as emotional or physical stress, extreme weight loss, over-exercise[449], or glandular disorders like polycystic ovary syndrome, hypothyroidism (underactive thyroid gland) and Cushings Disease (overactive adrenal gland).[450] Other causes include tumours, or diseases of the pituitary gland, Ashmerman's Syndrome (a uterine disease), as well as early menopause.[451]

Once any underlying causes have been investigated by your doctor, it's important to get your cycle going again as soon as possible due to the risk of osteoporosis (bone loss), infertility and early onset of menopause. The hormone oestrogen has an effect on peak bone mass, so if women don't ovulate regularly they are compromising their bone density. This is especially critical for younger women because, up to the age of 30, their bone tissue continues to grow.[452]

Yoga for Amenorrhea

Relieve the stress with Yoga Nidra and Restorative Yoga

Several of the common causes of amenorrhea point to a body under stress. In addition to mental and emotional stress, the body interprets being underweight[453] or engaging in overly vigorous exercise as stressors. If your amenorrhea is caused by these factors, you can be confident that yoga—the right kind of gentle, nourishing, feminine-focused yoga—will be a support in helping your body find balance again. As already mentioned, a study of young women with menstrual disorders, including amenorrhea, showed that regular practice of Yoga Nidra (the deep yogic relaxation practice over a six month period) had a positive impact on these girls.[454]

---

449   See: http://www.medicinenet.com/amenorrhea/page2.htm

450   See: Clennell, *The Women's Yoga Book*, p.219

451   See: www.medicinenet.com/amenorrhea/page2.htm

452   See: https://www.niams.nih.gov/health_info/bone/osteoporosis/bone_mass.asp

453   Menstruation only occurs when there is enough body fat in your body to support you, and potentially a growing foetus. 'Thus, menstruation will shut down in the female superathlete who has too little body fat, and menarche, the time of first menstruation, can be 4 years later for undernourished girls in poor countries as compared with that for well-fed girls in the more developed countries,' writes Mel Robin in, *A Physiological Handbook for Teachers of Yogasana* p.454

454   See: https://www.ncbi.nlm.nih.gov/pmc/articles/PMC3530296/

In addition to Yoga Nidra, regular practice of the Restorative Yoga postures (see Appendix 3) can help calm your nervous system and rebalance the reproductive system. If your amenorrhea is caused by too much rigorous exercise—for example, by athletics, gymnastics, dancing or even a really strong yoga practice—the gentle nature of Restorative Yoga will be a potential solution.

In summary, the first step to healing from amenorrhea is to substitute your overly dynamic exercise or yoga practice with regular Restorative Yoga practices.

Kickstart the ovaries with Inversions, Backbends and Twists

A regular practice of Inversions can help amenorrhea because they promote blood circulation to the endocrine (hormonal) glands— particularly the pituitary gland. According to Geeta Iyengar, Backbends also stimulate the pituitary gland,[455] but I would caution that if you know that your amenorrhea might be connected with over-activity and over-stimulation of the nervous system, it's best if you stick to the less rigorous backbends like the Bridge Pose (see Figure 16, p.92), the Bow Pose (see Figure 221, p.258), or the Camel Pose (see Figure 148, p.208). Even more restful for the nervous system, and therefore beneficial for the hormonal system, are the Restorative versions of the backbends—the Heart-Opening Postures—see Appendix 3—like the Supported Bridge Pose (see p.450).

Twists are also beneficial as they tone the digestive and reproductive organs; in particular, Bobby Clennell recommends Bharadvajasana (see Figure 8, p.87) for amenorrhea.[456]

Pacify your *vata*

Ayurveda considers that amenorrhea is generally caused by too much *vata* (see Appendix 1). Zoe Middlebrooks in her article, 'An Ayurvedic Approach to the Treatment of Secondary Amenorrhea,' suggests that this condition is an imbalance caused by 'vata-provoking lifestyle regimens that lead to depletion'. Middlebrooks goes on to say that this *vata*-overload can be caused by 'excessive motion such as a fast paced lifestyle filled with travel, stress and overwhelm.' She cites well known Ayuvedic specialist Dr David Frawley who says that along with showing signs of depletion, women with amenorrhea often exhibit the *vata*-like symptoms of 'constipation, dry skin,

---

455   Geeta Iyengar, *Yoga, A Gem for Women*, p.45

456   Clennell, *The Women's Yoga Book*, p.221

dry hair, weight loss, worry and anxiety'.[457] Dr Svoboda reinforces: 'Women who exercise excessively or who lose too much weight may aggravate their vata so much that they stop menstruating'.[458]

Viewing the condition through the lens of Ayurveda, it's clear that in order to pacify these elevated *vata* levels, a yoga practice for amenorrhea needs to calm, ground and slow you down. In addition to Restorative Yoga, I recommend practising the Women's Pawanmuktasana (joint-freeing) Sequence (in chapter nine), and also focusing on Supported Forward Bends and Seated Postures, particularly the Classical Women's postures (see Appendix 2). These practices will help to keep the ovaries healthy and promote a regular menstrual cycle, as well being as beneficial for calming and grounding your frayed nerves.

Even more than the postures you choose, it's your general approach that is important. You need to adopt an attitude towards your yoga practice, your body, and any other exercise that is slow and mindful. Dr David Frawley offers some helpful tips for practising yoga in a way that reduces your *vata*:

> They should never rush or hurry into asana practice. They should first put their minds in a calm space and place their emotions in a condition of rest. They should slow down and deepen their breath before beginning any postures. Vatas should warm up their bodies gradually, improving circulation and loosening their joints. They should be aware of overexertion or of attempting postures before their bodies are ready. A gentle attitude and gradually flowing movements are best for them.[459]

Literally move with the moon: fake it till you make it!

Even if you are not menstruating, or menstruating very infrequently, you can still follow the cycles of the moon in how you practise your yoga, i.e. adopt a literal Moving with the Moon approach. This applies especially during the new or dark moon phase of the month, which is when it's ideal to practise the gentle, Dark Moon menstrual practices (see chapter four) as if you were menstruating. This may help re-establish a natural, cyclical rhythm for your body.

---

457   See: http://www.ayurvedacollege.com/book/export/html/22

458   Svoboda, *Ayurveda for Women*, p.74

459   David Frawley, *Yoga and Ayurveda: Self-Healing and Self-Realization*, p.217

Premenstrual Syndrome

> *Hormones are witty messengers. "Female problems"*
> *such as PMS are often alleviated when we listen and*
> *give in to the call: "slow down, let go, drop in!" When*
> *we do get out of our heads, let go of "doing" and sink*
> *down into "being", it is a revelation and a great relief*

—CAMILLE MAURINE[460]

According to research by pioneering British gynaecologist Dr Katharina Dalton, women are more likely to injure themselves, have accidents, use alcohol, attempt suicide and commit crimes during the premenstrual phase of their cycles.[461] As discussed in chapter seven, Premenstrual Syndrome (PMS) is a common malady that is characterised by numerous physical and emotional symptoms. You will generally notice a pattern in which one or several PMS symptoms occur each month about 2–10 days before the onset of your period and that get better once menstruation begins.

If your symptoms are debilitating, especially if they include severe mood swings and interfere with your daily life, you may be suffering from Premenstrual Dysphoric Disorder (PMDD). In this case, it is worth seeking medical help to ascertain if there are any underlying causes and determine treatment options.

Treatment for PMS and PMDD

Since the jury is out as to the true cause of PMS and PMDD, there is no definitive cure for these conditions. The Western medical model treats a woman with PMDD with antidepressants or hormonal therapy

---

460 Camille Maurine and Lorin Roche, *Meditation Secrets for Women: Discovering your Passion, Pleasure, and Inner Peace*, p.149

461 As quoted by Maya Tiwari, *Women's Power to Heal*, p.107. Additional note: in 1953 Dr Dalton was the first person to coin the term PMS and carried out pioneering work in treating the condition with natural progesterone for 40 years. 'In the 80's, Dalton took PMS to court. She defended an 18-year-old named Anna Reynolds who was accused of murdering her mother and managed to get the girl's sentence reduced to manslaughter. She testified that Nicola Owen, an arsonist, had set fires during PMS plunges over which the teenager had little or no control.' See: http://query.nytimes.com/gst/fullpage.html?res=990DE2D81330F935A15751C1A9629C8B63

that may include the contraceptive pill.[462] Natural treatment for PMS in-cludes nutritional supplements like Vitamin B-6, magnesium and a herb called chasteberry, as well as diet and lifestyle changes.[463] In terms of diet, Dr Sarah Gottfried recommends eliminating sugar and caffeine from your diet.[464]

Yoga for PMS

Combined with diet and an awareness of reducing stress in your daily life, yoga can form part of an integrated, holistic treatment plan to help manage recurring PMS symptoms.

Chill out and get some perspective!

It has been postulated that PMS is not associated with abnormal hormone levels but rather an abnormal response to sex hormones which may be exacerbated during episodes of stress
—JEROME SARRIS AND JOHN WARDLE[465]

We have seen that stress can be associated with PMS symptoms[466] so that means your yoga practice needs to include plenty of gentle, supportive re-laxation practices to counteract the potentially harmful effects of stress. I recommend the deep, guided relaxation practice of Yoga Nidra. See page 268 for a beautiful Waning Moon Yoga Nidra especially conceived for your premenstrual phase. Also see chapter seven for my Waning Moon Pranayama

---

462   See: http://www.mayoclinic.org/diseases-conditions/premenstrual-syndrome/expert-answers/pmdd/faq-20058315

463   See: http://www.mayoclinic.org/diseases-conditions/premenstrual-syndrome/expert-answers/pmdd/faq-20058315 . In *Period Repair Manual*, location 3172 (kindle edition), Lara Briden offers comprehensive tips on supplements for different types of PMS.

464   'Women with PMS consume 275 percent more refined sugar than women who don't have PMS. Together with the data showing an association between caffeine and PMS, I advise women eliminate sugar and caffeine from their diets for ninety days when they have PMS,' recommends Gottfried in *The Hormone Cure*, location 2623 (Kindle edition).

465   Sarris and Wardle in *Clinical Naturopathy: an evidence based guide to practice*, p.425

466   Lara Biden provides further explanation as to how 'perceived stress' can cause PMS. See *Period Repair Manual*, location 3172 (Kindle edition).

and meditation practices—all designed for this premenstrual phase—to balance your nervous system, which should, in turn, positively impact on your hormonal system.

'Women who practise meditation or other methods of deep relaxation are able to alleviate many of their PMS symptoms,' asserts Dr Northrup. She goes on to say, 'Relaxation of all kinds decreases cortisol and epinephrine levels in the blood and helps to balance your biochemistry, including the reduction of inflammatory chemicals.'[467] Further, Dr Sarah Gottfried says that a guided visualisation has been shown 'to increase vaginal temperature, a proxy for a rise in progesterone, and to improve PMS'.[468]

An additional benefit of meditation, relaxation and positive visualisation practices is the perspective these can offer women at this volatile time of the month, when we tend to lose all sense of proportion. Miranda Gray uses the metaphor of a snowball[469] to describe how a premenstrual woman is likely to build one negative thought (and feeling) on top of another. I'm sure you've been there! It's when you find yourself ruminating on negative thoughts that feed off each other, causing you emotional tension or distress, and potentially negatively impacting your loved ones too!

Mindfulness Meditation for PMS

Mindfulness meditation can help in circumventing this monthly tendency to exaggerate the negative aspects in our lives.[470] By becoming aware of the patterns of your premenstrual mind, which have a tendency to carry you far beyond what is real and observable, you may be able to short-circuit a negative spiral, and instead gain some perspective, possibly avoiding destructive words or actions that spring from your hormone-clouded bias. One simple way to do this is to label the thoughts as they come into your mind, before they are able to take hold as an emotion.

---

467   Northrup, *Women's Bodies, Women's Wisdom*, pp.135-136

468   Gottfried, *The Hormone Cure*, location 2629 (Kindle edition)

469   Miranda Gray, *The Optimized Woman*, p.48, 'All these thoughts are creative extrapolations. They are messages, not reality, but we have emotionally bought-in to the thoughts we are creating, and we act on them as if they are real.'

470   See note 282 from chapter seven, regarding a study that was conducted that showed women are less likely to acknowledge positive words during their premenstrual phase.

How to do it

This meditation can be done sitting, but when I'm premenstrual or feeling particularly emotional, I sometimes do it whilst walking in nature.

Become aware of your breath. The sensations of your breath. In and out through the nostrils. Become aware of your environment. If you are doing this as an open-eyed, walking meditation, become aware of what you see around you—the trees, the birds, the sky and the ground beneath your feet. Become aware of the sounds around you. The sensation of the air or breeze against your skin. If you are sitting with the eyes closed, simply become aware of the various sounds around you. Name these sounds—for example: lawn mower, birds, cars etc.

Then become aware of your thoughts. Watch your thoughts like clouds passing through the sky. Notice a thought and try to just observe it without getting caught up in the whole narrative that might accompany it. Then, allow yourself to become aware of the next thought as it passes through the sky of the mind.

Here's another way to think about it: it's like you're watching all these crazy thoughts on TV—like they are played out in someone else's life.

As you notice the thoughts, see if a label spontaneously arises for each thought. For example, if I find myself projecting into the future—'He said this, which means he will now do this, and I will not be happy'—I try to stop this flow of interconnected thoughts and give this string of thoughts a label such as 'catastrophising' or 'worrying'. Or, if I find myself thinking, 'If I don't do X, then Y will happen, and I will be unhappy', I try to short-circuit this with a gentle label of 'planning' or 'projecting into the future'. Or, another common pattern is dwelling on the past: 'He said this, and I said that, and he did or didn't do what I wanted, and I am unhappy'. I label this thought pattern as 'hanging on' or 'stuck in the past'.

Ultimately, replace the various and many thoughts with the reminder that in the present everything is OK, just as it is; there is absolutely nothing to worry about or change in this present moment.

Continue this mindfulness practice as long as you like.

As you become more proficient you will find you can begin to bring this more fine-tuned awareness into your daily life, so that you are able to stop negative thoughts in their tracks, before they take hold too strongly.

Open Heart Meditation for PMS

This beautiful meditation is designed to bring you out of your head and into your heart, and can be another way to transform the potentially destructive energy of negative thoughts and emotions that can torture you during your PMS phase. It works well to go for a vigorous walk first to move the energy and then finish with this meditation to help settle and calm the mind and emotions.

How to do it

Sit or lie in a comfortable position. If you feel like it, play some soft, soothing, background music. Take a few deep breaths as you allow yourself to settle into your chosen position. Breathe deeply in through the nose and then let the breath sigh slowly and deeply out of an open mouth (Falling-Out Breath), perhaps accompanied with a soft, low and gentle 'aaah' or 'haaa' sound.

Place both palms on your lower belly, your womb-space, just below your navel. Take some deep breaths down into your belly (Soft Belly Breath). Feel your belly expand gently as you inhale and draw back softly away from the palms, towards the spine, as you exhale. Feel your whole abdominal area softening and relaxing with each deep breath in and out.

After a little while, place your left hand on your solar plexus area, on the lower ribs, above the navel and below the breasts. Take some deep breaths into your solar plexus area, behind your left palm. Feel this whole area, including your diaphragm, moving freely with each breath, softening and releasing any sense of holding or tightness there.

When you are ready, and you feel that your lower and upper belly are relaxed and soft, move your left palm up to the centre of your chest, between your breasts—your heart-centre (into the Heart-Womb Mudra, see Figure 154, p.222). Feel the subtle connection of energy between your heart-centre and your womb-space. As you breathe in, draw the breath down into the lower belly underneath the right palm and then continue to feel the inhalation move up into the solar plexus and all the way up into the centre of the chest behind the left palm. Exhale gently and fully—out of the mouth if you like—or just gently through the nose. Send the exhalation all the way back down out of the belly as you feel the navel gently draw back to the spine, belly drawing away from the right palm. Even feel the exhale descend right down to the pelvic floor, gently contracting there at the end of the out-breath. Do this deep full inhalation and exhalation a few times.

Then, move your right palm up to the centre of the chest—placing it on top of the left palm there (Hands to Heart Mudra—see Figure 152, p.212).

Bring all of your awareness to the space behind the palms, deep into the chest cavity, the heart-centre. Take a few breaths here. Imagine emer-ald-green light filling your heart-centre as you breathe in and out of this space. As you inhale, the glittering, crystal-green light at the heart-centre sparkles more brightly, and as you exhale, feel this beautiful green light overflowing out of your heart, outwards, like a river spilling its banks.

Continue to let your awareness stay settled in your heart-centre. Feel like you are smiling into this space. If your heart-centre could smile, what would that feel like? Keep smiling to your heart. If it helps, imagine some-thing that makes you really happy—a beloved child, friend or lover. Think of a happy memory. Or even visualise your favourite food. I think of dark chocolate and green tea (a combination I love!). Hold this image of undilut-ed happiness deep within your heart-space, smiling into your heart-centre. In addition to feeling your heart-centre smile, turn up the corners of your mouth into a smile. Don't worry if you feel silly, just keep physically smiling and energetically smiling into your heart a little longer.

Joy is overflowing from your heart-centre.

When you are ready—after about 5 more minutes of breathing and smiling physically and into your heart-centre—prepare to come out of the meditation by taking a few more breaths down into your belly, ground-ing yourself. Then place your palms together at your heart-centre (Anjali Mudra—see Figure 151 p.212). Finish by silently saying a little prayer of gratitude. Contemplate one or several things in your life for which you feel deep gratitude and let those feelings of gratitude emanate from your heart-centre outwards.

Namaste.

Be gentle with yourself coming out of the meditation. Have a cup of herb tea. Even take this time of softened-edges and extend it a little longer by running yourself a hot bath, or enjoying a swim in the ocean.

Inversions: a panacea for PMS

Inversions (practised throughout your cycle except when you're menstru-ating) play an important role in assisting with PMS as they help create balance and stability within your hormonal and nervous systems.

A wonderful feminine Inversion is Shoulderstand, 'the queen of all yoga poses'. For PMS, I recommend doing the Supported variations of Shoulderstand—with a bolster, block or chair (see p.454)—because they have a more calming effect on the nervous system.

Shoulderstand helps to balance the thyroid and parathyroid glands[471], which regulates the metabolism, and this posture opens the chest, elevating your mood. Halasana (the Plough Pose—see Figure 133, p.186) stimulates the adrenals and kidneys,[472] which can support the cleansing action needed to remove excess hormones from the body and regulate your cycle.[473]

Different types of PMS: yoga practices to match the specific symptoms

To address exacerbated PMS, it can be helpful to categorise the symptoms so that you can tailor your yoga practice to meet your specific needs.

From an Ayurvedic point of view, the kind of PMS symptoms a woman experiences is related to her constitution or *dosha* (see Appendix 1) and whether she is experiencing imbalances that can be caused by stress, poor diet, inadequate rest and unstable routines.

Vata Cycle

If you have a cycle that has an excess of *vata,* your PMS symptoms can include mood swings with a prevalence of anxiety as well as nervous tension and insomnia.[474]

Pitta Cycle

If you experience a cycle that is predominantly *pitta* in nature, you will experience premenstrual symptoms like irritability, anger, and food cravings.[475]

Kapha Cycle

If your cycle is dominated by the *kapha dosha,* you are more likely to experience fluid retention, swollen breasts and sluggishness, and you may feel tearful and emotional.[476]

---

471 'Savangasana has a direct effect on thyroid and parathyroid glands which are situated on the neck region, since due to the firm chinlock their blood supply is increased, helping them to function properly," B.K.S. Iyengar in *Light on Yoga,* p.171

472 See: Sparrowe, *Yoga for Healthy Menstruation,* p.57

473 See p.259 in chapter seven for more information on detoxing the liver and kidneys premenstrually.

474 See: Maya Tiwari, *Women's Power to Heal,* p.106

475 Ibid

476 Ibid

Dr Abraham's four types of PMS

Interestingly, we can also overlay this traditional, Ayurvedic way of viewing the differing symptoms of PMS with a modern, Western medical model of PMS that was laid out by Dr Guy Abraham in 1983.[477] Dr Abraham, an obstetrician and gynaecologist at UCLA, created a classification system that recognised four types of PMS.

Following are Dr Abraham's four types of PMS juxtaposed with their corresponding Ayurvedic imbalance.

Type A PMS

This is characterised by anxiety, irritability and mood swings. I suggest that this corresponds to a combined *vata* and *pitta* dominated cycle in Ayurveda.

Type C PMS

This type of PMS is manifested as cravings, especially for sweets, as well as fatigue and headaches. I suggest that this corresponds to a combined *pitta* and *kapha* dominated cycle.

Type D PMS

This type involves depression as well as confusion and even memory loss.[478] I suggest this corresponds to a combined *kapha* and *vata* cycle.

Type H PMS

Type H PMS exhibits with symptoms of water retention, weight gain, bloating and breast tenderness. I suggest this corresponds to a *kapha*-dominant cycle.

---

477   I first came across Dr Abraham's thesis for a 4-type model for PMS in Anna Rychner's 'Getting out from Under: Asana for Relieving PMS' at http://www.yogasite.com/pms.htm, which talks about the model in terms of yoga practices. Many naturopaths, such as Cassie Mendoza Jones (see: https://www.cassiemendozajones.com/4-subtypes-pms/) cite Dr Abraham's work in terms of nutritional and herbal supplementation. Read the original research study by Dr Abraham at: https://www.ncbi.nlm.nih.gov/pubmed/6684167

478   Research by pioneering British gynaecologist, Katharina Dalton showed that teenage girls' academic performance was lowest during their premenstrual phase. See: http://articles.latimes.com/2004/sep/28/local/me-dalton28

Yoga treatments for the four types of PMS

We can treat these different classifications of PMS symptoms with a more individualised approach to yoga, as well as with specific diet and lifestyle adjustments.[479]

Vata PMS and Type A symptoms

Try practising the Waning Moon Sequence for Nourishing the Nervous System (see chapter seven). This sequence involves beneficial soothing and grounding postures like the Supported Child Pose, and a supported Inversion that helps balance the hormones and instigates the parasympathetic (rest and repair) response.

Pranayama that can be helpful for this type of PMS includes the Feminine Nadhi Shodhana (see p.105), and a focus on a longer exhalation, for example, the Falling-Out Breath (see p.104). Also, Brahmari (the Humming Bee Breath—see p.267) can be very calming for the nervous system.

Pitta PMS and Type A symptoms

You can also practise the Waning Moon Sequence for Nourishing the Nervous System, and you can also try the Classical Waning Moon Premenstrual Sequence (see chapter seven). Both these sequences include supported Forward Bends, which are calming and pacifying for overheated emotions. Helpful Pranayama is the Sitali breath (see p.264) as it is has a cooling effect on the body, mind and emotions.

Type C PMS and combined pitta and kapha symptoms like headaches and tiredness

Try the Waning Moon Sequence for Exhaustion (see chapter seven), to address the symptoms of fatigue. In addition, try one or a series of Supported Forward Bending postures with the forehead supported, such as supported Pascimottanasana, (see p.451), Supported Prasarita Padottasana (see Figure 404, p.452) and Supported Down Dog (see Figure 409, p.453) to help calm and cool the mind and nervous system and alleviate premenstrual headaches or migraines.

---

479   See Appendix 1 for some dietary suggestions from the Ayurvedic perspective, as well as a helpful online article on nutritional tips to match Dr Abraham's four types of PMS here: http://www.health-and-natural-healing.com/PMS-4-Types.html

Also, you can practise the Falling-Out Breath (see p.104) whilst in any of the Restorative postures, to facilitate release of deep-held mental and emotional tension that can block the free flow of *prana*.

As mentioned, cravings, especially for sugar and chocolate, are a common characteristic for Type C PMS, and *pitta* dominated cycles. This is because the body can become more sensitive to insulin during the premenstrual phase, causing a potential drop in blood sugar and bringing on those cravings.[480]

If we indulge these cravings with sugary, high GI foods, we are likely to worsen the situation causing a further drop in blood sugar character-ised by a 'let-down feeling, fatigue and headaches'.[481] It's therefore best to work on balancing the body's systems by eating healthy, low GI snacks,[482] and also practising yoga that will support your digestion. Yoga teacher and registered nurse, Anna Rychner, in her article, 'Getting out from Under: Asana for Relieving PMS', recommends the Bow Pose (Figure 221, p.258) and Bridge Pose (Figure 16, p.92), because they stimulate blood flow to the abdominal and pelvic areas, which she says can help regulate your sugar metabolism. She adds that the Bridge Pose 'rejuvenates and tones the reproductive organs as well as the abdominal organs, thereby helping to relieve carbohydrate cravings.'[483]

---

480   See: Anna Rychner, 'Getting out from Under: Asana for Relieving PMS' at http://www.yogasite.com/pms.htm, and: http://www.huffingtonpost.com. au/2016/11/23/this-is-why-women-feel-more-hungry-around-their-period/ and: *Clinical Naturopathy: An Evidence Based Guide to Practice*. The authors, Jerome Sarris and Jon Wardle, mention a theory that hypoglycaemia may account for some premenstrual symptoms. And, here's a research study implicating changes in our insulin responsiveness throughout our cycle: https://www.ncbi. nlm.nih.gov/pubmed/17425444

481   See: Rychner, 'Getting out from under: Asana for Relieving PMS,' http://www. yogasite.com/pms.htm

482   For some healthy nutrition tips see the Cycle Diet Website: http://www. cyclediet.com. , and at: http://www.huffingtonpost.com.au/2016/11/23/ this-is-why-women-feel-more-hungry-around-their-period/

483   See: http://www.yogasite.com/pms.htm

Type D PMS and kapha dominated symptoms

For this type of PMS practise poses that elevate your mood, alleviating depression and stagnancy in the mind and body. Active Backbending postures like the Bow Pose and Bridge Pose, as well as more passive Heart-Opening postures like Supta Baddha Konasana (see Figure 395 p.449) and Supported Bridge Pose (see p.450) can all help balance these emotional symptoms.

In terms of Pranayama, try focusing on lengthening the inhalation as a way to build internal energy and joy.

Type H PMS and kapha dominated cycles

Inversions can be beneficial because they can help boost lymphatic flow, alleviating fluid retention and bloating. As mentioned, Shoulderstand balances the thyroid and parathyroid glands, which in turn, balances metabolism, and can therefore help with the symptom of weight gain that characterises Type H PMS.

The Classical Women's posture, seated Upavista Konasana (see Figure 384, p.442) can also be beneficial for relieving water retention and pelvic and abdominal congestion. Yoga teacher and doctor, Mary Pullig Schatz, M.D., says that the spreading effect of Upavista Konasana creates space in the pelvis that allows cleansing blood to enter and removes swelling and waste products.[484]

Twisting postures such as Bharvajasana (Figure 8, p.87) can also be good for Type H/ *kapha* symptoms as they flush out toxins from the liver aiding the cleansing process of eliminating excess hormones during this phase of our cycle.[485]

Additionally, practising slow Lunar salutes (see the Waning Moon Salutes p.278) helps to lift feelings of heaviness, congestion, fogginess and stagnancy caused by too much *kapha*.

---

484   Mary Pullig Schatz, M.D., *Back Care Basics: A Doctor's Gentle Yoga Program for Back and Neck Pain Relief,* p.184

485   Medical school instructor, Dr Ellen Kamhi writes, 'The liver is involved in a great many metabolic processes in the body, including breaking down excess estrogens. If the liver is working well, it will break down aggressive estrogen into less harmful varieties, leading to fewer PMS symptoms … The inability of the liver to properly detoxify estrogen leads to the overriding factor observed in PMS-Estrogen Dominance.' See: http://www.naturalnurse.com/2011/07/20/premenstrual-syndrome-pms/

MENSTRUAL MEDICINE: GO-TO POSTURES AND PRACTICES

Here are my 'go-to' postures and practices for some of the common menstrual complaints that many women tend to experience at some point in their cyclical lives.

Tired, aching legs

Legs up the Wall (Figure 410, p.453), Chair Savasana (Figure 414, p.455), Double Bolster Supine Savasana (see Figure 423, p.457), Chair Shoulderstand (Figure 411, p.454), Supported Supta Padangustasana II (Figure 387, p.444).

Fatigue

Viparita Karani (Figure 410, p.453), Supported Child Pose (Figure 401, p.451), Inclined Baddha Konasana (see Figure 388, p.444), Reclining Goddess Pose (Figure 421, p.457).

Irritability

Sitali (p.264), Supported Pashimottanasana (see p.451), Supported Prasarita Padottanasana (Figure 404 p.452), Viparita Karani (Figure 410, p.453), Supported Child Pose (Figure 401, p.451), Supported Cross-Leg Forward Bend (p.452).

Heavy or prolonged bleeding

Supta Baddha Konasana (Figure 395, p.449), Supta Virasana (Figure 397, p.450), Constructive Rest Position (Figure 418, p.456), Seated Baddha Konasana or Upavista Konasana against a Tall Bolster at the Wall (Figure 302, p.332),

Trikonasana supported with back against the wall (Figure 24, p.100), Ardha Chandrasana supported with back against the wall (Figure 25, p.100), Supported Uttanasana with chair (Figure 405, p.452), Supported Janu Sirsasana (Figure 408, p.453) and Trianga Mukha Ekapada Pascimottanasana (Figure 125, p.182) with head supported on chair, Supported Child Pose (Figure 401, p.451), T-Bolster Bridge Pose (Figure 57, p.138).

Lower Back Pain

Constructive Rest Position (Figure 418, p.456), Chair Savasana (Figure 414, p.455), Prone Savasana on Transverse Bolster (Figure 263, p.288),

Supta Padangustasana I—leg to ceiling (Figure 43, p.127), II—leg to the side (Figure 387, p.444), III—Leg across body (outer hip stretch—Figure 317), Gomukhasana (p.150), Cross-leg Twist (Figure 345, p.417).

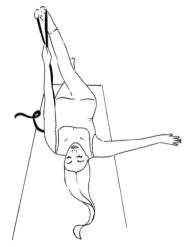

Figure 317

Menstrual Cramps

Supta Virasana (Figure 397, p.450), Supta Baddha Konasana, (Figure 395, p.449), Reclining Cross-Leg (Figure 396, p.449), Supported Pascimottanasana (can roll up a towel and place it between abdomen and thighs—Figure 318), Supported Child Pose (can place a folded blanket/heat-pack/hot water bottle on sacrum—Figure 296, p.321), Supta Padangustasana II with leg supported with a bolster (Figure 387, p.444).

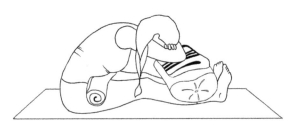

Figure 318

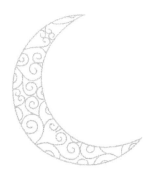

Part Five

Beyond the Four Phases

CHAPTER NINE

THE WISE WOMB: EMBRACING MENOPAUSE

Our menstruating years give us the opportunity to hone our power. And menopause is our graduation day! The woman who has crossed the menopause having understood the power of her menstruating years is truly a woman to be reckoned with. She has been offered, through the dynamics of her own body, a way to travel in both inner and outer worlds. She has stoked a fire inside which is now brilliant, fierce, enduring. She can warm herself on it, be powered by it. A power that allows her to know and love herself and the world as one, and to act accordingly.

—ALEXANDRA POPE[486]

THE SEASONS OF A WOMAN'S LIFE

So far, I have deconstructed the menstrual cycle: I have broken it down into four phases that can be likened to those of the moon. These phases can also be related symbolically to the four seasons. The Waxing Moon phase—from post menstruation to ovulation—is your spring; the Full Moon phase—around ovulation—is your summer; the Waning Moon phase—from post-ovulation to menstruation—is your autumn; and the Dark Moon phase—menstruation—is your dormant winter. Using this same seasonal symbology, we can also reflect upon the stages of a woman's life cycle. From girlhood until motherhood she is in the spring of her life, and viewed in terms of the ancient pagan archetypes, this is the phase of the 'maiden'. From motherhood until the onset of menopause she is in the summer, or 'mother' phase. Even if a woman doesn't nurture her own children as a biological mother, the mother life-stage is when she

---

486 Alexandra Pope, *The Wild Genie*, p.19

tends to nurture creative passions or projects (her career phase). Then, as her fertility winds down, from her mid-40s until her mid-50s, typically the perimenopause phase, she enters the autumn or 'maga'[487] phase of life. Finally, on the other side of menopause, in her elderly years she embodies the winter or 'crone' phase.

UNDERSTANDING THE PHASES OF MENOPAUSE

Menopause is diagnosed retrospectively—it's defined as the time when a woman no longer menstruates and has not done so for the last 12 months. The average age that a woman reaches menopause in Australia, the USA and the UK is 51.[488]

It's actually during the *perimenopause* when most of the action happens. Perimenopause, literally meaning 'around menopause', is the lead-up to menopause and can last anywhere from 4 to 10 years.[489] Women commonly enter the perimenopause from around the age of 45[490] when they begin to experience a number of emotional and physical symptoms.

One of the first signs that you are in the perimenopause is that your menstrual cycle changes. You may notice it becomes much shorter or longer, or more erratic in general, and you may experience heavier than normal bleeding or exacerbated PMS symptoms.

By the time you reach menopause, your oestrogen levels drop as much as 90%.[491] However, in the perimenopausal stage, women can often experience a depletion in progesterone that actually causes an oestrogen dominance. This initial under-supply of progesterone can cause several

487 Jane Hardwicke Collings builds on the traditional pagan 'triple goddess' framework of 'maiden, mother, crone' to add a fourth archetype, the 'maga', which she calls 'the Four Phase Feminine Way'. See: http://www.moonsong.com.au/honoring-rites-of-passage-in-a-womans-life/

488 See: http://www.mayoclinic.org/diseases-conditions/menopause/basics/definition/con-20019726 and https://www.justasjuicy.com/menopause-and-perimenopause/

489 See: https://my.clevelandclinic.org/health/articles/what-is-perimenopause-menopause-postmenopause and http://www.webmd.com/menopause/guide/guide-perimenopause#1

490 See: http://www.mydr.com.au/womens-health/menopause-what-you-can-expect

491 See: https://jeanhailes.org.au/health-a-z/menopause/about-menopause

symptoms in addition to the aforementioned changes in your menstrual cycle; these may include reduced libido, bloating, breast swelling and tenderness, mood swings, irritability, depression, weight gain around the belly and hips, and premenstrual headaches.[492]

During perimenopause, a woman will begin to experience anovulatory cycles (no ovulation) as her egg supply starts to run out leading up to the final stage of menopause when her body no longer ovulates. Along with progesterone, the production of oestrogen and androgens (male hormone precursors that can give us our sex drive) also eventually falls and their production is relegated from the ovaries to other organs like the adrenals and fat tissue.[493]

Approaching menopause, and even into post-menopause, women may experience the additional, stereotypical menopausal symptoms like hot flushes, night sweats and insomnia. According to Dr Northrup, 85% of women experience hot flushes (in the U.S. they are called 'hot flashes'), with approximately 40% considering these hot flushes to be intolerable.[494] Additionally, due to thinning of the vaginal tissue and lack of oestrogen, women may experience dryness (a lack of lubrication) in the vagina. Post-menopausal women are also more vulnerable to osteoporosis (thinning bones), which is caused by oestrogen deficiency.

492   See: Christiane Northup, M.D., *The Wisdom of Menopause: Creating Physical and Emotional Health during the Change*, p.121

493   See: http://med.monash.edu.au/sphpm/womenshealth/docs/androgens-in-women.pdf . Also see: https://canceraustralia.gov.au/affected-cancer/cancer-types/breast-cancer/treatment/what-does-treatment-breast-cancer-involve/hormonal-therapies/types-hormonal-therapy/menopause-and-oestrogen-production —'After menopause (post-menopause), monthly menstrual periods stop. The body still makes small amounts of oestrogen by changing hormones called androgens into oestrogen. Androgens are produced by the adrenal glands, which are above the kidneys. A hormone called aromatase changes androgens into oestrogen. Aromatase is produced mainly by fatty tissue.'

494   Christiane Northrup M.D., *Women's Bodies, Women's Wisdom*, p.551

Perimenopause: The Waning Moon phase of the feminine life cycle

She finds she has limits. Her energy falters, her mind drifts, her patience snaps. She begins to husband herself, to save herself for what really matters. She has seen enough to guess the trajectory of most events, to hold herself back from repeating old mistakes. She knows now that some energy is wasted. So sometimes she seems parsimonious, unwilling to expend in waste. But other times she is generous. That old coat? Give it away. That pretty pin? Oh, do take it. The half-finished book? No, it's yours. She does not need to cling to what she has outlasted. Things leave her: she does not need it all.

—PATRICIA MONAGHAN[495]

Perimenopause is a key transitional period, not only in the physical and emotional sense, as a woman's body gradually recalibrates its hormonal output, but also in terms of her whole value system that denotes where she stands within the matrix of her life.

Just as in the autumnal, premenstrual (Waning Moon) phase of your monthly cycle when your energy wanes as you prepare to shed your uterine lining, the stage in your life cycle as you move towards menopause represents a time of inward focus and ultimately of letting go of what is no longer serving you.

Elizabeth Davis and Carol Leonard, in *The Women's Wheel of Life*, further expand on the ancient pagan 'triple goddess' archetypes, and propose a total of 13 feminine archetypes to encapsulate a woman's life cycle. They offer the 'priestess' as one of the archetypes that represent an aspect of perimenopause, writing, 'Ultimately the Priestess finds she must shed her skin in order to truly wield power—a process that can be disorientating, and not a little painful if subject to outside scrutiny and criticism.'[496]

---

495 From *Seasons of the Witch*, quoted by Jane Hardwicke Collings at: http://www.moonsong.com.au/more-on-maga-the-autumn-season-of-our-lives/

496 Elizabeth Davis and Carol Leonard, *The Women's Wheel of Life*, p.45

Perimenopause: the great transformer

Become comfortable with the increasing darkness, creativity and inspired intuition of the Enchantress phase. Know that you are moving into a time of wild magic, sexual energy, inspiration and the opportunity to release past emotional baggage, to clear the decks and create a whole new you.

—MIRANDA GRAY[497]

Davis and Leonard suggest a pivotal archetype that threads throughout a woman's life cycle is that of the 'transformer'. This archetype can be understood as any transition phase within your life cycle. The transformer is a kind of 'cosmic washing machine' that you must churn through before embarking upon the next life stage. I suggest that we can view the upheaval a woman can encounter in the perimenopausal phase as an example of this 'transformer' archetype in action. When you realise you have hit uncharted territory within your life-trajectory, and you feel more than a little lost and disoriented by the unknown that is perimenopause, it is helpful to gain the perspective that out of this chaos comes the precious opportunity for a re-birth of your self, a self that can then carry you stronger, more self-aware, more compassionate, into the remainder of your 'maga' years, and into the final stage of the 'crone'.

In my early 40s, I found myself hurtling headlong into my own 'transformer' that catapulted me into the perimenopause phase. I suffered a health crisis that was precipitated by the exhaustion of holding all the pieces of my life together throughout my 30s. I had single-parented for almost a decade, run a busy, growing, yoga teacher-training business that had involved a lot of travel, and struggled to maintain a long term defacto relationship that had been on shaky ground for some time. I came crashing down with multiple health complaints including chronic fatigue, exacerbated PMS, heart arrhythmia and digestive issues (gut dysbiosis and multiple food intolerances). Whilst these health issues were obviously induced by years of compounded stress, not to mention too many antibiotics, there was a new ingredient here: an inner-voice that quietly yet persistently whispered to me that my life needed to change.

---

497   Miranda Gray, *Red Moon*, p.173. Gray uses her own archetype of the 'enchantress' for the menopausal life phase.

This is the voice of perimenopause.

As previously mentioned, the premenstrual phase can be viewed as a time of 'emotional housekeeping'. The perimenopausal life-phase can be regarded in the same way: if you are willing to listen to the signals of our body, you open yourself to the manifold gifts of this life phase. Dr Christiane Northrup has encapsulated his idea:

> Recall that the emotional and psychological changes of the peri-menopausal years are to the entire life cycle as the week before one's period is to the monthly cycle. All the issues that have been occurring premenstrually and which perhaps had been avoided previously—"Should I quit my job?" "Should I stay in this relationship"?—now come up and hit us between the eyes rather relentlessly, demanding that they be dealt with.[498]

Refreshingly, Traditional Chinese Medicine (TCM) views the menopause as a woman's 'second spring', reflecting the newfound life that is possible for her as she enters a stage where she is able to move her energies away from nurturing others and finally direct them towards nurturing herself.[499]

Dr Northrup also promotes this idea of menopause being the 'second spring', if only we heed the messages that our bodies and hormones are sending us. She writes, 'We must source our lives from our souls now. Nothing less will work. When we dare to do this, we truly prepare for the springtime of the second half of our lives.'[500]

---

498   Northrup, *The Wisdom of Menopause*, p.575

499   'So in Chinese culture and Chinese medicine, we regard this midlife time for a woman as second spring because we feel like, well, in the first half of your life if you are a woman, your life does not quite belong to you. Your life belongs to your family, your children particularly, and perhaps your community. You have obligations. You have biological and social obligations. However, the beginning of this kind of midlife creates tremendous shift in opportunity because by now most women will have older kids. They do not need to be there as much, meaning the kids are more self-sufficient and as well as that she now has life experience, she now has wisdom, she now perhaps also is more secure and confident of herself because of all the experiences she has had up to this point', says Dr. Mao Shing Ni, from Tao of Wellness. See: http://www.empowher.com/menopause/content/why-does-chinese-medicine-call-menopause-womans-second-spring-dr-mao-video

500   Northrup, *Women's Bodies, Women's Wisdom*, p.549

Now, in my late 40s, I feel that I am completing the massive life reassessment that perimenopause propelled me into five years ago. After finally letting go of a relationship that was draining my very life-force, I have now welcomed my husband into my life, and with his full support, I am joyfully undergoing a process of simplification within my life—sloughing off projects and commitments that are no longer serving me or my family.

As I continue to stabilise my health, ameliorating many of the stress-related symptoms with which I began this journey, I am able to discern the perimenopausal symptoms that continue, but my attitude towards these 'signs'[501] is imbued with gratitude rather than resentment, distress or denial. This attitude is fuelled by my deep appreciation of perimenopause as a vital process of transformation—the great 'transformer' at work in my life.

Strategies for navigating 'the change'

Strategies for moving through your perimenopause gracefully, and therefore more comfortably, echo those suggested for your Waning Moon, premenstrual phase (see some practical tips in chapter seven, p.253). Take time out just for you to reflect on what needs to change in your life. You may use various tools for this enquiry—meditation, journaling, Restorative Yoga, time in nature. I cannot stress enough the importance of carving out this reflective, solitary time that will help you gain perspective on what you *really* need to nourish yourself as you move forward and through the 'transformer' that is perimenopause.

The wise woman: honouring the menopause

> *When the Crone speaks her truth, she instils wisdom*
> *and initiates cross-generational understanding.*
> *The Crone is mother to many, not in a nurturing*
> *sense but as a universal point of reference.*

—ELIZABETH DAVIS AND CAROL LEONARD[502]

---

501 Anna Watts, spiritual healer and doula educator, prefers to call the 'symptoms' of menopause and perimenopause 'signs' as a way of positively reframing of our experience of menopause. See more about Watts' work at: https://www. spiritwayhealing.com.au

502 Davis and Leonard, *The Women's Wheel of Life*, p.175

In many indigenous and traditional cultures, menopausal women were respected and continued to play an important role well into their dotage. 'Crones have been revered for their Blood Mystery of menopause. By virtue of retaining their 'wise blood', with all its magical and visionary properties, they are considered ready to lead society,' write Davis and Leonard.[503] The political structure within particular Native American cultures included a 'Council of Grandmothers' that had the veto on all major decisions within the tribe, and also had the right to depose a Chief if he wasn't taking care of his people adequately. Such cultures also embodied the feminine in their nurturing approach to the earth, with an edict that all tribal decisions needed to be considered in terms of their implications for the next seven generations![504]

Mother Maya (Maya Tiwari) points out that Indian Hindu culture has traditionally exhibited a positive attitude towards the natural process of the ageing woman. She explains, 'The native women of my culture see this period as a harbinger of deep spiritual fortitude, a time to start loosening the grip on competitive partnerships with the world and to go within to commune with the greater power.'[505]

And, as already touched on, Chinese culture has always held a deep reverence for the elders of society including an appreciation of the gifts of menopause. Acupuncturist Dr Mao Shi Ning says of the menopausal woman, 'she now has life experience, she now has wisdom, she now perhaps also is more secure and confident of herself because of all the experiences she has had up to this point.'[506]

These ancient attitudes of honouring older women are in stark contrast to our 'ageist' contemporary society in which women become virtually invisible as they mature. Women often feel compelled by societal and media pressures around looks and body image to make artificial changes to their faces and bodies in a desperate and ultimately fruitless attempt to halt the ageing process. Perhaps related to these negative attitudes towards ageing, particularly towards older women, is the current dominant patriarchal and separatist approach to the earth and our environment—it's seen as something to be exploited for our own very short-term gain.

503 Ibid., p.172

504 Ibid., p.180

505 Maya Tiwari, *A Woman's Power to Heal*, p.206

506 See: http://www.empowher.com/menopause/content/why-does-chinese-medicine-call-menopause-womans-second-spring-dr-mao-video

Embracing the gifts of menopause

As she reweaves her identity apart from the
cycle of reproduction, she begins to weave
and mend the great Web of Life

—DAVIS AND LEONARD[507]

There seems to be a natural inclination in menopausal and post-menopausal women to be of service to society. They have entered a new phase in their lives—generally their child-rearing and active career-orientated days have passed—so their focus moves out beyond their immediate family or work environment. This broader focus of the older woman is reflected in the statistics: there are more women than men who volunteer, and more volunteers tend to be of perimenopausal and menopausal age.[508]

In Australia, we have a volunteer-run organisation called the 'Knitting Nannas against Gas and Greed', a kind of modern, self-appointed 'grand-mother council'. The Knitting Nannas protest against 'the destruction of our land and water' caused by coal-seam gas mining and 'other non-renew-able energy sources', and claim to 'draw on a broad history of knitting used as a tool for non-violent political activism'.[509] It's groups like this that represent invaluable social and environmental concern that is translated into action, and largely instigated by older women, who are invested in protect-ing the future environment for their children and their children's children. The Dalai Lama's assertion that 'the world will be saved by the Western woman'[510] should perhaps be amended to: 'The world will be saved by the *older* Western woman'!

---

507 Davis and Leonard, *The Women's Wheel of Life*, p.173

508 'In 2010, 38% of adult women volunteered (3.24 million women) and 34% of adult men volunteered (2.85 million men).' And, in the 45–64 age bracket, volunteers numbered 43–44 % compared to 27–42% in the 18–44 year old age range. See: https://www.volunteeringaustralia.org/wp-content/uploads/VA-Key-statistics-about-Australian-volunteering-16-April-20151.pdf

509 See: http://www.knitting-nannas.com/

510 This famous quote from the Dalai Lama (delivered at the Vancouver Peace Summit in 2009) is referred to here: http://www.dharmacafe.com/index.php/news-briefs/article/the-dalai-lama-the-world-will-be-saved-by-the-western-woman

I recently saw a news story about a distressing discrepancy between men and women in terms of the amount of superannuation accrued by retirement age. The poignant image of a 60-year-old woman forced to continue to work her low-paid childcare job into her dotage due to insufficient superannuation savings will stay with me forever. What I find so sad about this story is that, due to financial pressures, these older, post-menopausal women are not being permitted the natural rhythm of introspection that accompanies the 'wise woman' phase. It's our birthright within our feminine life cycle to be able to enjoy our 'crone' years as a quiet, inner time, freed up from the responsibilities of caring for a family and working a full-time job; a time that allows us to take our renewed energy and use it to benefit society at large. This is what these women, and ultimately our society, are being denied.

Societal change begins with ourselves: we need to reframe our own attitudes towards the menopause so that we see it as something to look forward to rather than dread; so we see it as another significant rite of passage in our feminine lives to be honoured; so that we enthusiastically inspire our sisters, daughters and granddaughters to do the same.

Here's what a woman interviewed by Davis and Leonard said about the positives she recognised in entering the post-menopausal crone phase:

> ...you no longer believe, in an ego related way, that you are the be-all and end-all, the source, the doer. I identify with a much more universal force and allow it to move you—for you are the only manifestation of the divine who can do what you do, and by surrendering to what that is and getting out of the way, you become capable of living in the most beautiful, graceful, efficient, effortless way possible.[511]

Having recently turned 60, my friend and colleague Anna Watts is 'on the other side' of menopause and recalls that, when she was heading into her climacteric, friends warned her about the negative aspects of growing older. 'One friend in particular said, "Wait till you turn 60, you'll notice a shift in energy levels, you won't be able to do the things you used to do".' On the contrary, Anna says that she has experienced an 'enormous creative surge' and feels 'juicy, alive and energised'. She goes on to explain, 'For me it's now about balancing that enormous creative flow without getting tired, and just being able to enjoy it.' This points to her innate, fine-tuned awareness of her evolving needs that is a defining characteristic of a Moving with the Moon approach to women's monthly phases and life stages.

---

511   Davis and Leonard, *The Women's Wheel of Life*, p.173

In the same way that I urge you to fall in love with your monthly bleed and honour it as your sacred 'red tent' time,[512] to support your health and wellbeing and to deepen your connection with your cycle and with nature, I also encourage you to draw inspiration from matriarchal practices and viewpoints that consider menopause as a positive life transition.

BUILDING A BRIDGE TO MENOPAUSE

How can you prepare for menopause?

*Until we take the small pauses at important junctures
along the way we will be quite unprepared as we
butt headlong into the big pause—menopause.*

—MAYA TIWARI[513]

If you're a younger woman wondering what you can do to prepare for this momentous next life stage, the primary thing to be aware of, which forms the very foundation of this book, is how to Move with *your* Moon. Learning to listen to your body's cues as you cycle through every month teaches you how to cultivate a healthy balance between activity and rest that will serve you well when you encounter some of the more challenging physical and emotional symptoms of perimenopause and menopause.

To enjoy a more positive connection with the middle-age years of per-imenopause, it is vital that as a younger, cycling woman, you learn how to honour your monthly bleed.[514] 'Womb Yoga' teacher and author of *Yoni Shakti: A Woman's Guide to Power and Freedom Through Yoga and Tantra*, Uma Dinsmore-Tuli agrees. She says of perimenopause, 'the harvest we begin to reap is the harvest of attitudes and experiences that we have brought to all our monthly cycles over the previous thirty years or more.'[515]

In addition to reframing and adapting your attitudes and practices around your menstrual cycle, it's also important that you enter the perimenopause

---

512   See p.18 in chapter one for more information on the idea of the 'red tent' as a way to honour your cycle and femininity.

513   Tiwari, *Women's Power to Heal*, p. 208

514   See p.80 in chapter four for ideas on how you can honour your menstrual Dark Moon phase.

515   Uma Dinsmore-Tuli, *Yoni Shakti: A woman's guide to power and freedom through yoga and tantra*, p.380

as healthy and robust as possible. Your nervous and hormonal systems need to be well balanced, which will minimise unnecessary depletion of progesterone that can cause the common perimenopausal condition of 'oestrogen dominance'.[516] Moreover, stress-related conditions involving cortisol (stress hormone) levels that are either too high or too low can negatively affect your hormonal system,[517] as Dr Libby Weaver explains:

> If a woman has been in SNS dominance (sympathetic nervous system— i.e: 'fight or flight' stress response) and then her sex hormone production starts to change, her menopause is far more likely to be challenging and potentially debilitating, with some of the major symptoms being hot flushes, interrupted sleep, and vaginal dryness.[518]

A critical benefit of a nourished, resilient nervous system is that your adrenal glands will be well prepared for the task of taking over much of the production of DHEA (androgen levels), and therefore oestrogen, that needs to take place post-menopausally. Ways to support your nervous and hormonal systems include diet, exercise and effective stress management techniques—yoga being an invaluable component, of course!

Promoting a healthy perimenopause and menopause

A healthy diet is an important ally on your journey into menopause and beyond. It is generally recommended to eat a whole-foods diet; reduce caffeine and alcohol; and limit or eliminate refined white flours and sugars, in order to ease your way into menopause. Women are also advised to boost their iron and calcium levels if necessary.[519] And making sure you eat plenty of fermented soy products may help with the symptoms of hot flushes.[520]

---

516 See p.74 in chapter four and p.306 in chapter eight for more information on how stress can upset our female hormonal balance.

517 See Sara Gottfried M.D.'s *The Hormone Cure*, chapter four, p..71, 'High and/or Low Cortisol: Stress Case? Is Life Without Caffeine Not Worth Living,' for more information on this condition.

518 Dr Libby Weaver, *Rushing Women's Syndrome*, location 5598 (Kindle edition)

519 See: http://www.webmd.com/menopause/guide/staying-healthy-through-good-nuitrition#2

520 Timothy McCall M.D., *Yoga as Medicine*, p. 456. Also see this helpful article 'What foods can ease menopause symptoms'— https://www.menopausecentre.com.au/information-centre/articles/what-foods-can-ease-menopause-symptoms/

Dr Michael Lam, M.D., a physician specialising in nutrition and anti-ageing, suggests that the oestrogen dominance that can occur in the perimenopause can be related to poor diet. He says, 'Studies have shown that the estrogen levels fell in women who switched from a typical high-fat, refined-carbohydrate diet to a low-fat, high-fiber, plant-based diet even though they did not adjust their total calorie intake.' Dr Lam goes on to explain that plants have 'progestogenic effects' and suggests that women in cultures who eat whole-food diets and exercise regularly seem to have fewer menopausal symptoms.[521]

For useful tips on diet for perimenopause and menopause I recommend Dr Christiane Northrup's holistic-bible for menopause, *The Wisdom of Menopause,* and Dr Sara Gottfried's *The Hormone Cure,* which also offers specific advice on nutrition and supplements for the various symptoms of perimenopause.

How yoga can help

> Yoga can help you pay attention to what your body
> and its changes have to tell you. It can realign your
> focus inward and teach you to love yourself and the
> process you're going through as it all unfolds.
>
> —LINDA SPARROW[522]

Exercise is a boon for women as we age. 'Properly performed exercises have been shown to modulate hormonal imbalance through the pre-menopausal years and beyond. Those who exercise regularly are also happier, less depressed, and have an optimistic outlook on life,' affirms Dr Lam.[523] Yoga postures, especially the more dynamic ones, represent a form of mindful exercise and combined with the stress-relieving aspects of yoga such as meditation, Restorative Yoga and relaxation (e.g. Yoga Nidra), make for a potent mix to support your overall health and wellbeing as you enter your menopausal 'maga' and 'crone' years.

---

521   Dr Lam: https://www.drlam.com/blog/estrogen-dominance-part-2/1781/

522   Linda Sparrowe, *The Woman's Book of Yoga and Health,* p.235

523   See: https://www.drlam.com/blog/estrogen-dominance-part-2/1781/ Dr Lam also writes, 'In another study reported in the Journal Cancer[sic], it was found that postmenopausal women who exercise 1 hour each day can significantly cut their breast cancer risk. Regardless of age, regular exercise is a proven key to reduction of breast cancer, not to mention the cardiovascular health benefits'.

Yoga has been shown to help in the reduction of hot flushes, night sweats and sleep disturbances[524] and, in a meta-study, it has been implicated in supporting women with psychological symptoms of menopause.[525]

Just like exercise, a more vigorous yoga practice will raise your endorphin levels leaving you feeling happy and energised. Plus, the stress-management benefits of yoga will not only support your hormonal system as it works to adjust to the fluctuations of perimenopause, but may also help with reducing your risk of osteoporosis (bone thinning).[526] This is because there is a connection between stress and osteoporosis—high levels of the stress hormone cortisol can draw the calcium from the bones and interfere with new bone growth.[527]

Yoga can also support women on the non-physical level by providing them with tools for self-acceptance. By understanding and integrating the key tenets[528] of yoga philosophy, you give yourself a better chance of finding peace amidst so much change so that you can learn to be content within your new menopausal-skin.

Ideally, a woman has grounded her entrance into menopause with years of dedicated practice so that she is able to blossom into her 'second spring'. In the same way that she used yoga to flow with the challenges as well as to appreciate the gifts of her previous feminine phases and stages, a woman with a solid yoga foundation can now fully embrace her experience of the 'maga' and 'crone' life stages. However, even if you're new to yoga at this later stage of life, there is still much to be gained by adopting a regular practice—yoga will meet you where you are *right now*. Some of the most

---

524   Research studies cited by Timothy McCall M.D. in *Yoga as Medicine* (p.446). See also a study reported in the *International Journal of Obstetrics and Gynaecology*.

525   See: http://www.hindawi.com/journals/ecam/2012/863905/

526   In *The Women's Book of Yoga and Health*, Linda Sparrowe cites a research study conducted at the California State University in 2000 that showed that yoga can increase bone density —p.329

527   'The body releases calcium from the bones to neutralise the ph balance of cortisol,' explains Dr Bhakti Paun Sharma at.:
http://www.thehealthsite.com/diseases-conditions/
heres-what-you-need-to-know-about-stress-induced-osteoporosis-bso316/

528   The concept of *ahimsa* is a helpful Feminine Yoga principle, which is discussed in chapter three p.50. Additionally, the idea of *isvara pranidhana*—translated loosely as 'surrender to the universal flow', can also help a woman be at peace with the changes and challenges of menopause and aging in general.

vibrant yoginis took the practice up late in life, to their own—and others'—great enrichment.[529]

Nourishing practices for your *vata* time of life

Hand in hand with the tools of yoga are those of Ayurveda that can support your health and wellbeing, and deepen your self-awareness, as you enter your 'wise woman' years. The Ayuvedic *dosha* of *vata* (see Appendix 1) is related to the season of autumn and becomes more predominant as you move into your perimenopausal phase of life. From an Ayurvedic perspective, many of the symptoms of menopause—thinning of the skin and hair, dryness of the skin, mood swings, anxiety, mental fogginess and insomnia—are typical '*vata*-deranged' symptoms.[530] Dr Robert Svoboda says that even hot flushes are ultimately a result of an imbalance in a woman's *vata*, and he recommends simple deep breathing to help to alleviate them.[531]

Therefore, as you transition into perimenopause, it's a good idea to focus on pacifying your *vata* in order to bring your body-mind into greater balance. This can be done by eating *vata*-nourishing foods (see Appendix 1) and taking care to keep a regular routine—eating, sleeping and resting regularly and sufficiently.

Your yoga practice may also need to emphasise *vata*-reducing postures and practices—depending on the menopausal symptoms experienced—which I elucidate later in the chapter.

Finally, Ayurvedic oil massage, or *abhyanga,* can also be very nourishing for women during this life-phase.

Ayurvedic oil massage: a healing daily practice for perimenopause and menopause

The Ayurvedic self-massage technique deserves special mention because of its balancing and regenerative power at this turbulent time of life. Shiva Rea enthuses that massage of warm oil on the body is 'one of the most

---

529   Influential Italian yoga teacher, pioneering yogini and author of the seminal book, *Awakening the Spine,* Vanda Scaravelli only took up yoga in her late 40s and practised well into her 80s. Here is an informative article on her life and yoga approach: http://www.relaxandrelease.co.uk/scaravelli-inspired-yoga/vanda-scaravelli/

530   See: Dr Robert E. Svoboda, *Ayurveda for Women,* p. 136, and Maya Tiwari, *Women's Power to Heal,* p.213

531   Dr Svoboda, *Ayurveda for Women,* p.136

nourishing, life-enhancing gifts of health you can give yourself for the rest of your life.'[532]

Ayurvedic oil massage works on a deep level to lubricate the joints. This has a powerfully healing effect on the typical dryness and stiffness of the joints, and depletion of the energy, characteristic of a person with high *vata*, and which naturally occur as women age. The warm sesame oil also moisturises dry, mature skin and, as you sit in meditation or contemplation for the 10 minutes or so while the oil soaks in, you can actually feel your nervous system being calmed and nourished.

How to do it

There are two important points for this daily self-massage technique. First, make sure you use cold pressed black sesame oil, available from health food stores and Ayurvedic suppliers—not the Chinese sesame oil you use for cooking. You can also get medicated black sesame oil that is infused with herbs to correct a particular imbalance in any of the *doshas*—*vata*, *pitta* or *kapha*. The second important point is that you warm the oil, as explained below.

If you are doing this practice in the colder seasons, start by heating the space where you will be doing your self-massage—usually your bathroom. Then, spread a large towel down on the floor. Place a small bowl or cup of the black sesame oil within another larger bowl of boiling water to gently warm the oil.

Take your clothes off and sit down to begin the massage. Take a few deep breaths to calm and ground yourself before you begin. Then, start by massaging the oil onto your feet—the soles then the tops of the feet and the toes. With long, flowing strokes, work your way up the legs to the outer hips and buttocks. Keep working up the body—with circular motions on your belly (always in a clockwise direction), into the sacrum, lower back and kidney area, on and around each of the breasts; and sweeping from the backs of the shoulders to the front, pectoral muscles and across the collar-bones. Then, work your way up the arms, from the palms of the hands and fingers and up into the armpits.

Breathe deeply and rhythmically throughout the massage, even working with some Falling-Out Breaths (see p.104) if that feels nice.

For the larger muscles and joints, use circular, sweeping motions with the palms—in an upward direction towards your heart. Pay particular attention to working into the major joints—ankles, knees, hips, wrists, elbows, shoulders. For the soles of the feet, you can use your thumbs and fists as you

---

532   Shiva Rea, *Tending the Heart Fire: Living in the Flow with the Pulse of Life*, p.171

massage into the insteps. Likewise, for the palms of the hands—use the fingers and thumbs and work into each finger joint as well as massaging into the palms.

Finish by massaging the face—focusing on any tense areas like the hinge joint of the jaw and eyebrow-centre—and using small circular motions with one or two fingers. Lastly, if you're planning to wash your hair, use a little of the oil to massage an Ayurvedic Marma Point on the very crown of your head with the tip of one or two fingers. Locate this point by measuring about eight of your finger-widths up from the eyebrow centre. This is an important 'stress-release point'. Conclude your massage with vigorous, heating rubbing motions with the palms of the hands up and down the thighs.

Wrap yourself up in an old towel or cuddly dressing gown and step into some old socks or slippers to protect your floors and carpets from the oil. Now it is time to for the oil to soak in and do its magic for about 10–15 minutes. If you have the time, sit quietly in meditation or do some gentle Pranayama (later in this chapter you will find recommended Pranayama for menopause).

Sometimes, I like to just sit in the morning sun with a cup of tea, thinking, breathing and doing nothing in particular; taking pause at the beginning of my day. If you are too busy to stop and need to get yourself or family members ready for school or work, that's fine too! I've sometimes made my son breakfast whilst wrapped up in my oil-dressing gown.

At least 10 minutes later, or when you're ready, take a hot shower to wash the oil off and complete your morning ablutions. As you wash the oil off, you can imagine you are sloughing off anything that is no longer serving you. I also like to imagine that when I do my oil massage I have created a kind of magical, good-vibes 'force-field' around me that sets me up for the day and keeps the 'good energy' in and any 'bad energy' out as I go about my day and interact with others.

YOGA FOR PERIMENOPAUSE AND MENOPAUSE

'The symptoms and timing of menopause are very individual, and your menopause will probably not look exactly like anyone else's'—so says Kate Bracy, a registered nurse who specialises in the area of women's health and family planning.[533] It follows that yoga for menopause is not a one-size-fits-all approach. There are no fixed rules for practising yoga during this stage of your life; the kind of yoga you do is going to depend on how you feel on any given day, which may change radically and unpredictably.

That said, there are some general yoga-principles that can help you navigate your 'maga' and 'crone' life stages so that you are as healthy and balanced as possible.

Perimenopause: move with *your changing* moon

If you're still menstruating fairly regularly, a good place to start is the Moving with the Moon approach detailed in this book—i.e., adapt your yoga practice (and expectations) according to the various phases of your menstrual cycle.

However, for many women, as they progress through perimenopause, their cycles become quite irregular and it becomes increasingly difficult to follow the Moving with the Moon template in a chronological and systematic way; you may often have no idea where you are in your cycle! I recently had a hiatus of 48 days without a menstrual period (the first ever!), and I really had no idea if and when I was next going to bleed. I would vacillate from one day feeling completely premenstrual to the next day feeling relaxed and calm—just like I do when I menstruate—even though I had not yet bled. Therefore, at my life-stage, my yoga practice needs to tune into my changing *daily* needs.

Unlike a younger woman, who can clearly follow (and predict) her menstrual phases because they form recognizable patterns over several days or even up to a week at a time, I now find that I need to apply a kind of daily 'yoga first aid' for perimenopause. If I notice that I am feeling decidedly premenstrual on one day, I may choose to practise any of the postures or practices from the Waning Moon phase (see chapter seven), or even specific PMS practices such as those described in the chapter eight (see p.357). The very next day, I may find that I shift to feeling quite energetic and focused, and therefore postures and practices from the Waxing Moon phase suit me better (see chapter five).

533   See Bracy's informative article on the types of menopause: www.verywell.com/what-is-menopause

By adapting your yoga practice to match the *changing* symptoms of perimenopause, you can give yourself a sense of control at a time when it feels like your body is rebelling against you—all the time!

Post-menopause: move with *the actual* moon

A question I'm often asked by women who have reached menopause and no longer have their own internal 'womb-moon' is, 'How can I still practise yoga in a feminine, cyclical way?'

This is where a literal Moving with the Moon approach can work well. Follow the phases of the moon so that you indulge in a more gentle, inward practice with the dark and new moons, practising the Dark Moon sequences from chapter four. As the moon waxes, practise the stronger, stabilising Waxing Moon sequences from chapter five. With the full moon, enjoy a more expressive, dynamic, heart-opening practice with the Full Moon sequences from chapter six; and as the moon wanes, begin to wind down and balance your energy with the Waning Moon sequences in chapter seven.

Post-menopausal women love this idea!

By enjoying a cyclical practice that ebbs and flows with the energies of the moon, a post-menopausal woman is able to maintain a sense of her own internal rhythm regardless of the fact that she no longer experiences the more obvious signs of bleeding and ovulating.

Interestingly, many post-menopausal women describe that they still register a subtle connection with their younger-woman womb-cycles: they report a monthly 'crampy' feeling in their womb, just as if they were premenstrual or bleeding. The body seems to echo those cycles it was so accustomed to following for decades before. If you do notice these subtle signs from your body, don't ignore them! Likewise, if your natural energy is at odds with the practices suggested for the relevant phase of the moon, first and foremost listen to your body (and emotions) and adjust your practice accordingly. It may mean that you need to change tack and follow your *internal* moon, rather than the external moon.

For example, if the moon is waxing or full, yet you feel quite tired and introspective, it will be more appropriate for you to practise the gentler and more nurturing Waning Moon or even Dark Moon practices. That's what the Moving with the Moon methodology is all about—a heightened sensitivity and responsiveness.

The same principle of flowing with the lunar cycles can apply to perimenopausal women who feel they've lost a connection to their cycle because it has become so irregular and unpredictable. When in doubt, and it feels like your own personal energy aligns, practise according to the current phase of the moon.

Practise *vata* reducing yoga

According to the Ayurvedic understanding of our life cycle,[534] a woman's twenties and thirties represent her *pitta*[535] phase of life—when she needs the drive and ambition offered by the fiery, *pitta*-energy to support her in building her career and/or mothering. During this life-stage, it's more appropriate to do a more dynamic yoga practice to harness the strong energy of *pitta* and also because a woman's body is stronger. However, as a woman ages, she moves into the *vata* phase of her life—she needs to go more gently and slowly, and use her yoga practice to nourish her nervous system and maintain overall agility and mobility.

An excellent yoga practice to balance your *vata* levels, and therefore help with many of the symptoms of perimenopause and menopause, is the Pawanmuktasana (joint-freeing) sequence. You will find my Women's Pawanmuktasana Sequence at the end of this chapter. This is a simple, gentle and well-rounded practice that you can do every day to keep your joints lubricated and mobilised, relieve general aches and pains, and nourish your nervous and hormonal systems. This sequence also has profound effects on your mental and emotional state—it is very calming and grounding (i.e., *vata* reducing), helping to counteract feelings of anxiety and agitation that are common during the menopausal journey.

An excess of *vata* causes depletion, so one of the best ways to balance your *vata* is rest—lots of it! According to Ayurvedic practitioner and naturopath Kester Marshall, regular rest nourishes both *vata* and *pitta*, which can be helpful as many of the symptoms of perimenopause—for example, premenstrual irritability—also represent a 'blow-out' in our *pitta*. 'Some Ayurvedic teachers recommend women should rest for at least 20 minutes a day, for a longer period once a week and then a day or more if possible each month (on the first day of their menstruation, if still menstruating),' writes Marshall.[536]

At least several times a week I like to take what I call a 'Yoga Nidra nap', which helps support my energy levels and fills me up physically and energetically during this, my perimenopausal phase. As already explored, Yoga Nidra is a guided relaxation practice that offers your body, mind and nervous system deep rest and rejuvenation. I invest time in this 20–30

---

534 See: http://www.muditainstitute.com/articles/ayurvedicmedicine/menopause.html

535 See Appendix 1 for more information on the *pitta dosha*, as well as all three *doshas* or constitutions.

536 Kester Marshall, 'Menopause: An Ayurvedic Perspective' at: http://www.muditainstitute.com/articles/ayurvedicmedicine/menopause.html

minute practice within my busy day, resting on my bed, an eye-bag on my eyes. Sometimes I fall asleep and sometimes I am awake throughout the practice. Either way, I feel more rejuvenated than if I just took a nap. Try it yourself! Choose from your favourite Yoga Nidra practices in this book: a Dark Moon Yoga Nidra on page 116, a Waning Moon Yoga Nidra on page 268 or a Full Moon Yoga Nidra on page 214. It is best not to try to take yourself through Yoga Nidra. Record yourself reading the scripts from this book, or there are audio recordings available of the Yoga Nidras that accompany this book.[537]

Nourish the adrenals with yoga

Nourishing your adrenal glands during the perimenopause and beyond can play a vital role in supporting your hormonal balance and therefore easing or minimising menopausal symptoms.[538]

Why are the adrenal glands so important? The adrenals, which sit on top of the kidneys, can over-produce the stress hormones, adrenaline and cortisol, when you are chronically stressed. Over time, if the stress persists and you do not adequately find ways to manage your response to it, your adrenals can become depleted. This ultimately affects the healthy balance of your whole hormonal system as discussed in chapters four and eight in regards to the potential of 'pregnelonone steal'—see pages 75 and 307. Maya Tiwari says that stress can be one of the major suppressors of healthy adrenal function. 'Anger, anxiety, worry, nervousness, fear, depression, insomnia, exhaustion, chronic pain, long-term illness, and malnutrition are the dominant factors that may contribute to adrenal dysfunction,' explains Tiwari.[539]

Since the adrenals also produce a hormone called DHEA, an androgenic hormone that can help increase the serum levels of oestrogen, it's necessary to encourage sufficient production of DHEA for optimal hormonal balance. Dr Christiane Northrup explains that the production of DHEA naturally declines in many women as they age, and if there's an

---

537 See my website: www.anadavis.com

538 Dr Northrup writes, 'If your adrenals are depleted from chronic overproduction of the stress hormones norepinephrine (adrenaline) and cortisol, you are much more likely to suffer from fatigue and menopausal symptoms'. See: *Women's Bodies, Women's Wisdom*, p.551

539 Maya Tiwari, *Women's Power to Heal*, p.232

imbalance in this hormone and an over-production of the stress hormone cortisol—caused by chronic stress—women become 'susceptible to fatigue and all manner of illnesses, as well as menopausal symptoms.'[540]

As I touched on earlier, once a woman reaches menopause, her adrenals take on a starring role instead of the ovaries, becoming responsible for the production of not only DHEA but also progesterone.[541] The androgens (DHEA and testosterone) act as weak oestrogens, and they are also associated with sexual response and libido, as well as general wellbeing. This all means that if you look after your adrenals you may have a better chance of moving more easefully and comfortably through menopause.

If you're tired all the time, or if you're not waking up refreshed and you need caffeine to get you through your day, you may be suffering from adrenal depletion. If left untreated, this is known as 'adrenal fatigue'.[542] Complementary therapies such as acupuncture and herbs (specifically adaptogenic herbs that nourish the adrenals) can help in the recovery from adrenal fatigue. It's also a good idea to give up coffee, alcohol and sugar as these all sap the adrenals. At the same time, take an honest look at your lifestyle as to how you might find better ways to manage your stress and to rest more.

Dr Libby Weaver talks at length about reframing your perception of stress as a way of bringing your body more into the healing parasympathetic nervous system dominance (PNS)—the rest, digest and repair response. An important technique for helping you *respond* rather than

---

540   Northrup, p.554. Among a number of its benefits, Dr Northrup explains that healthy levels of DHEA 'reverses many of the unfavourable effects of excessive cortisol', and that DHEA is also a 'precursor for testosterone', which is associated with libido.

541   'Going into menopause with SNS dominance sets you up to have poor adrenal production of progesterone, the hormone with significant antianxiety and antidepressant properties', writes Dr Libby Weaver in *Rushing Woman's Syndrome*, location 5598 (Kindle edition)

542   Northrup, p.551, details the symptoms of adrenal dysfunction. Note, in orthodox medical circles adrenal fatigue is still considered a 'myth'. A 2016 systematic review concluded 'there is no substantiation that "adrenal fatigue" is an actual medical condition'— https://www.ncbi.nlm.nih.gov/pmc/articles/PMC4997656/ Coming from the naturopathic-perspective, Lara Briden explains: 'Your doctor may not be familiar with the terms "adrenal fatigue" or "HPA axis dysfunction". If you mention adrenals to your doctor, she may test for Addison's disease, which is a rare autoimmune disease of the adrenal glands', location 1588 (Kindle edition), Briden, *Period Repair Manual*.

react to stressors in your life is instituting a gratitude practice—regularly acknowledging the many positives in your life—and this can set up a positive feedback loop, as Dr Weaver suggests:

> Exploring and resolving elements of your emotional landscape are also going to assist. And from the spaciousness that PNS dominance promotes, you cannot only see the magnificence and the wonder, but you can feel it within, just as you did as a very little girl. Your rituals create your life. Get some good ones![543]

There are two main ways you can use yoga to support your adrenals during the transition into and beyond menopause.

1. Cultivate self-compassion

The number one way to nourish your adrenals is to manage your stress levels by taking regular, mindful rest, and yoga can be one of your biggest allies in helping you do this. That's why it's so important, just as in any of the other key feminine life events and transitions—throughout the menstrual cycle, pre-conception, pregnancy and early motherhood—to use the tools of yoga to *go gently* on yourself. If your adrenal function is compromised, it is not helpful to undertake an overly challenging yoga practice. In fact if you overdo it with exercise or in your yoga practice, you may bring on an 'adrenal crash' in which you ultimately deplete your adrenals further and you end up feeling much worse!

I concur with the suggestions of Maisha Johnson and Nisha Ahuja, authors of a fascinating article in *Everyday Feminism*, who suggest that a mindful yoga practice needs to be sensitive and 'self-referencing', which ultimately embodies the key Feminine Yoga principle of *ahimsa*:[544]

> ...if it's stressing you out, then it's not what yoga is meant to be. There should be compassion, not ridicule, and a sense of internal ease, instead of poses that cause your body stress. You can honor the pace that's best for your body, instead of overexerting yourself.[545]

Your self-compassion-filled perimenopausal or post-menopausal yoga practice may look and feel very different from when you were a younger woman. And that's OK! If you're truly doing yoga, you will accept and

---

543   Dr Libby Weaver, *Rushing Woman's Syndrome*, location 1375 (Kindle edition)

544   See p.50 in chapter three for more information on this Feminine Yoga principle.

545   Maisha Z. Johnson and Nisha Ahuja: http://everydayfeminism.com/2016/05/yoga-cultural-appropriation/

embrace this change of pace, trusting that it will only serve to make you a kinder person towards yourself and towards those you love. Let's face it, your loved ones are often on the receiving-end when your hormones are out of balance!

This more gentle approach, reflecting the Moving with the Moon philosophy detailed in this book, will mean you'll listen and respond to the shifting needs of your body *every* time you step on your mat. Those days when you're exhausted because you've been tossing and turning the night before with menopausal insomnia you'll opt for a restful and rejuvenating Restorative Yoga practice, such as the Waning Moon Sequence for Exhaustion.

If you are suffering a menopausal headache, you will enjoy the Cooling (Forward Bending) Restorative postures (see Appendix 3) with your forehead supported.

And if you're feeling generally 'out of sorts', particularly with exacerbated premenstrual symptoms, you might try some of the Supported Inversions (see Appendix 3), or any of the Waning Moon practices that appeal to you from chapter seven.

2. Promote blood flow and energy to the adrenals

The other way that yoga can balance and nourish your adrenals is by promoting healthy blood flow and circulation of energy (*prana* or *chi*) to the adrenal glands. Tools to do this are movement, breath and visualisation.

The Adrenal Breath

The practice of Adrenal Breathing is designed to nourish and re-activate depleted adrenals. This Pranayama is based on the ancient Taoist technique of 'kidney breathing', or what Taoist sexology teacher Willow Brown calls the 'Turtle Breath'.[546] This breathing technique is said to help return essential energy, known as *jing* in traditional Chinese medicine (TCM), to the kidneys and adrenals. According to Chinese Medicine, your kidney energy can become depleted when there is an excess of fear.[547] The adrenal glands can become over or under-active[548] if your body labours under

---

546 Find out more about Willow Brown's work at: http://thetaoistway.com. The description of The Adrenal Breath that follows is inspired by Willow Brown's 'Turtle Breath' technique.

547 See: https://bodyecology.com/articles/kidney-health.php

548 In *The Hormone Cure* (chapter four), Dr Sara Gottfried explains how your body can become imbalanced by over or under producing the stress hormone cortisol. She writes, 'Stress causes high cortisol. But in later stages of long-standing stress, cortisol can swing too high and too low, and everything in between, sometimes in a matter of hours in the same day,' p.71.

chronic sympathetic nervous system (fight or flight) engagement—i.e., stress. Therefore, fear is just another way of describing this stress response, which helps us understand the necessity of nourishing the kidneys and adrenals, and of course, as I have mentioned, of reducing and managing our stress levels.

How to do it

Come into the Supported Child Pose (see Figure 401, p.451), with the knees apart, big toes touching, and torso supported along the bolster (see page 134 for detailed instructions for this Restorative Posture).

Allow your body to soften and relax for the first few breaths. Perhaps even taking a few Falling-Out Breaths (see p.104) in which you allow the exhalations to fall out of an open, relaxed mouth.

When you are ready, begin to deepen the inhalation and feel the breath filling up into the lower back, kidney area—on either side of the spine, about three inches above the top of the sacrum. Imagine your back-body is a big turtle shell, and as you inhale and breathe into your lower back, your turtle shell is lifting up and away from the front of the body, towards the ceiling. As you exhale, your turtle shell gently softens back towards the floor and your front-body. After a few breaths, add the refinement of a very gentle pelvic floor lift on your inhalations as you imagine you are drawing energy up from you perineum into the kidney area, into your turtle shell. As you exhale, you can relax the pelvic floor muscles.

Feel this 'turtle breath' circulating within and nourishing each of your kidneys and creating more space for your adrenals. Picture your adrenals as two spongy, pyramidal shaped organs that sit atop the kidneys, and as you inhale, the adrenals gently lift off the kidneys creating more space. After a few more of these 'turtle breaths', concentrate the awareness and the breath into the medulla (the very core or seed of the adrenals) and imagine you are charging each adrenal, right at its very core, with healing and energising energy, life-force or *prana*.

Continue for a 3–6 more breaths, and then come out of the posture in your own time.

Adrenal nourishing yoga postures

All of the Restorative postures (see Appendix 3) nourish the adrenals because they work to bring about parasympathetic nervous system dominance—the 'rest, repair and digest' or 'relaxation response'—giving the adrenals a break from pumping out the stress hormones.

According to yoga teacher Patricia Walden, Forward Bending, Twisting, and Backbending postures all work to 'pacify and then activate the adrenals'.[549] I would add the caveat that Supported Backbending (Heart-Opening) poses, such as Supta Baddha Konasana (see Figure 395, p.449) or the Supported Bridge Pose (see p.450) are the best options because they do not over-stimulate the nervous system in the same way that the Active Backbends do.

A simple Twist that replenishes your adrenals is the Sage Pose (Bharadvajasana—see Figure 8, p.87).[550] Paschimottanasana (see p.451) is also beneficial, especially if you consciously send the breath into the kidney and adrenal area.

Inversions are tonic for the adrenals, particularly Supported Inversions like Viparita Karani (Legs up the Wall Pose—see Figure 410, p.453). According to Iyengar Yoga teacher and research scientist Roger Cole, Viparita Karani, with the pelvis raised up on a bolster or folded blankets, stimulates the blood pressure sensors (baroreceptors) in the neck and upper chest. This, in turn, triggers reflexes that reduce the nerve input into the adrenal glands and slows down the heart rate and the brain waves, and relaxes the blood vessels, all serving to reduce the adrenal stress hormone, norepinephrine, in the blood.[551]

As a post-menopausal woman, my friend Anna Watts enjoys Supported Block Shoulderstand (see Figure 413, p.454) as her 'all time favourite yoga pose'. She says this is her 'go to' pose if she's feeling exhausted or just needs 'some time out'. 'I think it's the benefits of that slight inversion; I feel like it nourishes my adrenals,' explains Anna.

Inversions and menopause

In the same way that Inversions are beneficial for the premenstrual (Waning Moon) phase of our monthly cycle and for healing menstrual imbalances, they are also helpful for managing the symptoms of menopause. As I have pointed out previously, Inversions have a nourishing and balancing effect on our endocrine (hormonal) glands as well as our nervous system.

---

549   Patricia Walden and Linda Sparrowe, *The Women's Book of Yoga and Health*, p.209

550   Ibid., p.269

551   See the online article, 'Which Poses Treat Adrenal Exhaustion' by Roger Cole at:
      http://www.yogajournal.com/article/practice-section/treating-adrenal-exhaustion/

As women get older, their bones can become more brittle (osteoporosis), and their joints may degenerate with conditions like osteoarthritis. It therefore tends to be safer and more appropriate to practise supported versions of the traditional yoga Inversions. For some examples of Supported, Restorative Inversions see Appendix 3. These Supported Inversions allow greater comfort, alignment and ease within the posture, which, in turn, facilitates longer timings, potentially enhancing the many benefits available to the practitioner.

Pranayama for perimenopause and menopause

Ujjayi Breath

Slow, deep, regular breathing has been shown to reduce the incidence of hot flushes.[552] Therefore, the Ujjayi Breath that effectively helps you deepen your breath capacity is a good choice for menopause.

Ujjayi breath is a slightly sounded breath in which you create a soft, sibilant sound with the breath as it passes through the throat. It's by reminding yourself to follow this sound that you can help your mind stay present in the practice, calming an anxious, busy mind and over stimulated nervous system. See page 165 for instructions.

Extending the Exhalation

Anytime you lengthen the exhalation you are engaging the parasympathetic branch of the nervous system, and this has the effect of slowing the heart and calming the mind. Extending the Exhalation is a simple Pranayama practice that you can do in any restful posture, but it works particularly well in Viparita Karani (see Figure 410, p.453). See page 326 for instructions for this breathing practice.

Trusting in the Pause Pranayama

A significant contributing factor in easing your transition into menopause, and in fact, into any challenging feminine monthly or life phase, is practising the art of acceptance, and ultimately surrender. Trusting in the Pause Pranayama is a wonderful breathing practice to support the process of trust and letting go.

---

552 Timothy Mcall, M.D., in his book, *Yoga as Medicine*, (p.446) cites a research study—a randomized controlled study of 33 women with hot flashes, published in the *American Journal of Obstetrics and Gynecology* that concluded that 'slow, deep, regular breathing led to statistically significant reductions in the frequency of hot flashes'. And, Gottfried in, *The Hormone Cure*, says 'paced breathing' cuts hot flushes by 44%—location 3169 (Kindle edition)

How to do it

Lie in a comfortable supine position. You may want to position props underneath the thoracic spine to open the chest as in the Reclining Goddess Pose (see Figure 421, p.457). Make sure you feel completely comfortable and supported. Then, take some time to relax and soften here: scan your awareness around your body and breathe out and away any areas of tension in the physical body.

Gradually begin to deepen and lengthen your breath. Focus particularly on your exhalations. Begin to notice that there's a natural pause at the end of each exhalation, when your lungs are empty. It's a void, a complete emptiness. Increasingly become aware of this pause at the end of the out-breath. Can you let yourself linger in that pause, that emptiness? Can you completely surrender to and be present to this pause? Trust in that pause, and simply allow the inhalation to come of its own accord, in its own time, without any control on your part, to fill this space.

As you allow yourself to be in the pauses between the breaths, feel yourself drop more deeply into relaxation, into surrender, letting go of 'making things happen'. It's a liberating feeling, and deeply relaxing.

Stay with this practice for as long as you're comfortable and enjoying the process. Then, when you're ready, allow the breath to find its own natural rhythm for a few cycles—the exhalations returning to their natural length and pace—before rolling to the side and preparing to come up to sitting.

Complete the practice in a comfortable sitting position with the hands in Anjali Mudra (prayer gesture) at the heart-centre (see Figure 151, p.212), dedicating this practice to the divine within yourself and all living beings, and allowing this affirmation to sit in your heart:

Full of gratitude, I receive the good that waits for me.

The Falling-Out Breath

The releasing effects of this simple breathing practice are great for relieving the emotional tension that can accumulate during the passage to menopause. See page 104 for instructions.

Sitali

Sitali (and its variation, Sitkari) is an excellent breathing practice for cooling the mind and body and may help to counteract hot flushes. See page 264 for instructions.

Feminine Nadi Shodhana

This balancing practice is beneficial for the rocky times that can characterise the transition into menopause. Practise this breathing technique whenever you are feeling unsettled in order to focus and calm the mind and body and help balance your hormones and the masculine-feminine energies within your body-mind. See page 105 for instructions.

Ovarian Breathing

Ovarian Breathing is said to not only be beneficial for regulating the menstrual cycle but also for supporting menopause, and can help balance the energy and hormones in the body. See page 209 for more information and instructions on this ancient Taoist breathing practice.

Mudras for perimenopause and menopause

Yoni Mudra

Maya Tiwari says, 'Use this powerful practice to balance hormonal activity in the body even if you are no longer menstruating or sexually active'.[553] See page 327 for instructions and diagram.

Anjali Mudra

This simple gesture of deep honouring and gratitude can be helpful to begin or end your yoga practice and take the time to feel grateful for all of the blessings you have accumulated in your life. See page 212 for instructions and diagram.

DEVELOPING YOUR HOME PRACTICE FOR PERIMENOPAUSE AND MENOPAUSE

As discussed, the yoga practice that carries you into menopause needs to respond sensitively to your changing mental, emotional and physical needs, and this means that a *balanced* practice is key. So far I have emphasized being gentle with yourself and not practising in an overly vigorous way, especially if you're suffering from adrenal dysfunction. Of course it is always important to do a gentle, nurturing Restorative practice when you're feeling exhausted, under-slept or overwhelmed. However, it's equally beneficial to practise some of the more dynamic and strengthening movements from yoga to prevent and counteract weight-gain, osteoporosis and feelings of lethargy and depression—all potential symptoms of menopause.

---

553   Maya Tiwari, *Women's Power to Heal,* p.155

It all comes back to understanding the key Ayurvedic energies (*doshas*) and how they can become imbalanced, which can be a very useful way of assessing what your body-mind needs at any given time during your journey into menopause and beyond. In addition to assessing your current *doshic* imbalance—i.e., are you experiencing an imbalance in your *vata*, *pitta* or *kapha dosha*?[554]—it can also help to factor in the weather, season and time of day when you design your own home practice.

Here are some example scenarios that show how a yoga practice can be adapted according to how you're feeling physically, mentally and emotionally and in the context of the time of day, weather and season. In this way you can gain inspiration in crafting your own menopausal home practice to boost your health, energy and wellbeing.

Scenario One

It's summer, afternoon, very hot and humid and you feel tired and depleted. You haven't been sleeping well and on top of the hot weather you are experiencing regular hot flushes, and you have a premenstrual headache.

This would indicate that you are experiencing an excess of the *pitta dosha*, which means you'll need a gentle, cooling, soothing practice. Try starting with a Pranayama practice like Sitali (see p.264) and including plenty of restful, Restorative postures—particularly the Heart Opening Restorative Postures and the Cooling Restorative Postures (see Appendix 3).

Scenario Two

It's autumn, early in the morning; there's a cold erratic wind, and you feel anxious, flighty and ungrounded.

This would indicate that you are experiencing an excess of the *vata dosha*. You need a nourishing, grounding practice that lubricates the joints and gently releases dryness and the element of 'air' from your body-mind. Try the *vata*-reducing Women's Pawanmuktasana Sequence at the end of this chapter.

Make sure you include many of the more grounding, floor based postures—for example, the Classical Women's postures (see Appendix 2). Standing poses like the Standing Goddess (see Figure 394, p.447) and Warrior II Pose (see Figure 11, p.90), held for longer timings, can also feel very grounding.

---

554 See Appendix 1 for an understanding of the three Ayurvedic *doshas*.

Scenario Three

It's spring, mid-morning; you are feeling tired and sluggish, and you are craving a coffee to pep you up. You have gained weight around your middle and you are prone to depression.

This would suggest that you are experiencing an excess of the *kapha dosha*. You need to stimulate and move your energy and you probably need to nourish your adrenals. Try a dynamic Salute sequence, like the Full Moon Salutes (see p.225), or the Waning Moon Salutes (see p.278), to warm and energise your body and mind.

Also include some strengthening and dynamic postures that are in sequences like the Waxing Moon Post-Menstrual Sequence (see chapter five) and focus on the more active, Heart-Opening Standing postures like Virabhrasdana I (Warrior I, especially the heart-opening 'goal-post arms' variation—see Figure 84, p.149) and the Standing Goddess Pose (see Figure 394, p.447) to help boost your mood.

You could also try some passive, Heart-Opening postures—the Heart Opening Restorative postures (see Appendix 3)—that have the effect of uplifting you without over-stimulating the nervous system.

Finish with simple Half Shoulderstand (see Figure 132, p.186) or your favourite supported version of Shoulderstand (see p.454), and also try the Adrenal Breath in a Supported Child Pose (see p.451).

GO-TO POSTURES AND PRACTICES FOR PERIMENOPAUSAL AND MENOPAUSAL SYMPTOMS

PMS-like symptoms

- Waning Moon sequences (see chapter seven), and also see suggestions for different types of PMS in chapter eight (see p.362).
- Supported Inversions (see Appendix 3).
- Cooling Restorative poses (see Appendix 3).
- Nadi Shodhana Pranayama (see p.105).
- Sitali/Sitkari Pranayama combined with Nadi Shodhana (see p.265).

Hot flushes

- Ujjayi Pranayama (see p.165). You can integrate the Ujjayi Breath with Sara Gottfried's 'paced breathing'[555]—inhaling for a count of 5 seconds, holding the breath for a count of 10 seconds, and exhaling for a count of 5 seconds. Do this for 20 minutes, twice a day.
- Sitali/Sitkari Pranayama (see p.264).
- Supta Baddha Konasana (see Figure 395, p.449).
- Supported Bridge Pose (see p.450).
- Supported Inversions (see Appendix 3). Judith Lasater says that when we have a hot flush, *prana* moves from the core of the body outwards, heating your skin. Apparently Inversions draw the *prana* inward toward your organs and away from the skin surface, which cools you down.[556] Geeta Iyengar recommends Halasana (Plough Pose—Figure 133, p.186) for hot flushes.[557]
- Cooling Restorative postures (see Appendix 3).

Headache and Migraine

Covering your eyes with an eye-bag or even wrapping a crepe bandage around the eyes and forehead during the practice of Restorative postures can be very soothing for headaches.

- Cooling Restorative postures (see Appendix 3).
- T-Bolster Supported Bridge Pose (see Figure 57, p.138).

---

555 Gottfried, *The Hormone Cure*, location 3169 (Kindle edition)

556 As quoted by Linda Sparrowe in *The Women's Book of Yoga and Health*, pp. 238–239

557 Geeta Iyengar, *Yoga, A Gem for Women*, p. 181

- Supta Baddha Konasana (see Figure 395, p.449).
- Viparita Karani (see Figure 410, p.453).

Insomnia

- Reclining Goddess Pose (see Figure 398, p.450).
- Supta Baddha Konasana (see Figure 395, p.449).
- T-Bolster Supported Bridge Pose (see Figure 57, p.138).
- Supported Down Dog Pose (see Figure 409, p.453).
- Supported Cross Legged Forward Bend (see p.452).
- Supported Inversions, in particular, Shoulderstand (see Appendix 3).
- Yoga Nidra—choose from the Dark Moon Yoga Nidra on page 116, the Full Moon Yoga Nidra on page 214, or the Waning Moon Yoga Nidra on page 268.

Fatigue

- Waning Moon Sequence for Exhaustion (see chapter seven).
- Cooling Restorative postures (see Appendix 3).
- Constructive Rest Position (see Figure 418, p.456).
- Supported Inversions (see Appendix 3).
- Gentle Twists—Bharavadjasana (see Figure 8, p.87) and Cross-Legged Twist (see Figure 345, p.417). Patricia Walden says that these kinds of gentle Twists 'replenish your adrenal glands, restore your nervous system, and bring energy and stability to your whole system'.[558]

Heavy Bleeding

- See 'Yoga for Menorrhagia' in chapter eight, p.330.
- See the sub-section in chapter eight, page 367— 'Heavy or prolonged bleeding' under the 'Menstrual Medicine Go-To Postures'.

Stiff Joints

- Women's Pawanmuktasana Sequence (at the end of the chapter)— to loosen all of the major joints in both the upper and lower body.
- Heart Opening Restorative postures (see Appendix 3); the Dark Moon Late Menstrual Sequence (in chapter four), and the Vajrasana (kneeling) shoulder stretch sequence (Posture 1) from the Busy Days Nurturing Waxing Moon Sequence (see p.192)— to loosen the neck and shoulder joints.

---

[558] Walden and Sparrowe, *The Women's Book of Yoga and Health*, p.269

- Right Angle pose at the Wall (see Figure 307, p.338)—to loosen the shoulders, upper back and spine.
- Trikonasana (see Figure 24, p.100)—to loosen the hips, spine and upper back.
- Supta Padangustasana Series: Supta Padangustasana I—leg to ceiling (Figure 43, p.127), II—leg to the side (Figure 45, p.128), III—Leg across body (outer hip stretch—Figure 317, p.368); Gomukhasana (see p.150)—to loosen the hips.
- Seated Baddha Konasana (see Figure 383, p.441) and seated Upavista Konasana (see Figure 384, p.442)—to loosen the hips
- Supta Virasana (see Figure 397, p.450)—to loosen the hips, knees and ankles.

Weight-gain

- Waxing Moon Post-Menstrual Sequence (in chapter five).
- Shoulderstand (see Half Shoulderstand Figure 132, p.186).
- Dynamic Standing poses—Utkatsana (Figure 120, p.179), Warrior II (Figure 11, p.90), Warrior I (Figure 10, p.90) and Standing Goddess (Figure 394, p.447).
- Full Moon Salutes (see p.225) and Waning Moon Salutes (see p.278).
- Rolling Bridge Vinyasa (see p.295).
- Twists—Supine Twist on bolster (see Figure 415, p.455), Ardha Matsyendrasana Twist (see, p.236) and Twisting High Lunge (see p.281).

Depression

- The Heart-Opening Restorative postures (see Appendix 3).
- Bharadvajasana (Sage Twist—see Figure 8, p.87).
- Supported Inversions (see Appendix 3)—especially Shoulderstand and Supported Plough Pose (see Figure 319).
- Waning Moon Salutes (see p.278) and Full Moon Salutes (see p.225).
- Viloma Pranayama (see p.106) in Reclining Goddess (see Figure 421, p.457).

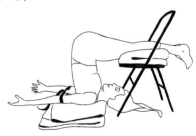

Figure 319

Brittle bones (Osteoporosis)

Patricia Walden says, 'the more bone mass you have going into menopause, the better off you'll be ten, twenty, or even thirty years down the line.' She suggests the keys to maintaining healthy bones and preventing osteoporosis are a healthy diet and lifestyle and a 'good weight-bearing exercise program'.[559] The following postures help give you maximum bone strength going into menopause.

- Plank Pose (see Figure 12, p.91)
- Down Dog Pose (see Figure 409, p.453)
- Dolphin Pose (see Figure 320)
- Dynamic Standing poses—Warrior I (see Figure 10, p.90), Warrior II (see Figure 11, p.90), Standing Goddess (Figure 394, p.447)
- Trikonasana (Triangle Pose—see Figure 24, p.100).
- Half Shoulderstand (see Figure 132, p.186)
- Modified Camel Pose with a bolster (see Figure 321)
- Yoga Nidra—choose from the Dark Moon Yoga Nidra on page 116, the Full Moon Yoga Nidra on page 214, or the Waning Moon Yoga Nidra on page 268—to help manage your stress levels as osteoporosis can be related to stress.

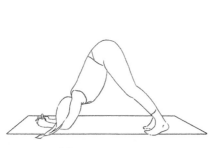

Figure 320

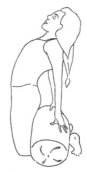

Figure 321

Important Safety Note

If you've been diagnosed with osteoporosis, check with your doctor first, as some of the above stronger postures may not be appropriate, and you may also need to work with a qualified yoga therapist for one-on-one attention.

---

559 Walden, *The Women's Book of Yoga and Health*, p.325

Digestive Sensitivities

- Supta Virasana (see Figure 397, p.450)
- Supported Child Pose (see Figure 401, p.451)
- Supine Single Knee to Chest Pawanmuktasana (see p.349).
- Supported Pascimottanasana (see Figure 402, p.451).
- Half Shoulderstand (see Figure 132, p.186) or Supported Shoulderstand (see p.454).
- Viparita Karani (see Figure 410, p.453)
- Supine Twist on a Bolster (see Figure 415, p.455)
- Yoga Nidra—choose from the Dark Moon Yoga Nidra on page 116, the Full Moon Yoga Nidra on page 214, or the Waning Moon Yoga Nidra on page 268. This practice can help because there is a connection between poor vagal tone and digestive issues.
- Sitali/Sitkari Pranayama (see p.264)

Prolapse

Important Safety Note

Avoid postures that have a bearing down effect like Malasana (the Squat Pose—see Figure 385, p.443)

- Kegels (pelvic floor exercises)
- Tadasana with block between the thighs (see p.178)
- Dandasana (see Figure 123, p.182)
- Down Dog with block between thighs (see Figure 121, p.180)
- Down Dog with feet on blocks (see Figure 322)
- Supported Inversions (see Appendix 3)—in particular Viparita Karani and Supported Shoulderstand variations
- Ardha Chandrasana (Half Moon Pose—see Figure 25, p.100)
- Urdvha Uttanasana—can have hands on bricks (Lifted Forward Fold—see p.177) and Ardha Prasarita Padottanasana (see Figure 323)
- Seated Upavista Konasana (see Figure 384, p.442)
- Supta Baddha Konasana (see Figure 395, p.449)
- Supta Virasana (see Figure 397, p.450)

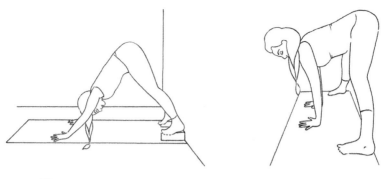

Figure 322   Figure 323

WOMEN'S PAWANMUKTASANA (JOINT-FREEING) SEQUENCE

Best time to practise

The Pawanmuktasana sequence is a wonderful perimenopausal and menopausal practice.

It is also a beneficial practice to do during the latter part of the Dark Moon (menstrual) phase of your cycle to gently mobilise the body and energy after the more static practices you will have done earlier in your menses.

This sequence can serve as a gentle yet comprehensive warm-up before you move into larger, stronger and more challenging postures. It can also be a self-contained practice to loosen up the major areas of tightness and stiffness throughout the body. When I'm seeking a gentle and time-efficient practice this is my go-to sequence.

The Women's Pawanmuktasana sequence is especially good as an early morning practice when your joints tend to be stiffer. I also love to do it as an anti-jetlag sequence to gently loosen and release stagnant energy throughout my whole body after a long flight.

Sequence duration

Anywhere between 25-40 minutes depending on how many repetitions you do for each movement, how slowly you breathe and move, and how long you stay in the static poses.

Sequence benefits

- Relieves stiffness in the joints—mobilises and lubricates many of the major joints in the body; good for arthritic conditions.
- Releases tension and tightness in many of the key muscles.
- Calming and grounding—relieves anxiety and mental agitation; meditative and relaxing—slows down the breathing.
- Balances an excess of *vata* (see Appendix 1 for an explanation of *vata* imbalance).
- The Classical Women's Postures and Womb Circling Movements help to nourish the reproductive organs, boosting your *shakti prana* (essential sacred feminine energy).

Props for this sequence

A folded blanket (if you're working on a hard floor and/or for sitting on if you find that you need support to sit up straight—good for beginners); a bolster to straddle in the Vajrasana (kneeling Thunderbolt) poses; and a folded blanket, small cushion or gertie ball to place under the front-leg-hip in Pigeon Pose.

1. Ankle flexion and circles

Benefits

Loosens and lubricates the ankles

Props for this posture

A folded blanket to stop you slumping if you have difficulty sitting up tall in Dandasana (Staff Pose—see Figure 325)

Recommended timing

Do 7-10 repetitions of the pointing/flexing of ankles (see Figure 326 and Figure 327); do 7-10 repetitions of the ankle circles in both directions (see Figure 328, Figure 329 and Figure 330).

How to practise

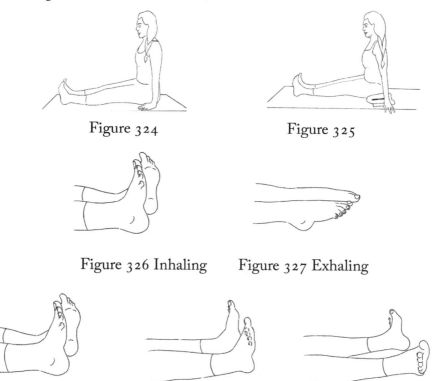

Figure 324   Figure 325

Figure 326 Inhaling   Figure 327 Exhaling

Figure 328   Figure 329   Figure 330

Start in Dandasana (Staff Pose) with the legs out in front of you (see Figure 324), sitting up on a folded blanket if you need help in sitting up tall (see Figure 325). Take a few breaths just to connect and check in before you begin the Pawanmuktasana sequence. Take some deep breaths down into your belly and feel the sitting bones descending into the earth with each exhalation, sensing into your body and preparing your mind for the single-focus of methodically and gently moving through your body to loosen and free up energy.

Then begin the ankle flexion movement. Inhale as you point your toes (plantar flexion—see Figure 326) and exhale as you flex your ankles (dorsiflexion—see Figure 327). Or, you can reverse the breathing (exhaling as you point and inhale as you flex). It doesn't really matter which way round you breathe, the main thing is to focus on slow breathing that coordinates with the slow, mindful movement, establishing a pattern for the rest of this practice. Repeat for 6-9 more times.

Moving into ankle circles. Circle your feet slowly away from each other, in circles (see Figure 328, Figure 329 and Figure 330). Do this 6-9 times one way, then repeat, circling the feet in the other direction—toes moving in towards each other and around. Work with full, deep breathing to accompany these slow, mindful circling movements.

2. Knee to chest and knee circles

Note

Do these postures—Knee to Chest and Knee Circles—and Postures 3—Stirring the Pot and Rock the Baby Hip Stretch—on the right leg. Then stretch your legs out into Dandasana (see Figure 324) before repeating the whole sequence on the left leg.

In a feminine approach to yoga, we usually start unilateral movements from the *left* side. However, the following movements are designed to stimulate and massage the digestive tract (especially the large intestine), so it is more therapeutic to start with the *right* leg.

Benefits

Warms up the leg muscles and lubricates the knee joints

Props for this posture

As for Posture 1 above.

Recommended timing

Do 5-10 repetitions of the Knee to Chest movement and 5 circles in each direction of the Knee Circles.

How to practise

Knee to Chest

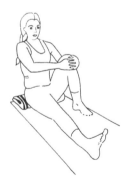 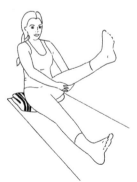

Figure 331 Exhaling   Figure 332 Inhaling

As you exhale, bend up the right knee, the hands around the outside of the knee at the top of the shin, and draw the knee in towards the right side of the chest, feeling the massaging action on the belly (see Figure 331). As you inhale, bring the hands (interlaced) behind the thigh and extend your leg, pushing the right heel away from you to stretch the back of the thigh, knee and calf (see Figure 332). Repeat up to another 9 times, moving slowly with the breath.

Knee Circles

Keep the hands interlaced at the back of the thigh, just near the back of the knee, and circle the shin. Imagine you are trying to trace a big circle in front of you with your big toe (see Figure 333). Do about 5 circles in each direction, keeping the breath even and deep.

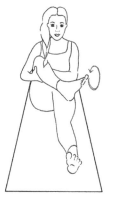

Figure 333

3. 'Stirring the pot' hip rotations and 'rock the baby' hip stretch

Benefits

- Stretches the outer hip muscles (rotators/piriformis), which is therapeutic for the lower back.
- Lubricates into the hip sockets.

Props for this posture

As for Posture 1 above.

Recommended timing

Do 5-8 circles in each direction for the Stirring the Pot movement; rock back and forth a few times for Rock the Baby, and do about 5 circles in each direction.

How to practise

'Stirring the Pot' Hip Rotations

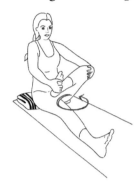

Taking the right foot in the left hand, the knee in the right hand, circle the right heel, like you're stirring a big pot with your foot—essentially stirring the head of the right femur (thigh) bone within the hip-socket joint (see Figure 334). Do another 4-7 circles and then change directions.

Keep the breath even and deep throughout and, if you like, work with some Falling-Out Breaths (breathing out through the mouth); this can help you release deep-held tightness in the hip and groin area—an area where a lot of emotional tension is stored.

Figure 334

'Rock the Baby' Hip Stretch

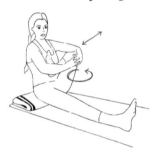

From Stirring the Pot, raise up the right foot so the shin is parallel to the floor (foot in line with knee) and, if you can, bring the foot and the knee into the crooks of the elbows, hands interlaced on the outside of the shin (see Figure 335). If that is not possible for you, just keep holding the foot and the knee in the hands. From here, do little rocking movements from side to side feeling how this gently loosens up the outer hip/buttock muscles. Then, play with circular

Figure 335

movements, about 5 in each direction. Breathe deeply the whole time. You might also like to perform some Falling-Out breaths here.

After completing Postures 2-3 on both sides, stretch your legs back out into Dandasana (Figure 324). Sit for a few moments with the eyes closed, breathing into your belly and hips, noticing already how you've moved *prana* (energy) within the lower chakras of the body.

4. Seated baddha konasana (bound angle pose) with heart-opening variation

Benefits

- Opens the hips—groins and inner thighs.
- This is a Classical Women's pose, which is beneficial for the health and vitality of your reproductive organs and balances your cycle. It energises the womb-space (Sacral Chakra) with *shakti* (feminine) energy.

- This Heart-Opening variation also brings energy to the other feminine centre—the heart-centre—and increases your breath capacity, releasing upper back and shoulder tension, uplifting you.

Props for this posture

A folded blanket to stop you slumping if you have difficulty sitting up tall.

Recommended timing

Stay here, breathing deeply into the heart and belly for up to 5 slow breaths.

How to practise

Bend up your legs into Baddha Konasana—soles of the feet together, heels close to the groin, knees opening towards the floor. From here, place the hands behind you and slightly out to the side. Press the hands into the floor to open the chest, rolling the shoulders back and lifting the chin to

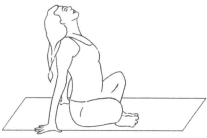

Figure 336

gaze upwards, opening the throat (see Figure 336). Take up to 5 slow, deep breaths here.

Safety Note

Do not force the knees towards the floor, and if you have SIJ (sacroiliac joint) sensitivity, you may want to place some support underneath each knee—such as folded blankets, cushions, or yoga blocks.

5. Seated upavista konasana (wide-legged seated pose) with variations

Benefits

- Stretches and opens the inner thighs, groins and hips.
- This is a Classical Women's pose which is beneficial for the health and vitality of your reproductive organs, and balances your cycle. It energises the womb-space (Sacral Chakra) with *shakti* (feminine) energy.
- The Heart-Opening variation increases your breath capacity, releasing upper back and shoulder tension, uplifting you.
- The Hands Clasped Overhead variation opens up the shoulders, stretches the spine, and limbers up the wrists and fingers.
- The Womb Circling variation loosens up the hips and torso, stretching the waist and releasing lower back and hip tightness.

Props for this posture

A folded blanket to stop you slumping if you have difficulty sitting up tall.

Recommended timing

Stay for 3-5 breaths in the Heart-Opening variation, a further 3-5 breaths in the Hands Clasped Overhead variation, and do about 5-8 circles of the torso in each direction for the Womb Circles variation.

How to practise

Heart-Opening Variation

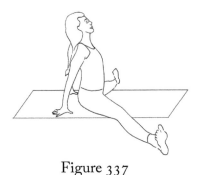

Figure 337

From Baddha Konasana, extend your legs out to the sides as wide as you can comfortably go. Activating the legs, flex the toes back towards you and roll the inner thighs up towards the ceiling. Place the hands behind you and slightly to the sides. Press the hands into the floor to lift and open the chest, shoulders rolling back, chin lifted, gazing up to open the throat (see Figure 337). Breathe deeply here, filling up the chest with the breath for 3-5 breaths.

Hands Clasped Overhead Variation

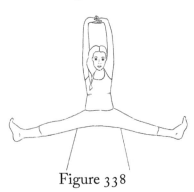

Figure 338

As you inhale, raise your arms overhead, clasping your hands so your palms face away from you (see Figure 338). Keep working the little finger side of the hands towards the ceiling and drawing the shoulder blades down your back to make sure you're not bunching up around the inner corners of the shoulders. Feel the extension through the spine and the sides of the torso. At the same time, ground your sitting bones down into the earth. Stay, and breathe deeply here for 3-5 breaths.

Womb Circling Variation

As you exhale, release the clasp of your hands (from the previous variation) and lower the hands to place them on your lower belly (womb-space). Begin to circle the torso, playing with small and then larger circles (see Figure 339). Spiral around in one direction about 5-8 times before changing direction.

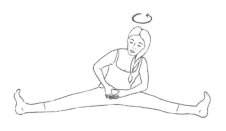

Figure 339

This is a good movement to work with some more Falling-Out Breaths (see p.104), feeling the whole spine, including the neck loosening and softening fluidly.

Note, instead of placing your hands on your belly as you circle, you can also bring your hands on the floor in front of your, for extra support for your lower back and sacrum.

6. Dandasana with legs internally rotated

Benefits

Provides a counterbalance to the hips by internally rotating them after the external rotation of the last two poses (Baddha Konasana and Upavista Konasana). In this way this movement lubricates the hip joints and provides full range of movement.

Props for this posture

A folded blanket to stop you slumping if you have difficulty sitting up tall.

Recommended timing

Roll the legs in and out about 6-8 times then hold in internal rotation for 3-5 breaths.

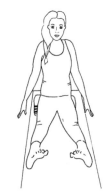

How to practise

From Upavista Konasana, bring the legs into Dandasana (see Figure 324, p.409) but have the legs apart—about hip-width. Roll the legs in so that the big toes move towards each other and the inner thighs spiral down to the floor (Figure 340). Then reverse and roll the legs out, heels moving towards each other, big toes moving away.

Figure 340

Do this rolling in and out action another 5-7 times. You can synchronise with the breath—for example, exhaling as you roll in and inhaling as you roll out—or you can simply keep the breath going smoothly. Then, hold the internal rotation position statically for 3-5 breaths.

7. Seated Cross-Legged Pose with Variations

Benefits

- The Chest Opening variation creates mobility in the upper back (thoracic spine) releasing tension there and freeing up the breath.
- The Side Bending variation limbers up the lateral body and releases tension in the spinal muscles; this movement also gently tones the waist and teaches how to move gently and subtly engaging the core.
- The Gentle Twisting variation releases tightness in the spinal muscles—lower and upper back, and gently tones the abdominal organs (kidneys, liver, spleen).
- The Womb Circling variation loosens up the hips and torso, releasing lower back and hip tightness

Props for this posture

A folded blanket to stop you slumping if you have difficulty sitting up tall.

Recommended timing

Do 5-8 repetitions of the Chest Opening variation movement. Repeat the Side Bending variation 3-5 times on each side and then hold the static stretch for up to 5 slow breaths. Do the Gentle Twisting variation 3-5 times on each side. And for the Womb Circling variation, circle 5-8 times in each direction.

How to practise

Chest Opening Variation

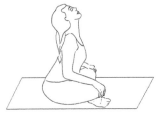 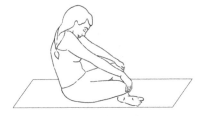

Figure 341 Inhaling   Figure 342 Exhaling

Cross your legs into an open, cross-legged position, so that when you look down there is a large triangle between the legs; the ankles are not crossed too close towards the groins but more towards the knees (see Figure 91, p.152). Sit up on a folded blanket for extra support if you find that your lower back slumps and you can't sit up tall. Place your hands on your knees and inhale as you tip forward through the pelvis rolling onto the front of your sitting bones (anterior pelvic tilt); lift your chest, roll your shoulders back, and lift your chin (see Figure 341). Then exhale as you round your upper back, pulling back against your knees, collapsing through your chest and spreading the shoulder blades, you can also suck in your belly towards the spine and tip your pelvis backwards (posterior pelvic tilt)—see Figure 342. Repeat this movement, synchronising the breath another 4-7 times.

Side Bending Variation

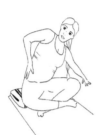

Figure 343

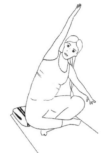

Figure 344

Change the cross-leg so the other leg is in front—just so you are working evenly through the hips as you continue on for this cross-legged series. Then, as you inhale, slide your left hand out to the side a foot or so and keep your right hand on your right hip, your right sitting bone grounded (see Figure 343). As you exhale, engage the pelvic floor and the abdominal muscles to bring your torso back up to upright with control. Repeat to the right side. And then repeat another 2-4 more rounds (to both right and left sides) in your own breath time.

Then hold statically in the side stretch—left hand out to the side, fingertips into the floor to maintain lift through the spine and reach up and over with the right arm, keeping the inner corner of the shoulder down by wrapping the shoulder blade into the back ribs (see Figure 344). Hold here for up to 5 deep breaths, sending each inhalation to expand into the side ribs (intercostal muscles) opening up into the right lung and right side of the diaphragm. Then repeat the stretch on the other side.

Gentle Twisting Variation

Working dynamically with your breath, inhale with your body in the centre, facing forward. Then, as you exhale, twist around towards your right, placing your right hand on the floor behind you and bringing your left hand onto your right knee (see Figure 345). As you inhale, come back to face forward, releasing your hands and lengthening up through the spine. As you

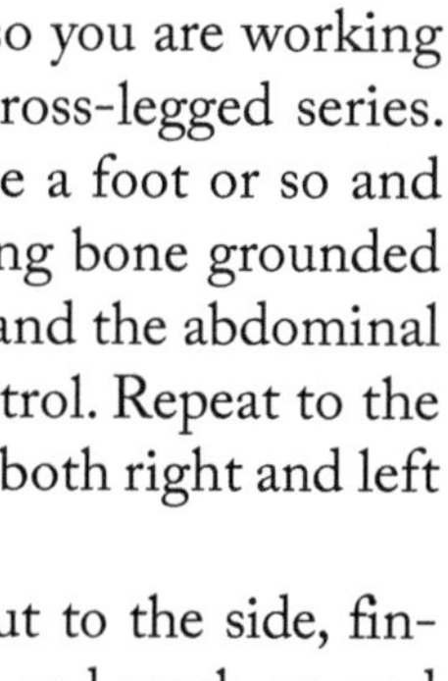

Figure 345

exhale twist around to the left and place the right hand on the left knee. Head gently following the direction of the twist and then inhale back to centre. Repeat another 2-4 rounds (twisting to the right and left), moving gently with the breath.

Womb Circling Variation

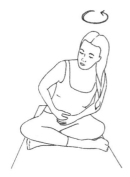

Place your hands on your lower belly, womb-space, and begin to circle the torso (see Figure 346) You can start with small circles and then spiral out to larger circles, working with some releasing, Falling-Out Breaths as you go. Circle 5-8 times in one direction then rotate the other way.

Figure 346

8. Cat-cow pose and hip circles

Benefits

- Mobilises the spine and releases tightness in the muscles of both the upper and lower back.
- Gently stretches the belly and front of the body.
- The Hip Circling variation releases aching hips and lower back, and brings energy into the lower energy centres (the Base and Sacral Chakras).

Props for this posture

Possibly a thin-fold blanket to rest your knees on if you are working on a hard floor.

Recommended timing

Repeat Cat-Cow 5-8 times and the Hip Circle variation for 3-5 times in each direction.

How to practise

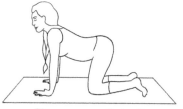

Figure 347 Inhaling

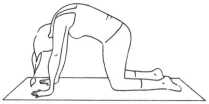

Figure 348 Exhaling

See Posture 5 in the Classical Dark Moon Menstrual Sequence on page 129, for instructions.

Hip Circling Variation

See the Posture 5 Variation from the Classical Dark Moon Menstrual Sequence on page 130, for instructions.

If you need to, take a rest into Child Pose (see Figure 283, p.297) before continuing on to the next posture, Sunbird.

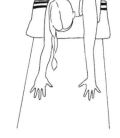

Figure 349

9. Sunbird

Note

- Do the following Postures 9-12 on the right leg. Then repeat the whole sequence on the left leg. Usually, in a feminine approach to yoga, we start unilateral movements from the left side. However, because these unilateral movements are designed to stimulate and massage the digestive tract (especially the large intestine) it is more therapeutic to start with the right leg.

Benefits

- Opens up the belly area and tones and massages the digestive organs—stimulates the digestive fire.
- Releases tightness through the back, particularly in the deep, lower back muscles.
- Strengthens and tones the hamstring and gluteal muscles, which can stabilize the pelvis and support the lower back.
- Subtly tones the abdominal muscles.

Props for this posture

Possibly a thin-fold blanket to rest your knees on if you are on a hard floor.

Recommended timing

Do about 6 repetitions on each side.

How to practise

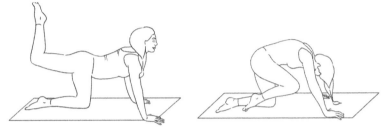

Figure 350 Inhaling   Figure 351 Exhaling

From the all-fours position, inhale as you raise the right leg behind you, in line with the hip, leg bent, toes moving towards the ceiling, chest opening forward and up, shoulders rolling back (see Figure 350). Exhale as you round the spine and bring the right knee in towards the forehead, sucking the belly in and up towards the spine (see Figure 351). Repeat another 5 times or so. Then move into the next pose on this side—Kneeling Lunge-Kneeling Hamstring Stretch.

10. Kneeling lunge-kneeling hamstring stretch

Benefits

- The Kneeling Lunge Pose stretches the groins and hip flexors, into the lower belly.
- The Kneeling Hamstring Stretch stretches the hamstrings, calf muscles and buttocks, and releases the lower back.

Props for this posture

Possibly a thin-fold blanket to cushion your knee if you're working on a hard floor.

Recommended timing

Do up to 5 repetitions of the lunge-hamstring stretch flow (Vinyasa). Then, hold the hamstring stretch for up to 5 slow breaths.

How to practise

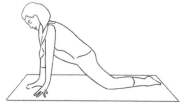

Figure 352 Inhaling

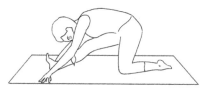

Figure 353 Exhaling

From the all-fours position step your right foot through the hands until the knee is in alignment with the ankle (the shin perpendicular to the floor). The fingertips are on the ground on either side of the front foot and the groins drop towards the floor as you lunge forward (see Figure 352). Inhale here. As you exhale, move your hips back and straighten out the front, right leg, resting on the heel as you draw the toes back towards you (see Figure 353). Relax the head and neck and position the hands closer towards your hips if you're less flexible and further away from you if you're more flexible and able to fold deeply into the stretch. Then repeat the two movements—inhale as you bend the front knee into the lunge and exhale as you move back again into the hamstring stretch—up to 4 more times, moving slowly and coordinating deep breaths with slow mindful movements.

Finally, hold the hamstring stretch for 5 deep exhalations, before moving on to the next pose Vinayasa—Calf Stretch-Gomukhasana Hip Stretch (see below).

11. Calf stretch-gomukhasana (cow-face) hip stretch

Benefits

- The Calf Stretch stretches the calf and Achilles and loosens the ankle joint.
- The Gomukhasana Hip Stretch releases the buttock/ hip (piriformis) area.

Props for this posture

Possibly a thin-fold blanket to cushion your knee if you're working on a hard floor.

Recommended timing

Do this Vinyasa (flow) of postures 3-5 times.

How to practise

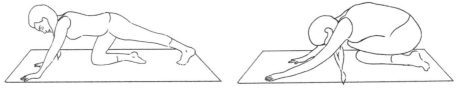

Figure 354 Inhaling   Figure 355 Exhaling

Flowing this pose from the previous Kneeling Lunge-Hamstring Stretch Vinyasa, bring the front right leg through an all-fours position until the foot is behind you, toes turned under, leg in line with the hip. Bring the hands slightly forward of the line of shoulders and push into the hands to help you deepen the calf stretch as you press the ball of the foot into the mat, lengthening the heel away from you (see Figure 354). Inhale here. Then, as you exhale, bring the right leg forward and wrap it around the left leg, letting the feet open to the sides, either side of the hips, as you sit back into Gomukhasana (Cow-Face) Hip Stretch (see Figure 355). Unravel the legs and go back into the Calf Stretch as you exhale. Continue the sequence for 2-4 more times.

12. Dynamic pigeon pose

Benefits

- Opens up the hips—stretches the outer hip area (buttocks and piriformis muscle) and also stretches the hip-flexor/groin and lower belly.
- This is another Classical Women's posture—it brings circulation to the pelvic area supporting hormonal health and balance, and is good for perimenopause and for boosting fertility.

Props for this posture

A folded blanket, cushion or gertie ball to place under the sitting bone of the front, bent-up leg.

Recommended timing

Do 4-6 repetitions of the Dynamic Pigeon.

How to practise

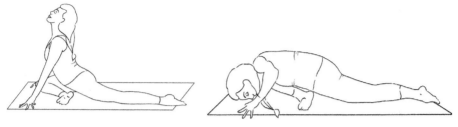

Figure 356 Inhaling   Figure 357 Exhaling

You can flow this pose straight from the Calf Stretch Position (previous pose—Posture 11), stepping the right knee forward to bring it behind the right wrist and opening out to the right side of the mat, right foot forward slightly. Extend the left leg behind you, in line with the hip, top of the foot resting on the floor.

It's a good idea to place a folded blanket or small cushion (or gertie ball) underneath the front, right sitting bone (see Figure 149, p.208). Have your hands on the floor in front of you, a little wider than shoulder-width, lifting up on your fingertips. As you inhale lift and open your chest coming into a slight backbend (in the upper back), shoulders rolling back, chin lifted, throat opening, spine curving back evenly (see Figure 356). As you exhale, fold forward, coming into Bowing Pigeon (see Figure 357), bending the elbows, and bringing the forehead on (or towards) the floor. Repeat this dynamic movement another 3-5 times.

Safety and Comfort Notes
- Take care in the upright, lifted version of this pose (Figure 356). Don't push back into the lower back so that you hinge too much from the lower vertebrae.
- It's very important that you adequately prop the front hip if you have SIJ (sacroiliac joint dysfunction); the hips must be level in this pose.
- If you can't easily rest your forehead on the floor in Bowing Pigeon (Figure 357), rest it onto a block.

13. Child pose (resting on forearms)

Benefits

A resting pose after the previous series of more dynamic movements.

Props for this posture

Nothing, just your body!

Recommended timing

Rest here for as long as you need

How to practise

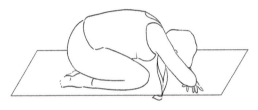

Figure 358

From the Pigeon Pose (previous pose—Posture 12) step the right foot back into all-fours and then move the buttocks back to the heels and bring the forearms in front of you—stacking one on top of the other—and rest the fore-head onto the stacked forearms into Child Pose (see Figure 358). Rest here for several breaths before rolling up to sitting and repeating the whole sequence on the other (left) leg—from Postures 9-12.

14. Vajrasana (thunderbolt kneeling pose) with variations for the arms, shoulders and neck

Props for these postures

A bolster or cushion to sit on.

Come into a kneeling position straddling your bolster (or large cushion) to perform the following arm, shoulder and neck mobilisation exercises.

Wrist Mobilisation: Flexion & Extension

Benefits

Lubricates and mobilises the wrists joints; may help alleviate carpel tunnel syndrome.

Recommended timing

Do 7-10 repetitions of the wrist flexion/extension movements.

How to practise

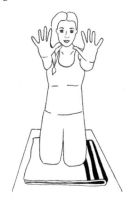
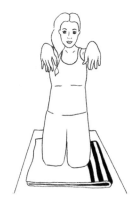

Figure 359 Inhaling   Figure 360 Exhaling

Bring your hands out in front of you at shoulder height, palms facing down. Inhale as you flex the wrists and pull you fingers back towards you, so they are pointing up towards the ceiling (see Figure 359). Exhale as you move the fingers down to point towards the floor, stretching the wrists the other way (see Figure 360). Repeat another 6-9 times, slowly and mindfully, with the breath.

Note, the breathing pattern doesn't really matter, the main thing is that you're synchronising each movement with a breath (inhalation or exhalation).

Wrist Mobilisation: Lateral Movement
Benefits

Lubricates and mobilises the wrists joints; may help alleviate carpel tunnel syndrome.

Recommended timing

Do 7-10 repetitions of the wrist flexion movements.

How to practise

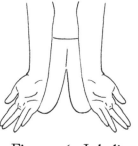
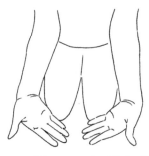

Figure 361 Inhaling   Figure 362 Exhaling

Bring your hands out in front of you, shoulder height, palms facing up. Inhale as you move your hands laterally, fingers moving away from each other (see Figure 361), exhale as you bring the fingers towards each other (see Figure 362). Repeat another 6-9 times, slowly and mindfully, with the breath.

Note, the breathing pattern doesn't really matter, the main thing is that you're synchronising each movement with a breath (inhalation or exhalation).

Wrist Mobilisation: Circles

Benefits

Lubricates and mobilises the wrists joints; may help alleviate carpel tunnel syndrome.

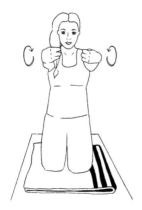

Recommended timing

Do 7-10 circles in both directions

Still with your arms out in front of you, wrap the fingers around the thumbs to make fists with your hands. Circle the wrists slowly, towards each other 7-10 times, and then away from each other for 7-10 times (see Figure 363).

Figure 363

Elbow Mobilisation

Benefits

Mobilises the elbow joint

Recommended timing

Do 6-8 repetitions of the extension/flexion movement of the elbow.

How to practise

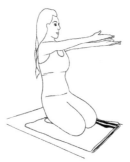

Figure 364 Inhaling

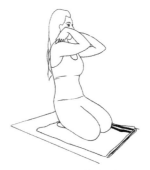

Figure 365 Exhaling

Begin with the arms out shoulder height, palms open and facing up (see Figure 364). Exhale as you slowly and mindfully bend your elbows to touch your fingertips to your shoulders (see Figure 365); inhale as you extend the elbows back to where you started (Figure 364). Repeat this movement another 5-7 times.

Shoulder Mobilisation: Elbow Open and Close

Benefits

Mobilises and lubricates the shoulder joint and scapula (shoulder blades); releases tightness in the shoulder muscles.

Recommended timing

Do 6-8 repetitions of this opening/closing movement

How to practise

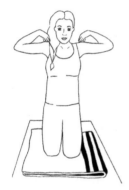
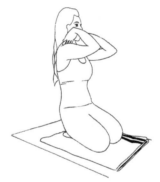

Figure 366 Inhaling   Figure 367 Exhaling

Start with your hands touching your shoulders, elbows out to the side at shoulder height (see Figure 366); inhale here. Exhale as you draw your elbows towards each other in front of you, touching them together if you can (see Figure 367).

Repeat this opening closing movement of the chest another 5-7 times, slowly and mindfully with the breath, focusing on feeling the chest expanding as you open the elbows out to the side and breathe into the top of the lungs (Figure 366). Then, exhale, moving the elbows towards each other. Feel the chest concaving as you open up the space between the shoulder blades in the upper back (back of the lungs), emptying the lungs completely (Figure 367).

Shoulder Mobilisation: Elbow Circles

Benefits

Mobilises and lubricates the shoulder joint and scapula (shoulder blades); releases tightness in the shoulder muscles.

Recommended timing

Do 6-8 circles in each direction.

How to practise

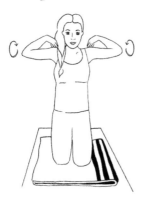

Start with your hands on your shoulders, elbows out to the sides, shoulder height. Slowly circle the elbows, circling them towards the back of the room first, and then reverse after 6-8 repetitions (see Figure 368). Make the circles big and even and take your time to really feel the shoulder joints loosening, the shoulder blades mobilising on the back ribs. Breathe evenly and deeply throughout.

Figure 368

Shoulder Mobilisation: Right-Angle Arms—up and down

Benefits

Mobilises and lubricates the shoulder joint and scapula (shoulder blades); releases tightness in the shoulder muscles.

Recommended timing

Do 4-6 repetitions of this rotational movement

How to practise

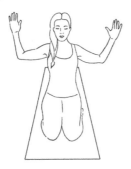

Figure 369 Inhaling

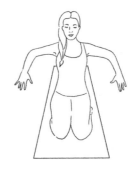

Figure 370 Exhaling

Bring the arms out to right angles, elbows in line with the shoulders palms facing forward (see Figure 369), inhale here. Exhale as you roll the shoulders forward, rotating the upper arm bones in the shoulder sockets, and bring the hands down to face behind you (see Figure 370). Repeat another 3-5 times, slowly with the breath.

Shoulder Mobilisation: Triceps Stretch Across the Body and Half Gomukhasana (Cow-Face) Shoulder Stretch

Benefits

Stretches the triceps muscle of the arm and also mobilises the shoulder joint and scapula (shoulder blade), releasing shoulder tightness and tension.

Recommended timing

Hold each stretch for 3-5 breaths.

How to practise

Triceps Stretch Across the Body

Bring the right arm across the body and hook the left elbow under the right forearm to draw the arm across the body, behind and towards the left (see Figure 371). Hold at a comfortable stretch for 3-5 slow breaths.

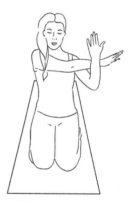

Figure 371

Half Gomukhasana (Cow-Face) Shoulder Stretch

Bring the right upper arm beside the right ear and bend the elbow so the hand reaches down between the shoulder blades. Use the left hand to draw the right elbow gently to point up towards the ceiling and a little behind the head (see Figure 372). Hold this stretch for 3-5 slow breaths.

Then release and do these two stretches with the other arm.

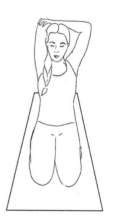

Figure 372

429

Shoulder Mobilisation: Arm Swings and 'Shoulder Wrench' Shoulder Opener

Benefits

Mobilises and lubricates the shoulder joint and scapula (shoulder blades); releases tightness in the shoulder and upper arm muscles.

Recommended timing

Do 6-8 repetitions of the arm swings; hold the Shoulder Wrench shoulder stretch for 3-5 deep breaths.

How to practise

Arm Swings

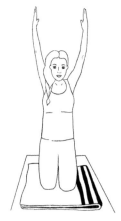
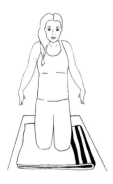

Figure 373 Inhaling   Figure 374 Exhaling

Bring your arms to the side to prepare. As you inhale, swing your arms forward, up and overhead, upper arms beside the ears (see Figure 373)—feel the spine extending and shoulders releasing tightness. As you exhale, swing the arms back down and bring them behind you, pressing the palms towards each other, rolling the shoulders back, spreading the chest, and squeezing the shoulder blades towards each other (see Figure 374). Repeat these two swinging movements a further 5-7 times, slowly and synchronised with the breath.

Shoulder Wrench Shoulder Opener

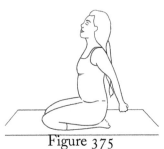

The last time you swing the arms behind you, keep them there and interlace the hands, palms squeezing together, knuckles facing the wall behind you (see Figure 375). Lift the interlaced hands as far as you can away from the body as you roll your shoulders back even further, spreading your chest and squeezing your shoulder

Figure 375

blades together. Hold this wonderful, tension relieving shoulder stretch for 3-5 slow breaths.

Safety Note

If you have a very flexible (hyper-mobile) joints, take care not to hyperextend into the elbow joints. You want to feel the stretch opening from the shoulder joints (not pushing through your hyper-flexible elbow joints).

Neck mobilisation: up and down

Benefits

- Mobilises and gently stretches the neck.
- Very calming for the nervous system.

Recommended timing

Do 6-8 repetitions of the up-down movement of the neck.

How to practise

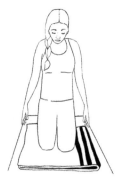
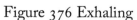
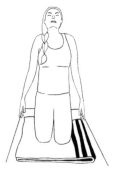

Figure 376 Exhaling   Figure 377 Inhaling

With your arms hanging by your sides, begin by having a sense of lengthening through the neck, crown of the head lifting; inhale here. As you exhale, slowly lower the chin towards the chest lengthening into the back of the neck (see Figure 376), and at the same time keep the chest lifted. As you inhale, raise your head up, chin lifting, looking up, feeling the throat stretching (see Figure 377); still see if you can maintain a sense of lift through the base of the skull here. Repeat another 5-7 times.

Note

Especially with these neck mobilisations, it's most beneficial to move really slowly and mindfully as you synchronise your movements with the breath. These simple, slow, mindful movements have a profoundly calming effect on your nervous system.

Neck Mobilisation: Side to Side

Benefits

- Mobilises and gently stretches the neck.
- Very calming for the nervous system.

Recommended timing

Do 6-8 repetitions of this side to side movement of the neck.

How to practise

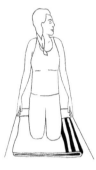 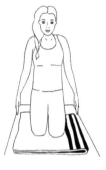 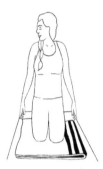

Figure 378 Exhaling   Figure 379 Inhaling   Figure 380 Exhaling

With your arms hanging to your side, begin by having a sense of lengthening through the neck, crown of the head lifting; inhale here. As you exhale, slowly turn your head to look over your left shoulder, at the same time keep the right shoulder rolling back (see Figure 378). Inhale and bring your head back to centre, lengthening up through the crown of the head (see Figure 379). As you exhale, turn your head to look over your right shoulder, keeping left shoulder rolling back (see Figure 380).

Continue another 5-7 repetitions of these side-to-side movements of the head.

Note

Especially with these neck mobilisations, it's most beneficial to move really slowly and mindfully as you synchronise your movements with the breath—these simple, slow, mindful movements have a profoundly calming effect on your nervous system.

Neck Mobilisation: Ear to Shoulder Trap Stretch

Benefits

- Stretches the trapezius muscle that runs along the side of the neck into top of the shoulder.
- Releases tension, very calming.

Recommended timing

Hold the stretch for approximately 5 breaths as you circle the hand about 3 times in each direction.

How to practise

Drop your right ear towards your right shoulder as you extend the left arm down, reaching the fingertips towards the floor. Bring your right arm up and wrap the hand and forearm over the head, right fingertips on left ear—bringing a little bit of gentle weight to deepen the stretch. Look down towards your right armpit. As you breathe deeply, consciously releasing the muscles along the left side of the neck and along the top of the shoulder, circle the left fingertips, as if you were tracing small circles on the floor, and keep

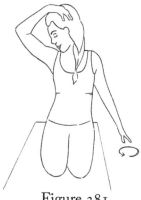

Figure 381

the left shoulder drawing down (see Figure 381). Do about 3 circles in each direction. Then slowly release the top hand and raise your head to the centre before repeating on the other side.

15. Womb-space mudra

To finish the Pawanmuktasana sequence, place your right palm and then your left palm on top, onto your lower belly—womb-space (see Figure 382). Take some time to sit quietly here breathing into your soft belly, your womb-space, and just notice how you feel at the end of this sequence. Hopefully you will feel more grounded and centred, as well as more open and joyful in your body, having moved *prana* (energy) throughout your entire body.

Namaste.

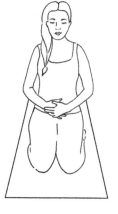

Figure 382

CONCLUSION
RECLAIMING YOUR FEMININE SOULSKIN

When a woman appreciates and honors her body
cycles she can awaken to a new level of the healing
power of her female nature. Female energy is creative
and spreading. What a woman heals within herself
permeates her life and affects others around her.

—KAMI McBRIDE[560]

One of the most gratifying aspects of my work with women is watching the 'light bulb' go off in their minds and hearts—a recognition of something untapped within them that opens up a more joyful, easeful and natural way of practising yoga, and ultimately of living their lives.

Recently, I taught my Full Moon Feminine Flow sequence to a group of women as part of a Women's Yoga teacher-training course. To a tapestry of feminine-tunes, we moved, flowed, sweated, groaned, sighed and softened into a yielding, more self-loving yoga practice. When we were done, an Asian woman whose cultural background is decidedly one of 'push' and 'strive', came up to me and declared excitedly, 'This is how I *always* want to practise yoga from now on!'

It reminds me of a richly-layered archetype-tale in Clarissa Pinkola Estes' *Women who Run with the Wolves*, about a woman who realises that somewhere along the way she has lost her 'soulskin' and must find her way back 'home'. Pinkola Estes employs this parable as a way of understanding the journey we must go on when we hit exhaustion-point, and life has drained our very 'soul', as she explains here:

When a woman is too long gone from home, she is less and less able to propel herself forward in life. Instead of pulling in the

---

560 Kami McBride, *105 Ways to Celebrate Menstruation*, p.15

harness of her choice, she's dangling from one. She's so cross-eyed with tiredness she trudges right on past the place of help and comfort. The dead litter is ideas, chores, demands that don't work, have no life, and brings no life to her. Such a woman becomes pale yet contentious, more and more uncompromising, yet scattered. Her fuse burns shorter and shorter. Pop culture calls it "burnout"— but it's more than that, it's *hambre del alma*, the starving soul. Then, there is only one recourse, finally the woman knows she has to— not might, maybe, sort of, but *must*—return to home.[561]

When you find your home, when you return to your self, your essential, *feminine* self, the elated certainty of it is intoxicating. 'When we breathe up that soul-state, we automatically enter the feeling state of "This is right. I know what I need",' affirms Pinkola Estes.[562]

It nourishes me so to see women switch-on to a whole new approach to their bodies, emotions and spirits. I am also gratified by the realisation that the more I focus on my own self-care, the more I inspire the women around me to do the same for themselves.

The impetus behind *Moving with the Moon* is therefore a personal journey that can be translated into the universal context. I propose a universal feminine paradigm that we can co-create, that supports us all in reclaiming our 'soulskins' and enjoying a juicy, fulfilling, creative life, no matter what point we have reached in the continuum of feminine experience.

My parting wish for you is to joyfully embrace your place in the trajectory of your uniquely feminine life in a way that celebrates its many gifts, as a way of making peace with yourself, and freeing up your gifts to share with others.

Namaste!

(The divinity in me salutes and honours the divinity within you).

---

561   Clarissa Pinkola Estes, *Women who Run with the Wolves: contacting the power of the wild woman*, p.280

562   Ibid., p.279

Appendix 1
UNDERSTANDING THE AYURVEDIC DOSHAS

According to Ayurveda, the ancient sister-science to yoga, everything in the universe consists of an amalgam of the five elements: air, ether, water, fire and earth. This means that all people, as individuals, exhibit their own unique synthesis of these elements; this, in turn, dictates their constitution or *dosha*.

There are three *doshas*, and each of us tends to consist of a combination of all three. Usually, one or two of these *doshas* predominates in how we present physically and in our personalities.

Vata Dosha

This *dosha* is governed by the elements of air and ether and, when it is in balance, a person manifests a lightness, quickness and creativity; when it is out of balance, she usually feel anxious and 'ungrounded'.

Remedies for balancing *vata*:
- Reduce your overall level of activity.
- Practise grounding, calming yoga: floor based postures (eg: the Classical Women's Seated Postures—Appendix 2), the Women's Pawanmuktasana sequence (from chapter nine), Restorative postures (see Appendix 3), and the Apana Breath (see p.102).
- Meditate to induce internal calmness.
- Maintain regular routines—take regular meal breaks and sleep regular hours.
- Do regular self-massage with warm black sesame oil. Dr Robert Svoboda says, 'Keeping your skin well oiled is one of the most reliable ways to keep vata under control.'[563] See page 386 for instructions on Ayurvedic Oil Self Massage.
- Eat warming, nourishing foods such as soups, stews, dhal; avoid raw, uncooked foods, particularly in colder weather.

---

563   Dr Robert E. Svoboda, *Ayurveda for Women: A Guide to Vitality and Health*, p.140

Pitta Dosha

The *pitta dosha* is governed by the elements of fire and water. When this *dosha* is balanced, a person is focused, pioneering, confident, and dynamic; when it is out of balance she may often feel angry or irritated and she can come across as overly strong and forceful—'fiery'.

Remedies for balancing *pitta*:

- Practise cooling yoga postures, such as the Cooling Restorative Yoga postures (see Appendix 3) and the Supported Inversions (see Appendix 3). Sitali Pranayama (see p.264) and relaxation practices like Yoga Nidra are also beneficial (see various Yoga Nidra practices on pages 116, 214, and 268).
- Eliminate stimulants (coffee and tea), alcohol and spicy foods. Eating a lot of red meat is also too 'heating'.
- Do the Ayurvedic self-massage with coconut oil (see p.386), especially on the head.
- Indulge in devotional practices such as chanting, singing, and prayer.
- Spend time in nature—especially cooling environments like the beach.

Kapha Dosha

The *kapha dosha* is governed by the elements of earth and water. When this *dosha* is in balance a person appears content, calm and grounded; when it is out of balance she can be sluggish, overly slow, and lacking in motivation.

Remedies for balancing *kapha*

- Increase/introduce stimulating activities—dynamic physical exercise.
- Practise dynamic yoga such as: Salutes to the Sun (see the Full Moon Salute on p.225 and the Waning Moon Salute on p.278). Dynamic Standing poses (eg: Warrior I—see p.90 and Warrior II—see p.90), unsupported Inversions, and Kapalabhati Pranayama (see p.268) are also beneficial.
- Avoid over-eating or over-sleeping; get up early and begin your day with an exercise or yoga regime.
- Enjoy a light diet with ample fruit and fresh foods, and minimise dairy.

For more information on Ayurveda and supporting your health and wellbeing as a woman, I recommend these books:

- *Ayurveda for Women: A Guide to Vitality and Health* by Dr Robert E. Svoboda*
- *A Woman's Power to Heal Through Inner Medicine* by Maya Tiwari*

*See Bibliography for full publication details

Appendix 2
THE CLASSICAL WOMEN'S POSTURES

These postures are universally beneficial for women of all ages and stages because they boost circulation in the pelvic, abdominal and hip areas, promoting reproductive health and hormonal balance.

BENEFITS OF THE CLASSICAL WOMEN'S POSTURES[564]

Seated postures and floor-based postures

Baddha Konasana (Bound Angle Pose)

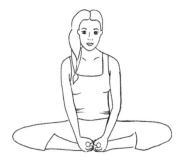

Figure 383

- Tones the abdominal and pelvic organs.
- Alleviates sciatica and varicose veins.
- Reduces menstrual pain, irregular periods, and leucorrhoea (vaginal discharge).
- Keeps the ovaries healthy.
- Helps to open blocked fallopian tubes.

---

564   Sources for these listed benefits include: BKS Iyengar, *Yoga the Path to Holistic Health;* Judith Lastater, Ph.D., *Relax and Renew: Restful Yoga for Stressful Times;* Bobby Clennell, *The Women's Yoga Book;* Linda Sparrowe and Patricia Walden, *The Women's Book of Yoga and Health*

- Can reduce vaginal irritation, relieving cystitis and pelvic inflammation.
- Promotes *apana* (downward moving energy beneficial for women's health).
- Mobilises the hip joints, releasing inner thighs and groins—beneficial for menopause. Bobby Clennell says, 'stiffness in the hip joints can cause abdominal tension which, in turn, can compress the pelvic organs.'[565]
- Tones the kidneys and 'exercises'[566] the abdominal organs.
- Tones the pelvic floor.
- Regulates and balances the menstrual cycle.[567]

Upavista Konasana (Wide-Angle Seated Pose)

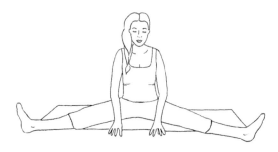

Figure 384

- Massages the reproductive organs.
- Relaxes and gently stretches the pelvic floor.
- Helps lift and tone the uterus.
- Stimulates the ovaries, regulates menstrual flow, and relieves menstrual disorders.
- Can unblock fallopian tubes and reduce pelvic inflammation.
- May reduce ovarian cysts.
- Can correct a prolapsed uterus or bladder.
- Relieves menstrual cramps—relaxes the abdominal and pelvic area and can relieve congestion in the uterus.

---

565 Bobby Clennell, *The Women's Yoga Book*, p.64

566 Ibid

567 Clennell says, 'Patient and focused practice of Baddha Konasana stabilizes menstrual cycles marked by either heavy bleeding or a scanty flow or where there is bleeding between periods,' Ibid

Malasana (Squat Pose)

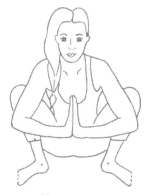

Figure 385

- Energises *shakti prana* (sacred, healing feminine energy) and draws *apana vayu (*downward moving, feminine energy*)* into rhythmic harmony.[568]
- Keeps the hip joints mobile and healthy—beneficial for menopause.
- Stretches and tones the pelvic floor.
- Supports healthy elimination.

Pigeon Pose

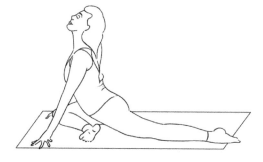

Figure 386

- Opens the hips, specifically the buttock/piriformis muscles; stretches the psoas muscle (particularly the upright version).
- The upright version opens the heart and deep-belly areas.
- Brings circulation to the pelvic area—blood circulation and *shakti* energy—boosting your reproductive health and feminine vitality; said to be beneficial for fertility.

---

568   Maya Tiwari, *A Women's Power to Heal*, p.254

Supine and restorative postures

Supta Padangusthasana II (Reclining Big Toe Pose)

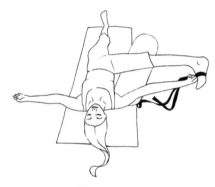

Figure 387

- Helps to relieve menstrual discomfort such as cramps, heavy bleeding or pain during menstruation.
- Keeps the reproductive organs healthy—beneficial for the prevention of uterine fibroids.
- Keeps the hips flexible—beneficial for menopause.
- May relieve hot flushes and prevent osteoporosis.

Supta Baddha Konasana (Reclining Bound Angle Pose)

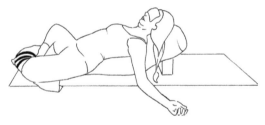

Figure 388

- Softens the abdominal area, boosting reproductive and digestive health, and takes the pressure off the pelvic area, easing pelvic congestion.
- Improves blood circulation in the ovarian region and is particularly beneficial during puberty and menopause.
- Beneficial for menstrual cramps and has a 'drying effect'[569], helping to reduce heavy menstruation.

569   Clennell, *The Women's Yoga Book*, p101

- Improves breathing.
- Revitalising and uplifting, and eases anxiety.
- Promotes *apana*—'helps the menstrual flow move down and out'.[570]
- Can help cystitis that can occur around menstruation as it relaxes the bladder.

Supported Upavista Konasana (Wide-Legged Forward Bend)

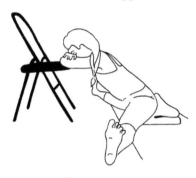

Figure 389

- See benefits listed for seated (unsupported) Upavista Konasana above.
- The Supported Forward Bending version calms the nervous system and can calm agitation and irritability.

Standing postures

Prasarita Padottanasana (Wide-Legged Standing Forward Bend)

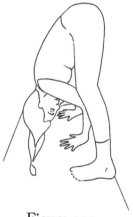

Figure 390

---

570   Lasater, *Relax and Renew*, p164

- Regulates menstrual flow and can also balance the cycle.[571]
- Soothes the brain and the sympathetic nervous system.
- Relieves stress-related headaches, migraine and fatigue.
- Tones the abdominal organs.
- Relieves lower backache.

Supported Prasarita Padottanasana
(Wide-Legged Standing Forward Bend)

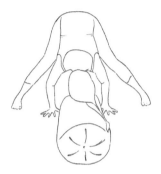

Figure 391

- See benefits listed above for (unsupported) Prasarita Padottanasana.
- The supported Forward Bending version (using a bolster—as pictured—or chair) calms the nervous system and can calm agitation and irritability; it also relaxes and softens the abdominal area, which is beneficial for digestive and reproductive health.

Trikonasana (Triangle Pose)

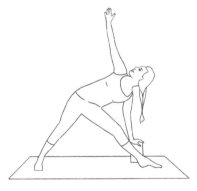

Figure 392

571 Clennell says, 'menstrual problems such as irregular periods, very light or very heavy periods, or spotting between periods, are corrected' by this posture—p.55, *The Women's Yoga Book*

446

- Can relieve backache and menstrual cramps.
- Supports the digestion and elimination.
- Can help with menstrual disorders.
- Relieves anxiety and nervous tension.

Ardha Chandrasana (Half Moon Pose)

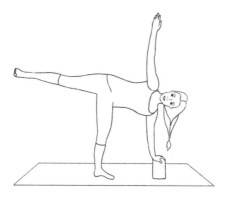

Figure 393

- Boosts circulation to the abdominal organs.
- Creates mobility in the hip joints—beneficial for menopause.
- Can correct a prolapsed uterus.
- Opens the chest—energising and uplifting.

Goddess Pose (Utkata Konasana)

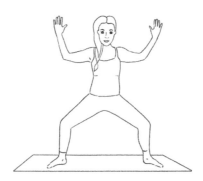

Figure 394

- Grounding and energising.
- Builds stamina and strengthens and tones the core muscles.
- Opens the hips and promotes circulation to the pelvic organs.

APPENDIX 3
RESTORATIVE POSTURES FOR WOMEN'S HEALTH

Heart-Opening Restorative Postures

These postures open the chest, refreshing the heart and lungs, facilitating deeper breathing.

The heart-opening effects of these postures help relieve tightness in the upper back, shoulder and neck areas. They also soften and open the belly, which boosts circulation to the digestive and reproductive organs, making them ideal postures for women's health.

The Heart-Opening Restorative postures are simultaneously relaxing and gently rejuvenating, boosting your physical energy and uplifting your mood.

- Supta Baddha Konasana (Reclining Bound-Angle Pose)

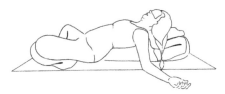

Figure 395

- Reclining Cross-leg Pose

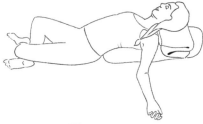

Figure 396

- Supta Virasana (Reclining Hero Pose)

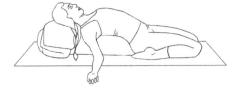

Figure 397

- Reclining Goddess

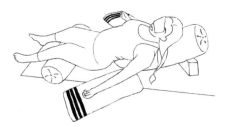

Figure 398

- Supported Bridge Pose
  - Supported Bridge pose with a bolster

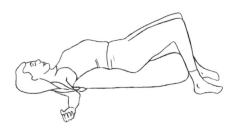

Figure 399

  - Supported Bridge pose with a block

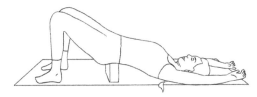

Figure 400

Cooling Restorative Postures

The Cooling Restorative postures cool the mind and body making them excellent postures to counteract premenstrual and menopausal agitation and irritation.

They have a calming effect on the mind and nervous system, and gently stretch the lower back, and can tone and support the kidney and adrenal function. These postures are also helpful in relieving fatigue and exhaustion.

- Supported Child Pose

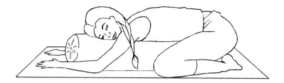

Figure 401

- Paschimottanasana (Seated Forward Bend)
  - Paschimottanasna with a bolster

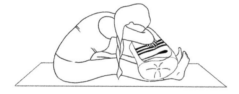

Figure 402

  - Paschimottanasana with a chair

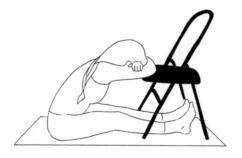

Figure 403

- Supported Prasarita Padottanasana (Standing Wide-Leg Forward Bend)

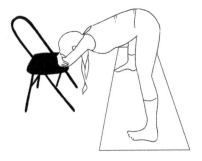

Figure 404

- Supported Uttanasana (Standing Forward Fold)

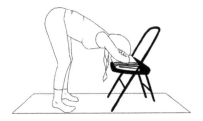

Figure 405

- Supported Cross-leg Forward Bend
  - Cross-leg Forward bend with a block

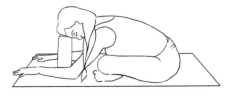

Figure 406

  - Cross-leg Forward bend with a chair

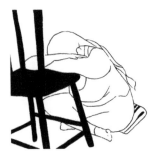

Figure 407

- Supported Janu Sirsasana (Head-to-Knee Forward Bend)

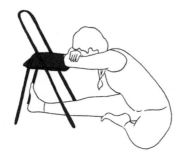

Figure 408

- Supported Dog Pose with block/bolster

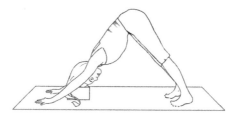

Figure 409

Supported Inversions

These postures help to balance and nourish the nervous and hormonal systems. They also boost the circulation and lymphatic flow supporting overall health and vitality.

The Supported Inversions simultaneously calm and energise you, and are particularly beneficial for counteracting fatigue, and relieving tiredness and heaviness in the legs.

- Viparita Karani (Legs up the Wall Pose)

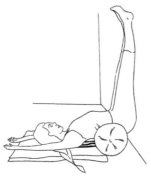

Figure 410

- Shoulderstand Variations
  - o Shoulderstand with a chair

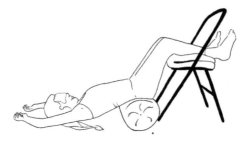

Figure 411

  - o Shoulderstand with a bolster

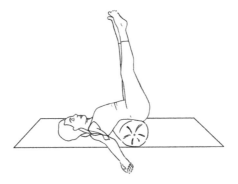

Figure 412

  - o Shoulderstand with a block

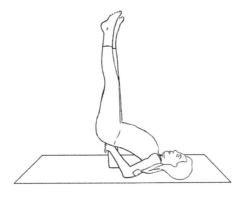

Figure 413

- Chair Savasana

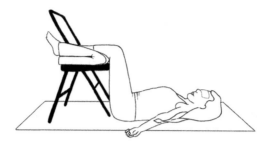

Figure 414

Detoxing Restorative Postures

These postures help detox the body by boosting circulation to the liver and kidneys, which is beneficial for supporting optimal hormonal balance.

- Ardha Jatara (Supine Twist) on a bolster

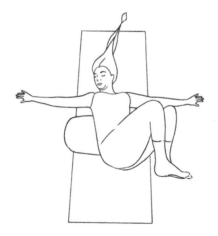

Figure 415

- Twisting Child Pose

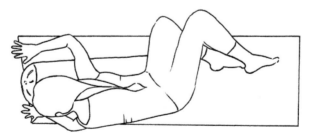

Figure 416

Relaxation Restorative Postures

These postures offer supported versions of the Savasana (Corpse Pose) relaxation pose that is typically practised at the end of a sequence. They help relax, balance and harmonise the body-mind.

- Simple Savasana

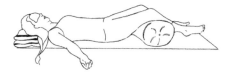

Figure 417

- Constructive Rest Position (CRP)

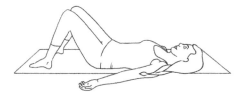

Figure 418

Note, this posture would be more typically used as a relaxing and centring posture at the beginning of your practice.

- Double Bolster Prone Child Pose

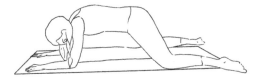

Figure 419

- Prone Savasana on Transverse Bolster

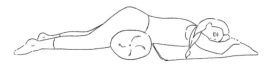

Figure 420

- Reclining Goddess Pose

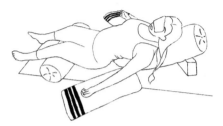

Figure 421

- Chair Savasana

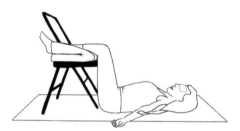

Figure 422

- Double Bolster Supine Savasana

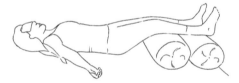

Figure 423

- Savasana with a bolster and wrapped blanket

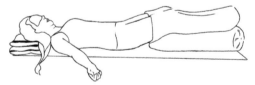

Figure 424

MOVING WITH THE MOON PLAYLIST SUGGESTIONS

DARK MOON PHASE

Music to support a meditative, Restorative practice

'Khumjung', 'Horizon of Gold' and 'Mother's Wingspan' by Ben Leinbach

'Zion Lullaby' and 'The Jasmani Garden' by Deya Dova

'Samba Sadashiva' by Donna De Lory

'Home' by Drala

'Devi Prayer' by Ananda

'Meditation of the Night' by Benjy Wertheimer

'Dream' by Peruquois

'Shehnai Song' and 'Kafi Noir' by Sheila Chandra

WAXING MOON PHASE

Feminine Pulse: music to support a dynamic practice

'Awaken the Snake' and 'I am She' by Peruquois

'Mystical Trance' and 'Shamanic Dream' by Anugama

'Isha' by Deya Dova

Music for balance and to support a Restorative 'Busy Days' Practice

'Alpha Relaxation System 1 and 2' by Jeffrey Thompson

'Farewell to Music' by Donna de Lory

Plus, choose from any of the tracks from the Dark Moon music selection above.

FULL MOON PHASE

Music to support a Feminine Flow practice

'Kafir Noir' by Sheila Chandra (centring at the start of practice)

'Bloom' by Deya Dova (warm-up/main body of practice)

'Samba Sadashiva' by Donna De Lory (warm-up/cool-down)

'I am She' by Peruquis (warm-up/main body of practice)

'Om Mantra: The Cosmic Yes' by Deva Premal and Mitan
        (main body of practice—Salutes)

'Café Mantra Theme—Song for Shiva' by Jo Kelly
            (main body of practice—Salutes)
'Mystical Trance' by Anugama (main body of practice—Salutes)
'I Bow to You' (main body of practice—Salutes)
'The Divine' and 'Fly so High' by Mel Dobra
            (main body or practice/cool-down)
'Ray Man Shabad' by Snatam Kaur (main body of practice—Salutes)
'Devaki' by Karnamrita (warm-up/main body of practice)
'Crystal Cave' (warm-up/cool-down)
'Zion Lullaby' (cool-down)
'Blood of the Earth' (warm-up/cool-down)

WANING MOON PHASE

Music to support Lunar Salutes and a reflective/cathartic practice

'Awaken the Snake' and 'Pool of Love' by Peruquois (Lunar Salutes)
'I Bow to You' by Mel Dobra (Lunar Salutes)
'Shamanic Dream' by Anugama (Lunar Salutes)
'Mia Chi Chi' by Peruquois (cool-down)
'Devaki' by Karnamrita (warm-up/cool-down)
'Moola Mantra—Invocation' by Deva Premal (warm-up/cool-down)
'Reunite' (warm-up/cool-down)

Music to calm the nervous system for a Restorative practice

'Alpha Relaxation System 1 and 2' by Jeffrey Thompson
'Om' by Peruquois
Plus, choose from any of the tracks from the Dark Moon music selection above.

ACKNOWLEDGEMENTS

This book has evolved into a much larger undertaking than I could ever have imagined. It has been at least five years in the making—a long, slow labour of love, and I could never have done it without the support of many.

I am indebted to the book's 'co-parent' Sophie Duncan who is responsible for the beautiful illustrations. Sophie has offered her unfailing support over the years that this project has unfolded, cheerfully meeting deadlines and putting so much love into her work.

I am so very grateful to my editors, Mark Gauntlett, Kirsten McGavin and Amanda Greenslade. To Mark I am especially indebted, not only for his patient grammatical lessons but also for his good-natured willingness to plough through my 140,000 words all about menstruation and uteruses—a true feminist man!

I am also grateful for the support of Amanda Greenslade from Australian eBook Publisher. Amanda's patient fielding of my endless questions about the publishing process, as well as her flexibility in accommodating my expanding, high-maintenance 'tome', has not gone unappreciated.

I am deeply grateful for the ongoing support of my friend and mentor Eve Grzybowski, who always believed in me and this crazy, ambitious project. I am so pleased that Eve has graced this book with her foreword. She is a constant inspiration to me as to how live and practise yoga joyfully into one's 'maga' and 'crone' years.

To my mother, I owe my gratitude for instilling in me a love of words, ideas and writing. And, in fact, my gratitude extends to my whole family— Miranda and Ray, George and Prukchika—for putting up with me carrying this project on my shoulders for so many years.

To my assistant and 'main-woman', Robyn Bell, I am beyond grateful. It is through her able management of Bliss Baby Yoga that I have been able to carve out the time to write and polish this book, knowing that my business was in her safe hands.

My appreciation also extends to all my students over the years who have taught me so much in their willingness to be vulnerable and to explore together this wonderful practice we call 'yoga'. Thank you all for so patiently waiting for me to birth my book, encouraging me on the way.

I am thankful to my husband, Peter, who has stuck by me in a new marriage while I laboured to finish this unwieldy project; his unconditional love and support—not to mention his IT expertise—means so much to me and frees me to write, and write, and write!

To my son Marley, I offer special thanks for tolerating his mother being so distracted for so many years and whose very existence has inspired the birth of my passion (and business!) around yoga for pregnancy, birth, motherhood, and now more broadly, for women's ages and stages. Marley, you are my greatest guru!

Lastly, I thank yoga. My yoga practice is like food and water to me; without yoga I feel I would be nothing. It is this wonderful art and science of yoga that inspires me to try to be a better person, every day.

Namaste!

ABOUT THE AUTHOR

Ana Davis (E-RYT 500, RPYT, Yoga Australia Registered Level 3 Senior teacher, qualified Doula, DRM, B.A. Honours) has been teaching yoga and training teachers since 1996.

With an Honours Degree in Japanese Feminism, Ana has long been passionate about working with women's experience and exploring the benefits of yoga and meditation for women's monthly and life cycles.

Ana is founder and director of Bliss Baby Yoga, which specialises in prenatal and postnatal, fertility yoga, women's yoga (menstruation and menopause), and restorative yoga. Visit the Bliss Baby Yoga website for more information on her specialised courses, workshops and online classes: www.blissbabyyoga.com

Ana lives in Byron Bay, Australia with her husband and teenage son.

BIBLIOGRAPHY

Armstrong, Alison A., *The Queen's Code*, Sherman Oaks: Pax Programs Incorporated, 2013

Bennett, Bija, *Emotional Yoga: How the Body can Heal the Mind*, New York: Simon & Schuster, 2002

Bobel, Chris, *New Blood: Third-Wave Feminism and the Politics of Menstruation*, New Brunswick: Rutgers University Press, 2010

Borysenko, Joan, *A Woman's Book of Life: The Biology, Psychology, and Spirituality of the Feminine Life Cycle*, New York: Riverhead Books, 1996

Briden, Lara, *Period Repair Manual: Every Woman's Guide to Better Periods*, (Kindle edition), Macmillan, 2018

Brizendine, Louann, *The Female Brain*, New York: Harmony Books, 2006

Buckley, Thomas and Gottlieb, Alma, *Blood Magic: The Anthropology of Menstruation*, California: University of California Press, 1988

Chia, Mantak and Wei, William U., *Chi Kung for Women's Health and Sexual Vitality: A Handbook of Simple Exercises and Techniques*, (Kindle edition), Rochester: Destiny Books

Chia, Mantak, *Healing Love through the Tao: Cultivating Female Sexual Energy*, (Kindle edition), Rochester: Destiny Books

Clennell, Bobby, *The Women's Yoga Book: Asana and Pranayama for all Phases of the Menstrual Cycle*, Berkeley, California: Rodmell Press, 2007

Davis, Elizabeth and Leonard, Carol, *The Women's Wheel of Life*, (Kindle, fourth edition) USA: Bad Beaver Publishing, 2012

Delaney, Janice, Lupton, Mary Jane and Toth, Emily, *The Curse: A Cultural History of Menstruation*, Chicago: University of Illinois Press, 1988

Dinsmore-Tuli, Uma, *Yoni Shakti: A Woman's Guide to Power and Freedom Through Yoga and Tantra*, London: YogaWords, 2016

Devi, Nischala Joy, *The Secret Power of Yoga: A Woman's Guide to the Heart and Spirit of the Yoga Sutras*, New York: Three Rivers Press, 2007

Diamant, Anita, *The Red Tent*, (Australian edition), St Leonards: Allen & Unwin, 1998

Elias, Jason and Ketcham, Katherine, *In the House of the Moon: Reclaiming the Feminine Spirit Healing*, New York: Warner Books, 2009

Farhi, Donna, *The Breathing Book*, New York: Henry Holt and Company, 1996

Farhi, Donna, *Yoga for Women Therapeutic Practice Sequences* (e-book), 2009

Frawley, David, *Yoga and Ayurveda: Self-Healing and Self-Realization*, Wisconsin: Lotus Press, 1999

Gottfried, Sara, *The Hormone Cure: Reclaim Balance, Sleep and Sex drive; Lose Weight; Feel Focused, and Energised Naturally with the Gottfried Protocol*, New York: Scribner, 2013

Gray, Miranda, *Red Moon: Understanding and Using the Creative, Sexual and Spiritual Gifts of the Menstrual cycle*, (revised edition), Dancing Eve, 2009

Gray, Miranda, *The Optimized Woman: Using your menstrual cycle to achieve success and fulfilment*, Park Lane: O Books, 2009

Groover, Rachael Jayne, *Powerful and Feminine: How to Increase your Magnetic Presence & Attract the Attention You Want*, Colorado: Deep Pacific Press, 2011

Gurupremananda Saraswati, Swami, *Mother as First Guru*, Numbugga: Swami Gurupremananda Saraswati, 2002

Hirschi, Gertrud, *Mudras: Yoga in your Hands*, Boston: Weiser Books, 2000

Huffington, Arianna, *Thrive: The Third Metric to Redefining Success and Creating a Happier Life*, London: WH Allen, 2014

Iyengar, B.K.S., *Yoga, The Path to Holistic Health*, New York: Dorling Kindersley, 2001

Iyengar, Geeta S., *Yoga, A Gem for Women*, Canada/England: Timeless Books, 1990

Kent, Tami Lynn, *Wild Feminine: Finding Power, Spirit & Joy in the Female Body*, Oregon: Atria Paperback & Beyond Words, 2011

Kittson, Jean, *You're Still Hot to Me: The Joys of Menopause*, Pan MacMillan, e-book (Kindle) version

Koch, Liz, *The Psoas Book* (Updated and Expanded Edition), Felton: Guinea Pig Publications, 1997

Kraftsow, Gary, *Yoga for Wellness: Healing with Timeless Teachings of Viniyoga*, New York: Penguin Putnam Inc., 1999

Lasater, Judith, *Relax and Renew: Restful Yoga for Stressful Times*, (First Edition), Berkely: Rodmell Press, 1995

Manitsas, Katie, *The Yoga of Birth*, Katie Manitsas, 2010

Maurine, Camille and Roche, Lorin, *Meditation Secrets for Women: Discovering your passion, pleasure, and inner peace,* New York: Harper One, 2001

McBride, Kami, *105 Ways to Celebrate Menstruation*, Vacaville: Living Awareness Publications, 2004

McCall, Timothy, *Yoga as Medicine: The Yogic Prescription for Health and Healing,* New York: Bantam Books, 2007

Miller, Richard *Yoga Nidra: The Meditative Heart of Yoga*, Boulder: Sounds True, Inc., 2010

Muktananda, Swami, *Nawa Yogini Tantra: Yoga for Women*, (reprint of revised edition from 1983), Bihar: Yoga Publications Trust, 1998

Naish, Francesca, *Natural Fertility: The Complete Guide to Avoiding or Achieving Conception*, (revised edition), Bowral: Sally Milner Publishing, 1999

Northrup, Christiane, *Women's Bodies, Women's Wisdom: Creating Physical and Emotional Health and Healing*, New York: Bantam Books, 2006

Northrup, Christiane, *The Wisdom of Menopause: Creating Physical and Emotional Health During the Change*, (E-book edition— newly revised and updated), Christiane Northrup, Inc. www.DrNorthrup.com, 2012

Ohlig, Adelheid, *Luna Yoga: Vital Fertility and Sexuality*, Woodstock: Ash Tree Publishing, 1994

Owen, Lara, *Her Blood is Gold: Awakening to the Wisdom of Menstruation,* Dorset: Archive Publishing, 2008

Pearce, Lucy H., *Moon Time: A Guide to Celebrating your Menstrual Cycle,* CreateSpace, 2012

Pinkola Estes, Clarissa, *Women who Run with the Wolves: Contacting the Power of the Wild Woman,* London: Random House, 1993

Pope, Alexandra, *The Wild Genie: The Healing Power of Menstruation,* Bowral: Sally Milner Publishing, 2001

Prakasha, Padma and Anaiya Aon, *Womb Wisdom: Awakening the Creative and Forgotten Powers of the Feminine,* Toronto: Destiny Books, 2011

Pullig Schatz, Mary, *Back Care Basics: A Doctor's Gentle Yoga Program for Back and Neck Pain Relief,* Berkley: Rodmell Press, 1992

Raman, Krishna, *A Matter of Health: Integration of Yoga and Western Medicine for Prevention & Cure*, (Kindle edition), Chennai, India: Helios Books, 1998

Raman, Krishna and Suresh, S., *Yoga and Medical Science FAQ,* (Kindle edition), Chennai: Helios Books, 2003

Rea, Shiva, *Tending the Heart Fire: Living in the Flow with the Pulse of Life,* Boulder: Sounds True Inc, 2014

Reichard, Joy F., *Celebrate the Divine Feminine: Reclaim your power with Ancient Goddess Wisdom,* USA: Joy F. Richard, M.A., C.C.H.T., 2011

Robin, Mel, *A Physiological Handbook for Teachers of Yogasana,* Arizona: Fenestra Books, 2002

Roche, Lorin, *The Radiance Sutras: 112 Gateways to the Yoga of Wonder and Delight,* Boulder, Colorado: Sounds True, 2014

Rodrigues, Dinah, *Hormone Yoga Therapy: To Reactivate Your Hormone Production and Eliminate Symptoms of Menopause, TPM, Polycystic Ovaries, Infertility,* Sao Paulo: Dina Rodrigues, 2009

Roth, Gabrielle, *Sweat Your Prayers: Movement as a Spiritual Practice,* Tarcher, 1997

Sarris, Jerome and Wardle, Jon, *Clinical Naturopathy: an Evidence-Based Guide to Practice,* Chatswood: Elsevier, 2010

Satyananda Saraswati, Swami, *Yoga Nidra,* Bihar: Yoga Publications Trust, 1998

Shuttle, Penelope and Redgrove, Peter, *The Wise Wound: Menstruation and Everywoman,* London: Marion Boyars Publishers Ltd, 1999

Singer, Katie, *Honoring our Cycles: A Natural Family Planning Workbook,* Winona Lake: New Trends Publishing, Inc., 2006

Singer, Katie, *The Garden of Fertility,* New York: Avery, 2004

Sparrowe, Linda with Yoga Sequences by Walden, Patricia, *The Women's Book of Yoga and Health: A Lifelong Guide to Wellness,* Boston: Shambhala Publications, 2002.

Sparrowe, Linda, with Yoga Sequences by Walden, Patricia, *Yoga for a Healthy Menstrual Cycle,* Massachusetts: Shambhala Publications, Inc., 2004

Stein, Elissa, and Kim, Susan, *Flow: The Cultural History of Menstruation,* New York: St. Martins Press, 2009

Svoboda, Robert E, *Ayurveda for Women: A Guide to Vitality and Health,* Vermont: Healing Arts Press, 2000

Tiwari, Maya, *Women's Power to Heal Through Inner Medicine,* New York: Mother Om Media, 2007

Trickey, Ruth, *Women, Hormones and the Menstrual Cycle: Herbal and Medical solutions from adolescence to menopause*, (Revised edition), Crow's Nest: Allen & Unwin, 2003

Weaver, Libby, *Rushing Woman's Syndrome: The Impact of a Never Ending To-Do List on Your Health*, (Kindle edition), Green Frog Publishing, 2011

Wilson Schaef, Anne, *Meditations for Women Who do Too Much*, New York: Harper & Row, Publishers, 1990

Lightning Source UK Ltd.
Milton Keynes UK
UKHW031012270919
350574UK00007B/658/P

9 781925 764499